Clinical Dermatology

2

Clinical Dermatology

HARVEY BAKER, M.D., F.R.C.P. (LONDON)

Consultant Dermatologist,
The London Hospital

FOURTH EDITION

Baillière Tindall
London Philadelphia Toronto Sydney Tokyo

Baillière Tindall
—————————
W.B. Saunders

24–28 Oval Road
London NW1 7DX, England

The Curtis Center, Independence Square West
Philadelphia, PA 19106–3399, USA

1 Goldthorne Avenue
Toronto, Ontario M8Z 5T9, Canada

Harcourt Brace Jovanovich Group (Australia) Pty Ltd
32–52 Smidmore Street, Marrickville, NSW 2204, Australia

Harcourt Brace Jovanovich Japan Inc.
Ichibancho Central Building, 22–1 Ichibancho
Chilyoda-ku, Tokyo 102, Japan

First published 1964
Second edition 1970
Third edition 1979
Reprinted 1986
Fourth edition 1989

Typeset by Colset Pte. Ltd., Singapore
Printed in Singapore

British Library Cataloguing in Publication Data

Baker, Harvey
    Clinical dermatology.—4th ed.
    1. Medicine. Dermatology
    I. Title
    616.5

ISBN 0–7020–1359–5

Contents

Preface   vii

Introduction   ix

1   The Biology of the Skin   1
2   Symptoms and Signs in Dermatological Diagnosis   11
3   Simple Investigations in Dermatological Diagnosis   19
4   Principles of Treatment and the Use of Drugs   22
5   The Skin and Systemic Disease   29
6   Cutaneous Manifestations of Malignant Disease   36
7   Viral Diseases   39
8   Bacterial Diseases   52
9   Fungous Diseases   63
10   Parasitic Infections and Insect Bites   75
11   Dermatitis   82
12   Psoriasis, Reiter's Disease and Lichen Planus   98
13   Neonatal and Childhood Disorders   109
14   Genetic Diseases   115
15   Sunlight and the Skin   123
16   Vascular Disorders   130
17   Autoimmune Diseases and Other Diseases of Collagen and Elastic Tissue   141
18   Bullous Diseases   151
19   Tumours of the Skin   157
20   Acne Vulgaris, Rosacea, Perioral Dermatitis   171
21   Disorders of Pigmentation and Pigmented Naevi   178
22   Diseases of the Scalp, Hair and Nails   185
23   Adverse Reactions to Drugs   196
24   Tropical Diseases Imported into Temperate Countries   200
25   Psychogenic Disorders   203

Appendix I: Sport and the Skin   205
Appendix II: Drug Interactions Important to the Dermatologist   206
Appendix III: A Formulary of Useful Topical Preparations   207

Index   211

Preface

This volume succeeds and replaces the long-lived third edition (1979) of *Dermatology* by J.S. Pegum and H. Baker in Baillière Tindall's Concise Medical Textbooks series.

Unlike its predecessors it is written by a single author, so the writer can blame no-one but himself for errors, omissions, etc. It has been totally rewritten and reorganized and the 198 figures include 145 colour pictures as well as many black and white ones and diagrams.

A departure is the addition of 96 tables of very basic information intended primarily for medical students, but which may also be useful for graduate readers. Enough concise information has been included in the text to satisfy the appetites of junior hospital physicians, especially those reading for higher degrees, and to provide a basic introductory text for entrants to the specialty, as a stepping stone to the larger but more formidable textbooks.

A substantial amount of therapeutic detail has been included in the hope that the volume will prove useful for physicians, whether family practitioners or generalists, who do not have ready access to expert specialist dermatologists outside the U.K. in English-speaking countries. In addition, a formulary has been added as an appendix, together with an appendix of drug interactions of importance to the dermatologist.

The common infectious exanthemata of childhood (viral diseases) have been included, as well as sexually transmitted diseases, neither of which were well covered in the previous edition. The chapter on genetics has been expanded to include pre-natal diagnosis, and a chapter on photodermatoses has been added.

The author has had the benefit of detailed criticisms of the previous edition, commissioned by the publishers. He has also gained enormously from the support, encouragement and guidance of Sean Duggan and Alison Campbell on behalf of the publishers.

Virtually all the clinical photographs were taken in the Department of Medical Illustration of the London Hospital, and I am indebted to Mr Ian Berle, its Director. Dr Cicely Blair, Dr Irene Leigh and Dr J.S. Pegum kindly allowed certain material to be used.

Finally, the efforts of those who converted the author's illegible manuscripts into elegant typescripts were heroic; without their help, nothing would have been achieved.

HARVEY BAKER

Dedication

To my wife, Adrienne

Introduction

It has been estimated that the care of skin disease in the United Kingdom absorbs more than 600 million pounds annually, some 3% of the National Health Service budget. Not less than 7 million working days are lost annually as a result of skin disorders and 15% of family practitioner consultations arise from cutaneous complaints.

No longer is dermatology a Cinderella subject. The last decade has seen enormous advances in understanding of the basic mechanisms of skin disease, founded on increasing knowledge of skin biology and the dramatic advances in many fields, particularly biochemistry and immunology.

A new generation of young clinical scientists, trained in clinical dermatology, but skilled in fundamental investigative techniques, is slowly transforming the practice of dermatology. At the same time, the imperatives of the market place have generated massive pharmaceutical research and the arrival of innovative drugs targeted at skin disease.

The old descriptive dermatology is melting away under the onslaught of new knowledge, but in the clinic the classical principles of detailed history-taking and careful physical examination of the patient remain paramount as the starting points of successful diagnosis and management. No dermatological equivalent of a chest radiograph has swept away our equivalent of percussion and auscultation; molecular biology and its applications must be focused by the findings of the ears, the eyes and the fingertips if they are to achieve relevance for the individual patient who, when all else is put aside, should be the first and final concern of the physician.

1

The Biology of the Skin

The Functions of Skin

Skin is a complex structure with many functions (Table 1.1). It is a frontier and protects the body against losses and incursions. It prevents the loss of water, electrolytes, proteins and other substances and thereby assists in keeping the internal environment constant; likewise, it prevents potentially dangerous micro-organisms and other foreign substances, be they solid, liquid or gaseous, from entering the body. Light too is screened by the horny layer and absorbed by *melanin* pigment. With regard to radioactivity it is a complete barrier only against alpha particles. The skin protects against mechanical injury by the toughness and plasticity of the *stratum corneum* (horny layer) and by the resilient strength of the collagen and elastin of the dermis. Bacterial proliferation on the skin surface is discouraged by its dryness. Micro-organisms are actively dislodged by the constant shedding of the horny layer. The dry surface also restricts electrical conductivity by virtue of its high impedance. Its frictional resistance is important, allowing 'grip', par-ticularly on the palms and soles. The epidermis is also the frontier of the immune system by virtue of the antigen-presenting function of Langerhans' cells and the various immunomodulatory cytokines secreted by these cells and keratinocytes.

Its other central role is in thermoregulation; heat is conserved by controlling cutaneous blood flow and dissipated by the secretion of eccrine sweat and dilata-tion of blood vessels. It is the frontier of the sensory nervous system, containing nerve endings sensitive to heat, cold, pain, itching and touch. Via the autonomic nervous system our skin may also signal various emo-tions, such as fear, anger or lust. Finally, it may contri-bute vitamin D to the body's economy by allowing sun-light to convert dietary sterols.

The appendages have lost a good deal of their impor-tance. The nails are small in man but highly developed in other animals as claws. They function as tools to pick up and manipulate fine objects. The hair has an important heat conserving function in furry animals but not in man. The hair that does remain on the scalp, however, protects against ultraviolet light, thereby lessening the hazard of skin cancer, and acts as a helmet against minor injury. The hair roots and the appen-dageal glands serve as a source of epidermal cells for regeneration after injury.

The Structure of Skin

Figure 1.1 illustrates the gross histopathological features of normal skin. The outer layer or *epidermis* is of ectodermal origin. The underlying layer or *dermis* is of mesodermal derivation. The skin appendages, i.e. hair follicles, sebaceous glands, eccrine and apocrine sweat glands, are derived from epidermis, i.e. are ecto-dermal. Their structure and function are described at the beginning of the Chapters dealing with their diseases.

Regional variation

Skin may be hairy or non-hairy (glabrous). Thus glab-rous skin is found on the palms, soles and glans penis.

Table 1.1 The functions of skin.

Maintains thermoregulation
Protects against mechanical injury
Prevents entry of noxious chemicals and micro-organisms
Screens and reduces penetration of radiation
Prevents loss of body contents
Provides a frictional surface for grip
Discourages microbial growth
Restricts electrical conductivity
Serves as the outpost of the immune system
Serves as the outpost of the sensory nervous system
Signals emotions via the autonomic nervous system
Synthesizes vitamin D

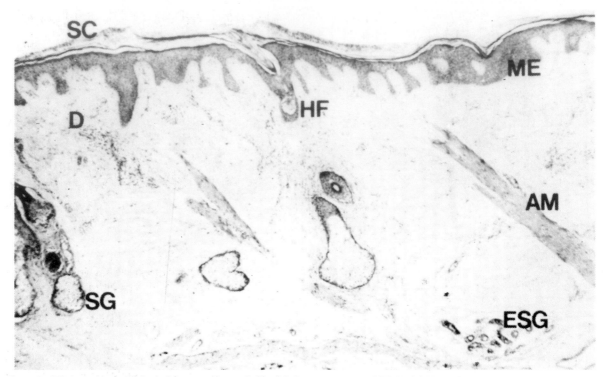

Fig. 1.1 The gross histopathological features of normal skin. SC, Stratum corneum; ME, Malpighian epidermis; D, dermis; SG, sebaceous gland; AM, arrector muscle; ESG, eccrine sweat gland; HF, hair follicle.

Sebaceous glands are most profuse and active on the face, scalp and upper trunk; apocrine sweat glands are found in the axillae, about the nipples and the ano-genital region. Eccrine sweat glands, in contrast, are most profuse and active on the palms and soles.

The surface of the skin is very variable. Its barrier function varies widely; thus insensible water loss is much greater from scrotal skin than from the back. This may be related to a need to maintain the most appropriate temperature for testicular function.

The Epidermis

The majority cell of the epidermis is the ectodermal keratinocyte but at least three other cell populations are present (Table 1.2). The epidermis is organized in distinct layers (Fig. 1.2) which really represent the stages of maturation of keratinocytes.

The basal (keratinocyte) layer

This is the germinative layer. Keratinocytes divide by

Table 1.2 Cell populations in the epidermis.

Cell	Product	Function
Keratinocyte	Stratum corneum	Barrier
Melanocyte	Melanin	Ultraviolet screen
Langerhans' cell	—	Antigen trapping and presentation
Merkel cell	—	Sensory nervous system

mitosis, a proportion of the resulting daughter cells moving outwards. Every keratinocyte at this early stage has a phase of association with an adjacent mela-nocyte from which it receives a donation of subcellular organelles, melanosomes, which contain melanin (see Chapter 21). The basal cells contain keratin filaments (keratins 5 and 14) arranged in bundles (tonofibrils). Hemidesmosomes anchor the cells to the basement membrane (see Fig. 1.6).

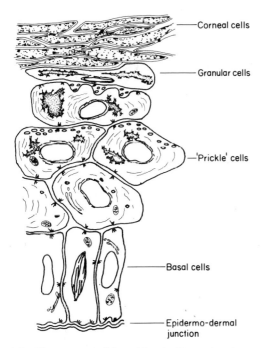

Fig. 1.2 The structure of the epidermis. The various layers represent the keratinocyte population at different stages of maturation.

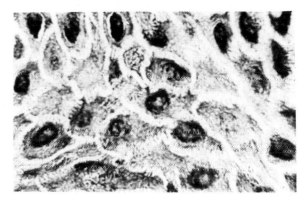

Fig. 1.3 Malpighian 'prickle' cells in the epidermis. The 'prickles' are intracellular desmosomal attachments.

The prickle cell layer

Immediately above the germinative basal layer, the keratinocytes lose their columnar shape and become polyhedral. Under the light microscope their desmosomal attachments can be seen clearly (Fig. 1.3). In the upper parts of this layer the keratinocyte is synthesizing soluble proteins (such as involucrin) which are the precursors of the cross-linked envelope of the stratum corneum. The tonofibrils form a network filling the cytoplasm of the cell and are mainly keratins of types 1, 5, 10 and 14.

The granular layer

The appearance of keratohyalin granules in the keratinocytes signals a further stage of maturation. These are amorphous protein particles (filaggrin) which are not bound to membranes. Equally or more important, are the lipid Odland bodies, sometimes called lamellar or membrane-coating granules. The lipid contents of these lamellar granules are now known to be extruded into the intercellular spaces of the deeper stratum corneum where they are incorporated into the sphingolipid sheets which are a crucial component of the

epidermal barrier (see below) as well as having a role in preventing epidermal dessication and influencing the cohesion and dyshesion of stratum corneum cells.

The horny layer (stratum corneum)

This is the final product of keratinocyte division, differentiation and maturation. It consists of 10–20 layers of flat polyhedral cells slightly overlapping each other (Fig. 1.4) and sometimes stacked like the chips of the gambler (Fig. 1.5). The cells have lost their nuclei and are dead. The cell envelopes are thickened and the cells are packed with keratin, i.e. tonofibrils encased in an amorphous matrix derived from the keratohyalin granules. The cells are cemented together by the intercellular lipid which contains enzymes related to lipid

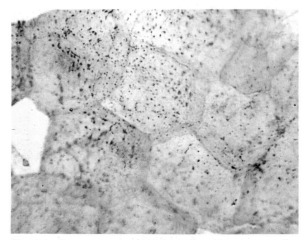

Fig. 1.4 Stratum corneum cells in horizontal section: anuclear overlapping cells containing keratin and melanin granules.

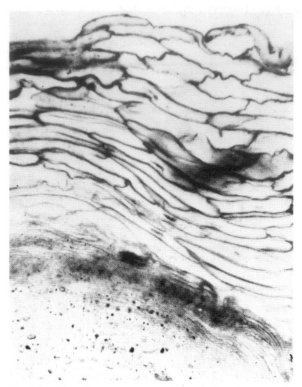

Fig. 1.5 Cleared stratum corneum in vertical section; note the 'stacking' and thick cell envelopes.

metabolism. The interior of the keratinocytes (corneocytes) is an aqueous milieu, but the intercellular area is lipid and hydrophobic. By weight, the stratum corneum is mostly protein with 10% of lipid. The intercellular material is 50% lipid and constitutes 10–30% of the stratum corneum by volume.

As the horny layer cells approach the skin surface they gradually lose their cohesion and are shed singly or in clumps.

Epidermal Barrier Function

It was thought until very recently that most percutaneous absorption was transcellular and that the whole stratum corneum made up the barrier layer. Now it is increasingly clear that most penetration is intercellular, particularly of lipid-soluble molecules, and that it is the composition of the intercellular lipids in the deeper stratum corneum which crucially influences barrier efficiency. Thus, in essential fatty acid deficiency the lamellar bodies are empty, the

corneal intracellular lipid sheets are grossly abnormal and barrier impairment is substantial.

In life, the stratum corneum is a fine, flexible plastic-like membrane. If its water content falls below about 10%, pliability is lost and 'chapping' may result. Conversely, it can take up to 300% or more of its own weight in water under immersive conditions. Its strength depends upon the strong disulphide bonds in the keratin, the thick cell envelopes and the lipid intercellular cement.

Vitamin D Metabolism in Skin

Provitamin D3 (7-dehydrocholesterol) is metabolized to vitamin D3 (cholecalciferol) under the influence of ultraviolet light. Sequential hydroxylation in the liver and kidney subsequently produces the metabolically active form of vitamin D3 which enhances intestinal calcium transport and mineral mobilization in bone. The presence of vitamin D3 receptors on keratinocytes and activated lymphocytes suggests a role in epidermal differentiation and immune responses.

The epidermodermal junction

Figure 1.6 shows the epidermodermal junction in diagrammatic form. Light microscopy shows only a 'basement membrane' between the basal keratinocytes and the dermis. Electron microscopy reveals a sub-basal plasma membrane with periodic hemidesmosome attachment plaques. Deep to this is a clear zone, the lamina lucida, traversed by anchoring filaments. Below this is a lamina densa. Anchoring fibrils extend from the lamina densa into the papillary dermis.

These various layers have great importance in relation to the precise level of the cleavage which occurs in inherited epidermolysis bullosa (p. 120) and various acquired blistering diseases (Chapter 18). The junctional area is now known to be highly antigenic: at least 18 antigens have been identified, the most important of which are listed in Table 1.3.

The melanocyte

This cell, its structure and function are described in Chapter 21.

The Langerhans' cell

The Langerhans' cell (Table 1.4) is a dendritic cell which, unlike the melanocyte, is found in the supra-

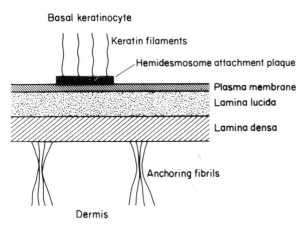

Fig. 1.6 Epidermodermal junction at electron microscopic level in diagrammatic form.

Table 1.3 Some 'basement membrane' antigens in normal human skin.

Antigen	Localization
Laminin (basement-membrane protein)	Lamina lucida
Bullous pemphigoid antigen	Lamina lucida
Cicatricial pemphigoid antigen	Lamina lucida
Type IV collagen	Lamina densa
Acquired epidermolysis bullosa antigen (Type VII collagen)	Lamina densa
Entactin (nidogen) (a laminin-binding protein)	Lamina lucida

Table 1.4 Characteristics of the Langerhans' cell.

Dendritic cell
Suprabasal localization
Mesodermal (bone marrow) origin
Racquet-shaped (Birbeck) cytoplasmic granules
ATP-ase positive
Expresses HLA-DR (CD1) and CD4 membrane antigens
Surface receptors for C3 and Fc fragment of IgG
Can secrete interleukin-1

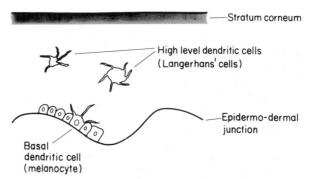
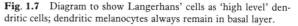

Fig. 1.7 Diagram to show Langerhans' cells as 'high level' dendritic cells; dendritic melanocytes always remain in basal layer.

basal layers of the epidermis (Fig. 1.7). It was described by Paul Langerhans when he was a medical student in 1868. It does not synthesize melanin and only in the last 15 years have its origin and role become clear. It is a bone-marrow derived mesodermal cell. Desmosomes and keratin filaments are absent and its cytoplasm contains tennis-racquet shaped granules. On its surface it expresses HLA-DR and the membrane antigens CD1 (T6) and CD4 (T4). It has surface receptors for the complement fraction C3, and the Fc fragment of IgG. The Langerhans' cell is a non-phagocytic mononuclear cell which functions as an antigen-trapping and antigen-presenting cell and is thus the outpost of the immune system. It also cooperates with lymphocytes in eliciting immune responses. Histiocytosis X (p. 114) is now known to be usually a proliferative disorder of Langerhans' cells.

The Merkel cell

This cell is thought to be involved in sensory touch reception. It is found in the basal epidermis associated with nerve endings and in the dermis close to Schwann cells. Unlike the melanocyte and Langerhans' cells it has desmosomal connections with keratinocytes but, unlike keratinocytes, its basal plasma membrane is devoid of hemidesmosomes. It has characteristic inclusion granules in its cytoplasm which contain the neuropeptides bombesin and metencephalin. The cytoplasm has neurofilaments as well as keratin filaments.

The Dermis

The dermis is the 'underfelt' of the epidermal carpet.

It is a matrix of fibrous collagen and elastin filled in with ground substance. It supports the epidermal appendages, vascular and lymphatic networks, nerves and various immunocompetent and inflammatory cells. The papillary dermis is the superficial part, extending to the depths of the epidermal rete ridges; below it is the reticular dermis.

Collagen

Collagen is a protein formed of three polypeptide chains coiled in a rope-like triple helix. Cross-linking between molecules makes this structure even stronger. Proline and lysine are the two main amino acids in the chain and also form hydroxyproline and hydroxylysine which stabilize the helix. Vitamin C is involved in this conversion.

Collagen is synthesized within ribosomes in the fibroblast as a precursor molecule, procollagen. Outside the cell this is converted enzymatically to tropocollagen, molecules of which aggregate into fibrils, strengthened by cross-links.

The collagen 'pool' is constantly being metabolized and replaced, collagenase being the principal enzyme of degradation, a process accelerated by ultraviolet light (p. 124).

There are 8 main types of collagen according to the amino acid sequences in the polypeptide chains. Those found in skin are listed in Table 1.5. Deeper dermal collagen is Type I but the papillary dermal collagen is finer (Type III). Basement membrane collagen is Type IV but a Type VII collagen is present in lamina densa and anchoring fibrils. Type VIII collagen is found in endothelium.

Elastic tissue

Elastic tissue consists of elastin, a protein similar to collagen, in which are embedded microfibrils. Like collagen, it is derived from fibroblasts but is made up of different amino acids (e.g. desmosine) and is more elastic. Ageing leads to slow loss of elasticity.

Ground substance

This, too, is secreted by fibroblasts and contains acid mucopolysaccharides, hyaluronic acid and chondroitin sulphate in an aqueous gel. It is increased in myxoedema.

Blood vessels

The skin has an arterial input and a venous drainage. A deep network of vessels lies close to the subcutis and a more superficial one of smaller vessels high in the dermis, the two being interconnected. From the superficial plexus, capillary loops occupy the dermal papillae and are responsible for epidermal nutrition. The loop consists of an ascending 'arterial' capillary and a descending 'venous' capillary.

In the extremities there are richly innervated arteriovenous anastomoses deep in the dermis concerned with thermoregulation, called glomus bodies. An afferent arteriole runs into a convoluted thick-walled anastomosis, called the Sacquet–Hoyer canal (Fig. 1.8), where characteristic glomus cells are found. Solitary benign tender glomus tumours may arise from the glomus body.

Table 1.5 Collagens in human skin.

Collagen	Localization
Type I	Reticular dermis
Type III	Papillary dermis
Type IV	Basement membrane
Type V	Interstitial tissue
Type VII	Anchoring fibrils
Type VIII	Endothelium

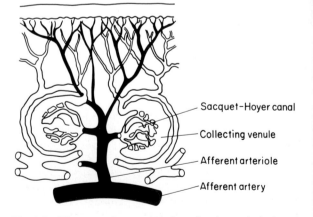

Sacquet-Hoyer canal

Collecting venule

Afferent arteriole

Afferent artery

Fig. 1.8 Diagrammatic representation of a glomus body in the deep dermis.

Lymphatics

Terminal lymphatics are present in the papillary dermis and drain into interconnecting lymphatic spaces deeper in the dermis and thence into the lymph nodes.

The cutaneous nerves

It has been estimated that the skin contains at least a million afferent nerve fibres. The hands, feet, face and genitalia are richly supplied; other areas such as the back or outer thigh are sparsely served. The cell bodies of these fibres are in the dorsal root ganglia. The axons are surrounded by Schwann cells and are of both myelinated and non-myelinated type.

Afferent receptors may be corpuscular or free. The former involve non-nervous tissue and may be encapsulated (e.g. the Pacini and Meissner corpuscles), ending in the dermis, or non-encapsulated, ending in the deep epidermis in relation to a Merkel cell. Free nerve endings are found in both epidermis and dermis and subserve itch, pain and temperature sensation. The hair follicle has its own nervous network. Meissner's corpuscles transmit touch sensation and are profuse in the dermal papillae of the hands and feet. Pacinian corpuscles lie much deeper in the dermis or even the subcutis and detect pressure and vibration.

The Cell Population of the Dermis

The fibroblast

This term embraces a heterogeneous family of cells with differing characteristics and products. These cells probably all originate from a primitive mesenchymal cell. They are active in the synthesis and secretion of collagen precursors, dermal ground substance and probably elastin. In the inactive non-secreting phase they are called fibrocytes.

The mast cell

Mast cells (Table 1.6) are also of mesenchymal origin. Their cytoplasm is full of granules. Human dermis contains many mast cells, mostly near small blood vessels. The mast cell is a secretory cell, capable of releasing various mediators of inflammation, which originate from the granules and which stain with toluidin blue. The cell membrane has high-affinity receptors for IgE, and mast cells play a critical role in IgE-mediated (Type I) immediate hypersensitivity

Table 1.6 Characteristics of the mast cell.

Mesenchymal origin
Found in dermis (and other connective tissue)
Dense cytoplasmic granules
Secretes mediators of inflammation, e.g. histamine
IgE receptors on cell membrane

Table 1.7 The interleukin cytokines.

Factor	Origins	Actions
IL-1	Macrophages Lymphocytes Keratinocytes	Induces B-cell proliferation and differentiation, lymphokine release from activated T cells
IL-2	Activated T cells	B-cell proliferation; potentiates release of lymphokines by T cells
IL-3	Activated T cells	Growth factor for haematopoietic cells; stem cell stimulation
IL-4	Activated T cells	Growth factor for T cells
IL-5	T cells	IgM and IgA secretion by B cells; induces differentiation of eosinophils
IL-6	Monocytes Fibroblasts Myeloma cells	Induces Class I HLA expression on fibroblasts; B-cell stimulation

reactions (see below). However, degranulation can be induced by other mechanisms, for example directly by drugs, by physical agents such as cold or light and by complement fragments (e.g. C5a).

The mediators released include histamine, eosinophil and neutrophil chemotactic factors, heparin, various proteases and metabolites of arachidonic acid. Mast cells are probably heterogeneous, varying in their products.

Mast cell production and regulation may depend on a T-lymphocyte derived growth factor, interleukin-3 (Table 1.7).

The lymphocyte

The lymphocyte is discussed below.

Immunological (Allergic) Hypersensitivity

Immune responses are essential and beneficial when they generate antibodies to micro-organisms and vaccines. They are harmful when they result in anaphylaxis, delayed (cell-mediated) contact sensitivity or cytotoxic reactions.

Classification

Immunopathology has become extremely complicated but the simple Coombs' classification of immune reactions still has merit.

Type I responses (immediate hypersensitivity)

Here, specific IgE (reaginic) antibody is bound to mast (and other) cell receptors. When the antigen (e.g. a food, pollen or drug) encounters such cells, release of inflammatory mediators is provoked. Anaphylaxis is a fierce Type I reaction due to massive histamine release. Hayfever, urticaria and bronchial asthma may be induced in this way.

Type II responses (cytotoxic reactions)

Here, antibody reacting with cell surface antigen provokes complement activation leading to cell damage or destruction by lysis. The classical Type II response is haemolysis following a mismatched transfusion. In the skin, drug-induced vascular reactions and homograft rejection are examples.

Type III responses (Arthus reactions)

This reaction results from the formation of 'immune complex', i.e. antigen plus antibody aggregates which precipitate in very small blood vessels, activating complement and attracting neutrophils. Various forms of cutaneous vasculitis may involve this immune reaction.

Type IV lymphocyte-mediated responses (delayed hypersensitivity)

Here, antibody bound to circulating lymphocytes responds to antigen by releasing lymphokines which initiate complex inflammatory responses. Allergic contact dermatitis is a Type IV response.

The lymphocyte is the body's central weapon in coping with invasion by foreign substances, i.e. antigens, such as viruses. The 'immune response' encompasses the ability to engage, recognize and neutralize antigens. It must discriminate 'self' from 'foreign' and must be subject to precise regulation.

Engagement (encounter)

Engagement of the antigen depends upon various 'accessory' cells (not lymphocytes) which 'capture' or 'trap' antigen, break it down into a form suitable for reaction with lymphocyte surface receptors and hold it on the cell surface ready for 'presentation' to passing lymphocytes. In the epidermis, the Langerhans' cell is the main 'accessory' cell; in the dermis, monocytes, macrophages and fixed histiocytes serve the same function. Accessory cells and lymphocytes can meet anywhere in the body, including the skin, but most such encounters probably take place in the lymphoid organs. Thus 'accessory' cells are obligate intermediates in the engagement of antigen by lymphocytes.

Recognition

Immune recognition depends upon antigen receptors on the surfaces of lymphocytes, each cell expressing only one such receptor. The T and B lymphocytes have similar receptors but B-cell proteins can be secreted into the plasma as antibodies, whereas T-cell receptors cannot.

The recognition units are proteins coded for by genes. All cells possess genes coding for receptors but these are organized as separate chromosomal segments. Only in B and T lymphocytes do these segments undergo 'shuffling' or assortment. These random gene translocations result in a huge repertoire of lymphocytes, each with its own unique specificity. This is the pre-antigenic stage of immune readiness resulting from antigen-independent lymphocyte differentiation.

Activation

The lymphocytes migrate actively so that antigen captured by accessory cells soon encounters a B or T cell with a receptor that happens to 'fit'. Thus, once a B cell is activated it secretes large amounts of immunoglobulin antibody for which its translocated genes code. This activation requires the collaboration of T 'helper' cells (T4 cells with a surface membrane protein called CD4) and accessory cells. In addition, a second cycle of multiplication and differentiation produces more identical cells. This is the postantigenic phase of immunity.

T-cell receptors differ from B-cell antibody in only recognizing antigen in association with a membrane protein, i.e. part of the T-cell itself, called a 'restriction element'. One, known as CD8 (T8), provides a marker of a suppressor/cytotoxic T-lymphocyte subset; the other, called CD4 (T4), defines a helper/inducer lymphocyte subset. CD4 and CD8 can be recognized with suitable monoclonal antibodies. A single lymphocyte carries CD4 or CD8 but never both. They are thought to aid binding of antigen to its receptor.

B antibodies and T receptors are thus located on the outside surfaces of the lymphocytes. These proteins are attached to the cell surface by a 'constant region'. The part of the protein which engages the antigen is the 'variable region' which is free on the cell surface. Effector function, i.e. telling the cell to multiply, etc, is encoded by the constant region. Thereafter a complex series of reactions occurs. CD4 T cells secrete cytokines which are chemical (protein) messengers. B cells divide and secrete antibody. T and B cell functions are closely interrelated and a cytokine called interleukin-1 (Table 1.7) released by accessory cells is also important in activation. Cytokines are released which mobilize neutrophils, macrophages and eosinophils. Another T-cell cytokine, γ-interferon, also stimulates macrophages. A cascade of inflammatory events follows. At least 15 cytokines have now been recognized. Those now called interleukins are listed in Table 1.7. Other cytokines include interferons, tumour necrosis factors, colony stimulating factors, and lymphotoxin.

Monocytes and Macrophages

Monocytes are formed in the bone marrow from monoblasts derived from stem cells. They leave the blood after a few days, entering the tissues to become macrophages which are found throughout the body but particularly in the spleen, lymph nodes and dermis. Epidermal Langerhans' cells are derived from these cells.

The monocyte–macrophage system is phagocytic and is also involved in activation of the immune and coagulation systems, defence against micro-organisms and cancer cells and in tissue repair.

Inflammation

When tissues are injured, the consequent damage and its repair are called 'inflammation'. Clinically, the process is marked by redness due to increased vascularity, increased local temperature as a consequence, swelling due to oedema and pain (or itching), probably due to chemical mediators.

The cellular and chemical events involved are of great complexity. Neutrophil polymorphonuclear leukocytes are of central importance, invading the site of damage, ingesting and killing micro-organisms and removing debris. They have surface receptors for a variety of mediators such as complement fragments and are capable of synthesizing various mediators. Eosinophils are also phagocytic and are summoned by a variety of chemotactic mediators. The roles of mast cells and lymphocytes have already been described.

Monocytes and tissue macrophages are able to ingest and break down micro-organisms, foreign material and tissue debris, secreting enzymes and mediators, such as arachidonic acid derivatives (Fig. 1.9).

Chemotaxis is clearly crucial in mobilizing all types of leukocytes and the cleavage products of complement are particularly chemotactic (e.g. C5a). Finally, the repair stage of inflammation depends on fibroblast stimulation and collagen synthesis.

Mediators of inflammation

Only the arachidonic acid system, the interleukins and the complement pathways are briefly mentioned.

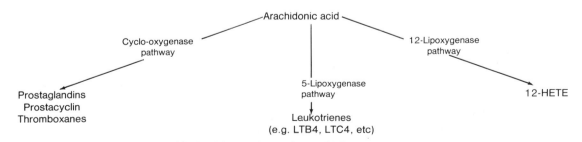

Fig. 1.9 Metabolic pathways from arachidonic acid generating mediators of inflammation.

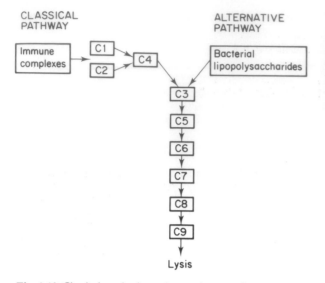

CLASSICAL PATHWAY

ALTERNATIVE PATHWAY

Lysis

Fig. 1.10 Classical and alternative pathways of complement activation.

Table 1.8 Interpretation of changes in serum complement.

C3	C4	Significance
↑	↑	Acute inflammation
↓	↓	Classical pathway activation
↓	N	Alternative pathway activation

Complement. This is the name given to an interacting group of plasma proteins which normally exist as inactive precursors. Activation involves a series of enzymatic cleavages. Two pathways of activation seem to be possible (Fig. 1.10). The *classical* pathway is triggered by immune complexes involving IgG or IgM. Other immunoglobulins cannot activate this pathway. In the *alternative* pathway, activation of C3 is achieved without the intervention of antibody or C1, for example by bacteria. This pathway thus provides an immediate defence against micro-organisms.

Either pathway causes sequential activation of C5, C6, C7, C8 and C9 leading to lysis of cells or micro-organisms, anaphylotoxin production, chemotaxis and coating of organisms by C3b leading to phagocytosis (opsonization). Throughout, activation of complement is modulated by specific inhibitors. Very rapid decay of complement fragments also confines their effects. The most easily measured fragments are C3 and C4. The commonest changes in C3 and C4 and their significance are summarized in Table 1.8.

Arachidonic acid pathways. Arachidonic acid is a fatty acid derived by enzyme action from cellular phospholipid. It can be degraded in three different ways (Fig. 1.9) by different enzymes, resulting in prostaglandins or leukotrienes.

Interleukins. These are cytokines synthesized by macrophages, lymphocytes, keratinocytes, etc, with a variety of functions. Present knowledge is summarized in Table 1.7.

Symptoms and Signs in Dermatological Diagnosis

As in every branch of medicine, diagnosis in dermatology is based on history and examination. However, skin disease can sometimes be recognized at a glance, so a brief preliminary look at the skin can save time.

The History

As in internal medicine, the history is made up of several components.

The present complaint

How long ago and where on the body did the condition start? Was the onset abrupt or gradual? How did it spread? Has its course been phasic or continuous? Is it now getting better or worse?

Itching is a valuable pointer. 'Does it itch?' should always be asked. All dermatoses can be classified into three groups: a handful which itch intensely, those which never itch and an intermediate group where itching is variable (Table 2.1). In addition, itching (pruritus) in the absence of rash may be an important clue to internal disease (Table 2.2).

'Does it weep or is it dry?' is the other crucial question. Exudation is characteristic of several common

Table 2.1 Does it itch?

Common conditions which always itch	Variable itching	Never itch
Dermatitis	Psoriasis	Vitiligo
Urticaria	Impetigo	Neurofibromatosis
Insect bites	Tinea	Warts
Scabies		
Pediculosis		
Lichen planus		

Table 2.2 Main systemic diseases causing pruritus.

Renal failure	Neoplastic disease
Hepatic disease	Anxiety
Thyrotoxicosis	Depression

Table 2.3 Common 'weeping' dermatoses.

Dermatitis	Herpes zoster
Impetigo	Acute tinea
Herpes simplex	

conditions (Table 2.3) and virtually all patients immediately understand questions phrased in this way.

Simple analysis of the combination of three variables—itching, 'weeping' and duration—often points straight to the diagnosis. Specific enquiry should always be made about certain areas in assessing the spread or distribution of a rash, particularly the scalp, eyelids, genitalia and nails. Some diseases are mucocutaneous (Table 2.4), so enquiry about the mouth, lips, conjunctivae and anogenital mucosae is important.

Eliciting provocative factors may be informative. Is the condition influenced by the menstrual cycle? Is it seasonal? Do sunlight, heat, cold, pressure, etc, worsen it? Does it worsen from Monday to Friday only to improve at weekends or holidays (implying an occupational cause), or the reverse sequence (implying that a hobby can be blamed)?

Previous medication

In an age of iatrogenic and medicament-induced disease, information about recent oral, parenteral or topical treatment is crucial. What drugs were being taken *before* the onset and for how long? (Most drug

Table 2.4 Some mucocutaneous diseases.

Common

Candidosis

Primary herpes simplex

Uncommon

Lichen planus

Erythema multiforme

Secondary syphilis

Rare

Pemphigus vulgaris

eruptions begin 7–10 days after treatment is started.) What oral or topical medication has been used *since* onset? Have any clearly aggravated the condition? Some applications are notorious irritants or sensitizers and their use immediately rouses suspicion of medicament-induced or worsened dermatosis. An eminent teacher of the author was fond of saying that he had made his reputation (and his fortune) 'stopping other doctors' treatment'!

Previous medical history

Enquiry should elicit major previous illnesses or operations. Previous skin disease is particularly relevant, for example eczema (dermatitis) in childhood, psoriasis decades ago, asthma, etc. Known allergies should never be forgotten—to drugs such as penicillin, or external exposures such as perfume, rubber or metal (nickel). Prolonged immobilization or leg injury decades ago may have led to deep venous thrombosis underlying present symptoms in a leg.

Occupational history

Some detail may be required, for example in a manual worker with dermatitis of the hands. What chemical exposures are known at work or in hobbies? Has a man's working life been mainly outdoor or indoor? (Sunlight is an important carcinogen.) Has the patient ever lived in the tropics or sub-tropics? Does a housewife do gardening or keep indoor plants?

Not all chemical exposure is occupational or hobby-related. Women—and increasingly men—use cosmetics and toiletries which may contain sensitizing chemicals (see Chapter 23).

Family history

This is important in both genetic disease (e.g. psoriasis) and infections (such as tuberculosis or leprosy). Enquiry is mandatory about first-degree relations, i.e. parents, siblings and children. In addition, information about sexual contacts, intimate social contacts and work contacts may provide important clues.

Social history

Smoking and drinking (alcohol) habits should be noted, as should other drug addictions or exposures. Where mood is altered or psychogenic disease is suspected, detailed enquiry about life-style, stresses (e.g. bereavement), anxieties, responsibilities, marital harmony, sexual life, etc, may be needed. It should be remembered that most diagnostic mistakes would never have been made if the history had been thorough.

The Examination

Certain principles are of prime importance. 'Peephole' diagnosis should be avoided. The whole organ should be examined. If the patient is not fully undressed, relevant lesions can be missed. Thus a widespread dermatitis may be due to sensitization by a medicament applied to a chronic leg ulcer swathed in bandages which the patient assumes is irrelevant and may not mention. Never examine an eruption of the hands and neglect to look at the feet. In a baby always look at the napkin (diaper) area.

Good light is essential and natural light is best. Anaemia, slight jaundice, scabetic burrows, etc, can easily be missed in poor light.

The examination has two components which should be studied separately:
- Distribution
- Morphology

Distribution

Is the eruption widespread or localized? Is it unilateral or bilateral? If the latter, is it symmetrical or asymmetrical? Symmetry favours internal causation (Fig. 2.1); asymmetry suggests external causation (unilateral herpes zoster or, conversely, a symmetrical photodermatosis are exceptions to an otherwise valuable rule). Is it predominantly flexor (as in atopic eczema)

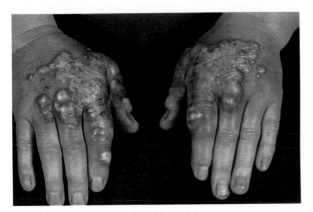

Fig. 2.1 Drug-induced erythema multiforme; note the perfect symmetry.

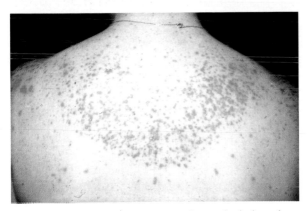

Fig. 2.2 Psoriasis affecting sun-exposed upper back above dressline.

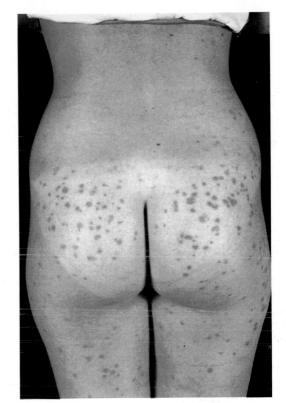

Fig. 2.3 Psoriasis remaining on covered skin where sun-exposed areas have largely cleared.

or extensor (as in psoriasis)? Is it confined to light-exposed areas (Fig. 2.2) or protected areas (Fig. 2.3), are shadow areas (such as the upper eyelids, upper lip, under chin and earlobe (Fig. 2.4)) spared? Is it predominantly centrifugal, affecting the extremities, or centripetal (sparing the extremities and concentrated on the trunk (Table 2.5))? Lastly, note hair, scalp, nail or mucosal involvement.

Morphology

A rapid inspection will determine whether the eruption is monomorphic or pleomorphic. If the former, description of a small area describes the whole. If the latter, each different lesion must be analysed in turn (see below). Palpation of skin lesions is vital; both the eyes and fingertips are needed for dermatological diagnosis.

Table 2.5 Centripetal and centrifugal dermatoses.

Centripetal	Centrifugal
Varicella	Granuloma annulare
Pityriasis rosea	Erythema multiforme
Morphoea	Erythema nodosum
Pemphigus vulgaris	Bullous pemphigoid

Other relevant examination

Palpation of regional lymph glands if neoplasia is suspected, abdominal examination to detect hepatic or splenic enlargement, palpation of peripheral arterial pulses where ischaemia is suspected and auscultation where relevant are obvious examples.

Terminology

It is impossible to record or describe the morphology of

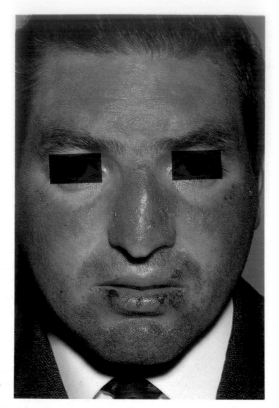

Fig. 2.4 Photodermatitis of face; note sparing of 'shadow' areas.

an eruption succinctly without the use of terms with an accepted conventional meaning. The following are used.

Erythema. Erythema is redness due to vascular dilatation. It may be transient or chronic. It can be blanched by pressure. It may be localized, diffuse or even universal. Flushing is a form of acute, transient erythema.

Purpura. Purpura is also red, usually darker and cannot be blanched by pressure. It is discoloration of the skin due to extravasation of blood. Capillary leakage produces punctate purpura, whereas leakage from torn venules produces larger areas of purpura, seen in senile and steroid-induced purpura. The degradation of haem within phagocytes induces the colour changes observed in purpura, dark red giving way to yellow-green shades and later to brown haemosiderin over a period of days or longer. In the elderly, purpura always lingers longer and changes colour more slowly (owing to diminished phagocytic responses).

Telangiectasia. Telangiectasia is a condition of dilated blood vessels in the skin. Redness is apparent but (unlike in erythema) individual dilated vessels are discernible. In the *spider naevus*, a dilated central arteriole has branches like the legs of a spider.

Flat impalpable lesions have to be distinguished from raised palpable ones and several terms accomplish this.

Macule. A macule is a circumscribed area of skin of any size which is discoloured. It may be erythematous, purpuric, pigmented (haemosiderin or melanin) or depigmented, uniform or speckled but is not palpable, being neither raised nor depressed nor thickened.

Papule. This is a small solid elevation of the skin less than 0.5 cm in diameter. A papule may be epidermal (due to local hypertrophy) and scaly ('papulo-squamous') or dermal due to increased cells, fluid or metabolic deposition in the dermis.

Wheal. This is a transitory pink or white papule or plaque of dermal oedema (seen for example in urticaria).

Nodule. This is a solid mass, greater than 0.5 cm in diameter. It may be epidermal, dermal, a mixture of both, or even subcutaneous (as in rheumatoid nodules) (Fig. 2.5). Nodules may be of any colour or consistency. For instance, the nodule of dermatofibroma is typically hard, whereas that of neurofibroma is soft.

Plaques. These are essentially flattened nodules of any size over 2 cm.

Vesicle. This is a circumscribed elevation of the skin less than 0.5 cm in diameter and containing fluid.

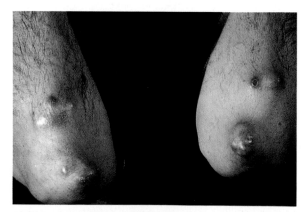

Fig. 2.5 Subcutaneous nodules at elbows in rheumatoid arthritis.

Bulla (blister). This is a circumscribed elevation of the skin larger than 0.5 cm containing fluid. Bullae may form within the epidermis or by separation of the epidermis and dermis. The precise level of cleavage may be of great diagnostic importance (see Chapter 18 on blistering diseases).

Pustule. This is a visible collection of pus in the skin. Pustules are not necessarily infective. Sterile pustulosis may occur in psoriasis and acne, for instance.

When the surface of the skin is loose and detachable it is important to distinguish between scale and crust (scab).

Scale. Scales consist of flat plates or flakes of abnormal stratum corneum, indicating disordered epidermal maturation and keratinization. Their shedding is called *exfoliation*. Scales may be very fine and bran-like or large and polygonal like fish-scales (in ichthyosis) or silvery and white (in psoriasis).

Crust. In contrast, crust is dried exudate and implies inflammatory exudation. Serum crusts are yellow or honey-coloured; purulent crusts are yellow–green and haemorrhagic crusts are dark red or black.

Blackheads (comedones). These are small pin-head plugs of pigmented stratum corneum cells and sebum in dilated pilosebaceous orifices. They are the primary lesions of acne vulgaris. Occasionally, gross comedones are occupational in origin, as from oil exposure for example in ships' engineers (Fig. 2.6).

Various 'breaks' in the skin surface have to be described and their depths distinguished.

Erosions. These are lesions where there is partial loss of skin, for example loss of stratum corneum or even loss of the whole epidermis, but leaving dermis in the base. Erosions heal without scarring.

Fissures. These are small, fine, linear gaps or splits (i.e. erosion) in the skin surface.

Excoriations. An excoriation is any loss of substance of skin due to scratching. It is usually linear.

Ulcers. These are defects formed by the loss of the entire epidermis and dermis due to trauma, sloughing or necrosis. The base of an ulcer may be granulation tissue or any subcutaneous structure according to ulcer depth (Fig. 2.7).

Atrophy. The recognition of atrophy (i.e. tissue diminution) is important. *Epidermal atrophy* may be due to ischaemia. *Dermal atrophy* is due to loss of collagen, for example in striae or corticosteriod abuse.

Scars. A scar (cicatrix) is the fibrous tissue replacing normal tissues destroyed by injury or disease. Scars may be atrophic, thin and wrinkled, or hypertrophic due to excessive collagen tissue (fibrosis).

Lichenification. This is a chronic thickening of the epidermis with exaggeration of its normal markings due to scratching or rubbing.

A few other miscellaneous definitions are appropriate here.

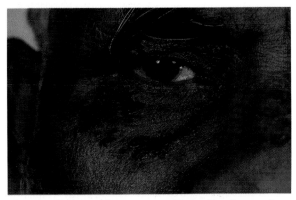

Fig. 2.6 Giant comedones on upper cheeks of face in an engineer.

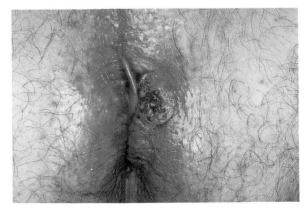

Fig. 2.7 Perianal ulcer. This was a squamous cell carcinoma but, if acute, primary chancre should be considered in differential diagnosis.

Abscess. This is a localized collection of pus formed by tissue necrosis and disintegration.

Alopecia. This is simply abnormal loss of hair.

Burrow. This is a tunnel in the stratum corneum made by a parasite.

Callus. This is a localized hypertrophy of the stratum corneum, especially of the palm or sole, caused by physical pressure.

Cyst. This is any closed cavity, lined with epithelium or endothelium and containing liquid or semi-solid material.

Furuncle. This is a follicular pyogenic infection.

Folliculitis. This is inflammation of hair follicles, whether chemical or microbial.

Gangrene. This is tissue death due to ischaemia.

Horn. This is a keratosis which is taller than it is broad.

Infarct. This is an area of coagulation necrosis due to ischaemia.

Papilloma. This is a papule or nodule with multiple nipple-like projections from its surface.

Regional Differential Diagnosis

In many areas of the body a few common conditions cause most clinical disease. A grasp of these short-lists aids accurate diagnosis enormously. Tables 2.6–2.13 summarize the relevant differential diagnoses.

The foot

Tinea usually involves the toe clefts initially. Endogenous dermatitis favours the insteps, whereas psoriasis favours the heels as well as insteps. Contact dermatitis due to footwear affects the heels and balls of the feet (if due to soles) and the dorsa of the feet (if due to the uppers).

The hand

Contact dermatitis favours the backs of the hands, finger clefts and fingers. Endogenous dermatitis

Table 2.6 Differential diagnosis of eruptions of the feet.

Tinea
Psoriasis
Contact dermatitis
Endogenous dermatitis

Table 2.7 Differential diagnosis of eruptions of the hands.

Contact dermatitis
Endogenous dermatitis
Psoriasis
Tinea

Table 2.8 Differential diagnosis of eruptions in the anogenital folds.

Candidosis (in females)
Tinea (in males)
Seborrhoeic dermatitis
Psoriasis

Table 2.9 Differential diagnosis of eruptions of the axillae.

Seborrhoeic dermatitis
Psoriasis
Contact dermatitis

Table 2.10 Differential diagnosis of eruptions of the glans penis.

Candidosis
Psoriasis
Lichen planus
Scabies
Intraepidermal carcinoma

Table 2.11 Differential diagnosis of eruptions of the face.

Acne vulgaris	Contact dermatitis
Rosacea	Lupus erythematosus
Atopic dermatitis	Perioral dermatitis

Table 2.12 Differential diagnosis of eruptions of the scalp.

Pityriasis capitis
Seborrhoeic dermatitis
Psoriasis
Tinea capitis
Discoid lupus erythematosus

Table 2.13 Differential diagnosis of abnormalities of the nails.

Trauma
Psoriasis
Chronic paronychia (fingers only)
Tinea
Lichen planus
Secondary to nail fold dermatitis

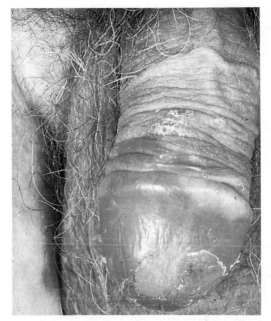

Fig. 2.8 Psoriasis of glans penis.

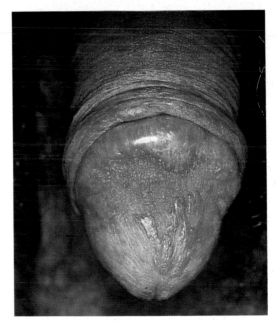

Fig. 2.9 Lichen planus of glans penis.

usually involves the palms. Psoriasis can be anywhere. Tinea may be unilateral.

The groin

Tinea is much more common in males; candidosis is more common in females. Psoriasis is symmetrical about the flexures and natal cleft.

The axilla

Psoriasis and seborrheic dermatitis involve the vaults of the armpit. Contact dermatitis from clothing tends to spare the vault, involving the axillary margins.

The glans penis

Psoriasis (Fig. 2.8) and lichen planus (Fig. 2.9) form plaques. Candidosis is diffuse and inflammatory.

Scabies causes pruritic papules or nodules (often also on the scrotum). Intraepidermal carcinoma should be considered in men over 50 years. Plasma cell balanitis of Zoon is typically purpuric (Fig. 2.10). The normal mucous glands of the rim of the glans penis may attract

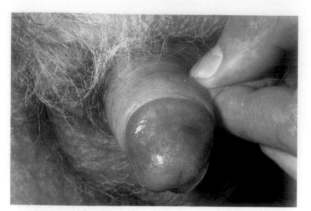

Fig. 2.10 Plasma cell balanitis of Zoon.

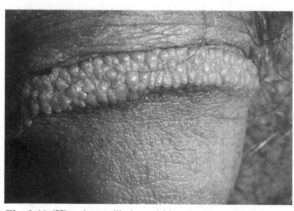

Fig. 2.11 'Hirsuties papillaris penis' in a healthy young man.

the attention of anxious young men in fear of sexually transmitted disease. This 'hirsuties papillaris penis' (Fig. 2.11) is normal anatomy.

The face

Contact dermatitis particularly affects the eyelids. Rosacea and lupus erythematosus spare the eyelids (although rosacea can cause blepharitis). Age is a crucial discriminating factor.

The scalp

The presence or absence of alopecia may be important.

The nails

Psoriasis is very common. Chronic paronychia is common in the fingers but rare in the toes.

Differential Diagnosis of Linear Lesions

Psoriasis, contact dermatitis and lichen planus (Fig. 2.12) may include linear lesions due to the Köbner phenomenon. When an extensive solitary linear lesion is seen, the diagnosis is likely to lie between the conditions listed in Table 2.14.

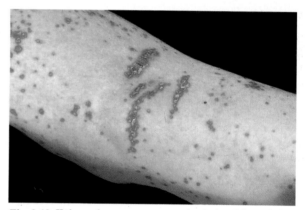

Fig. 2.12 Köbner phenomenon; trauma has induced linear lesions of lichen planus.

Table 2.14 Differential diagnosis of linear lesions.

Epidermal naevus	Morphoea
Lichen planus	Plane warts
Lichen striatus	

— 3

Simple Investigations in Dermatological Diagnosis

The following techniques are of great value in diagnosis.

Swabbing

This is a method of obtaining material for bacteriological or virological examination. Aspiration from an intact vesicle or pustule after the surface has been gently sterilized with alcohol is usually more valuable than swabbing an open surface, although the latter may be needed, for example in ulceration.

Stratum corneum scrapings for mycology

When tinea is suspected, material for direct microscopy may be obtained by scraping the surface of the lesion with a scalpel blade moistened in 10% potassium hydroxide (KOH) solution and transferring it directly to a microscope slide. After maceration in more KOH and mounting under a cover slip, the specimen is examined unstained under low illumination and low power after the material has been pressed down to obtain a monolayer of cells (Figs 3.1–3.3). For culture, a dry blade is used to transfer scrapings onto a piece of black paper (8 × 8 cm) (for ease of visualization) which is folded and sealed for transmission to the laboratory. The material is inoculated onto a layer of

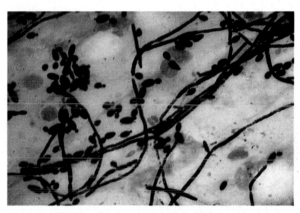

Fig. 3.2 *Candida albicans*: microscopic preparation.

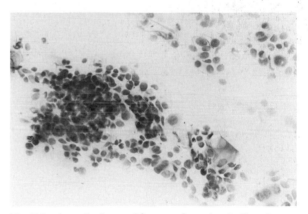

Fig. 3.3 An easily disrupted fragment from a basal cell carcinoma. Individual cells have only scanty cyteplasm. Toluidine blue × 400 (courtesy of Dr C. Browne).

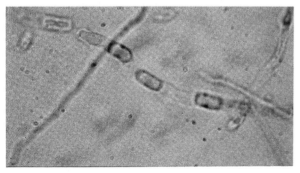

Fig. 3.1 Dermatophyte fungus: microscopic preparation.

agar containing glucose and peptone (Sabouraud's medium) in a Petri dish. Bacterial growth is prevented by addition of antibiotics and growth of saprophytic moulds by adding cycloheximide. Culture may be continued for up to 3 weeks.

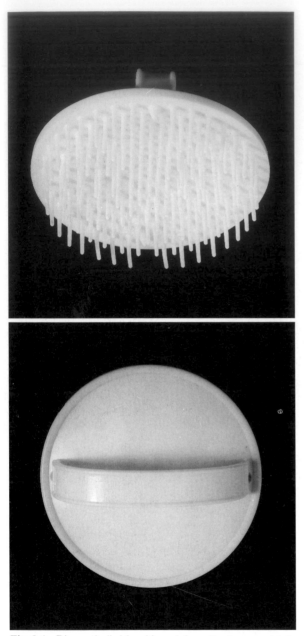

Fig. 3.4 Diagnostic 'hairbrush' used for collecting material for culture for tinea capitis.

'Hair brushings' for mycology

Sterile round plastic hair brushes which fit into a Petri dish (Fig. 3.4) are valuable to obtain material for fungal culture in suspected tinea capitis. The scalp lesions are 'brushed' and the brush returned to its plastic bag. In the laboratory the brush is pressed into the agar in a dish to produce multiple inoculations.

Brushes can be reused by sterilizing in Hycolin for 30 minutes, washing in detergent, drying at 60°C and reinserting into a plastic bag which is sealed and heated at 60°C.

Wood's light examination

This is a special lightbulb in which an ultraviolet source is enclosed in a special cupro-nickel glass which prevents emission of short-wave ultraviolet B. Scalp hairs infected with certain microsporum species of fungus fluoresce bright green, allowing instant recognition and removal of infected hairs for culture. Wood's light is invaluable for mass screening in outbreaks of tinea capitis in institutions, schools, camps, etc, and in following treatment through to cure.

Cytology

Expert cytological examination of scrapings stained supravitally is invaluable in the quick diagnosis of basal cell carcinoma, pemphigus vulgaris (Tzanck test) and herpes simplex or zoster (Fig 3.3).

Surgical biopsy

Obtaining three-dimensional tissue by punch or ellipse skin biopsy provides material for histopathological examination, culture (e.g. for *Mycobacterium tuberculosis*) and immunofluorescence (Fig. 3.5) or immunoperoxidase studies which detect the deposition of immune globulins in the skin. Using the immunoperoxidase method, monoclonal reagents can be applied to formalin-fixed, paraffin-embedded tissue but are not specific. Monoclonal antibodies are more specific but work best on frozen sections. The main antibodies used are shown in Table 3.1. In addition, antibodies to cutaneous antigens may be detected in blood samples by indirect immunofluorescence methods.

Hair plucking and root analysis

Chapter 22 lists the techniques available in this area.

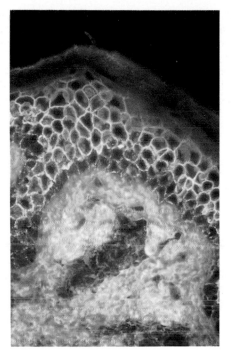

Fig. 3.5 Intercellular intraepidermal immunofluorescence in pemphigus vulgaris.

Table 3.1 Principal monoclonal antibodies in immunoperoxidase studies

Tissue	Antibodies
Epidermis	Antibodies to IgG, IgA, IgM Antibodies to complement C3, fibrin Various basement membrane antibodies Various antibodies to keratins
Melanocytes, melanoma	S100 antibody
Nerve fibres, nerve sheath tumours	S100 antibody
Blood vessels, vascular tumours	Factor VIII antibody
Lymphoid cells, lymphoma	T and B cell antibodies Heavy and light-chain antibodies
Macrophage/ histiocytic cells	$\alpha 1$ antitryspin antibody $\alpha 1$ antichymotrypsin antibody
Langerhans' cells	S100 antibody

Hair shaft microscopy

This is essential for the diagnosis of certain hair disorders, particularly congenital and hereditary ones. Transmission or scanning electron microscopy are sometimes very useful.

Other important techniques

Electron microscopy

When available, electron microscopic studies can be valuable in the rapid diagnosis of herpes simplex, for example in eczema herpeticum in babies, in the detection of wart viruses and the precise identification of certain blistering diseases and genodermatoses.

DNA probes

Nucleotide sequences in wart (HPV) viruses can be analysed using DNA probes, allowing 'typing' of these viruses. This technique has been invaluable in studying the relationship between genital warts and cervical dysplasia, and indeed in the study of the epidemiology and routes of transmission of various types of warts.

Principles of Treatment and the Use of Drugs

Although some skin diseases are treated systemically, dermatological treatment has the added dimension of topical, i.e. external therapy. This Chapter is a brief attempt to explain systemic and topical therapy of skin diseases on a rational basis.

Systemic Therapy

The principles of systemic therapy of skin disease do not differ from those appropriate for internal disease.

Analgesia

Itching is generally more important than pain and it is rarely necessary to use analgesics stronger than aspirin, paracetamol or ibuprofen.

Antipruritic drugs

Our antipruritic weapons are unsatisfactory, only antihistamines and sedatives being available. Older antihistamines with sedative side-effects, such as promethazine hydrochloride or mepyramine maleate, may be useful, especially at night, but vehicle drivers or those handling dangerous machinery should be particularly warned about the sedative effects. Two modern antihistamines rarely cause sedation: terfenadine does not cross the blood–brain barrier so rarely causes drowsiness, while astemizole does cross the barrier but has little affinity for central receptors. However, its half-life is over 100 hours so there is some risk of accumulation with daily dosage.

If sedatives are used, diazepam or nitrazepam in low dosage are safest.

Antibiotics

Only a few antibiotics have a regular place in the treatment of skin disease. In streptococcal infections penicillin is the drug of choice, initially benzyl penicillin G by injection followed by phenoxymethyl penicillin (V) orally. If the patient is allergic to penicillin, erythromycin or fusidic acid can be used. In serious *Staphylococcus aureus* infection, erythromycin and flucloxacillin are the drugs of choice and only rarely will fusidic acid, gentamicin or cephalosporins be needed. Vancomycin is very toxic but may rarely be needed for serious infections due to multiple (and methicillin) resistant strains of *S. aureus*.

Antifungal antibiotics

Griseofulvin is the only antibiotic active against the dermatophytes which cause tinea. It is inactive in *Candida albicans* infections, where mycostatin (nystatin) or, rarely, intravenous amphotericin B can be used.

Anti-infective chemotherapeutic agents

Dapsone (a sulphone) is used in the treatment of leprosy, as are rifampicin and clofazimine. Co-trimoxazole may be useful in Gram-positive and Gram-negative skin infections. Tuberculosis of the skin, as of other organs, is treated with isoniazid, rifampicin or ethambutol.

Ketoconazole, an imidazole, given orally is a valuable second-line drug in tinea and is the drug of choice in serious resistant *Candida albicans* infections (for example in immunocompromised patients). Rarely, it causes serious hepatotoxicity.

Acyclovir is an important recent advance in the management of herpes zoster and herpes simplex. Used intravenously, it may be life-saving in severe eczema herpeticum and herpes simplex infections in severely immunocompromised subjects.

Retinoids

This important new class of drug is derived from vitamin A. Retinoids are synthetic analogues of vitamin A and two are now widely used. Etretinate is valuable in psoriasis and certain other disorders of keratinization. Isotretinoin has profound suppressive effects on the sebacous gland and is used in severe intractable acne vulgaris. All retinoids are teratogenic. Fortunately, isotretinoin has a short half-life but etretinate may remain in the body for 2 years or even longer and should be used in women of child-bearing age only in exceptional circumstances. These retinoids cause mucocutaneous dryness and may have serious skeletal consequences, including hyperostosis, premature epiphyseal closure and ligamentous calcification, if treatment is maintained long term.

Corticosteroids

These suppress but never cure disease. Their disadvantages include a lowering of resistance to many infections, and metabolic disturbances particularly in regard to electrolytes (leading to sodium and water retention and potassium loss) and carbohydrate metabolism, aggravating any diabetic tendency. The fluid retention may lead to oedema (moon face, buffalo hump), increase in weight and a steady increase in blood pressure. Catabolic effects on collagen slowly lead to osteoporosis, skin atrophy and striae formation (Fig. 4.1). Purpura may follow. Androgen-like effects encourage acne and hirsutism in the female. Dyspepsia is common and pre-existing peptic ulceration may perforate. Aseptic necrosis of the femoral head rarely follows prolonged treatment. In children growth may be retarded. In the eye, increased pressure in the anterior chamber may cause glaucoma. Rarely, cataracts form. Emotional disturbance is not uncommon on high dose therapy. Euphoria and even hypomania can occur, and rarely depression follows.

Obviously, patients must be carefully selected for corticosteroid treatment and as carefully supervised when under treatment. The minimum care demands an initial radiograph of the chest to exclude pulmonary tuberculosis, and regular recordings of weight and blood pressure and regular urine examinations for glycosuria; the latter should be done at least once a month in ambulant cases. X-ray examination of the thoracic spine should be undertaken every 2 years in long-term treatment to ensure that osteoporosis is not occurring.

Deviations from the normal in any of these investigations demand careful attention and appropriate action on the part of the physician. Sometimes iatrogenic abnormalities discovered by these tests necessitate abandoning steroid therapy. Patients must be warned never suddenly to stop taking steroids, for intense fatigue, prostration, and even collapse from adrenal insufficiency are likely unless they are weaned slowly. Patients must also be told that, should they have to have an anaesthetic, even 'gas' for the removal of a tooth, they must warn the anaesthetist, and this caveat must be remembered for 2 years after ceasing to take the drug. The patient should carry a steroid record card.

Prednisolone is the drug usually used. Initial dosage depends on the disease being treated. It may be quite small (10–15 mg daily) in a chronic dermatitis, rather higher in very acute urticaria, lichen planus, contact dermatitis or pompholyx eczema (30–40 mg daily) and still higher in dermatomyosis, systemic lupus erythematosus or bullous pemphigoid (40–80 mg daily). Even higher doses, up to 360 mg daily, may be needed for short periods in pemphigus vulgaris.

The dose is reduced as soon as the disease comes under control. Where maintenance therapy is necessary, the smallest possible dosage should always be used. There is some evidence that alternate-day therapy is a safer schedule for long-term treatment; certainly it causes much less growth retardation in childhood.

Corticotrophin has largely been superseded by its synthetic analogue, tetracosactrin zinc (Synacthen Depot, U.K.). Both have the disadvantage of having to be given by injection. They also have a greater sodium-retaining potential than prednisolone. The author does not favour the intramuscular use of triamcinolone acetonide (Kenalog, U.K.). It is less flexible than oral prednisolone and cannot be withdrawn if steroid complications occur. Its effects last 2–4 weeks.

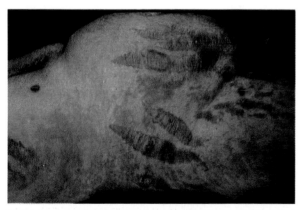

Fig. 4.1 Gross striae induced by prolonged oral and topical corticosteroid therapy in a patient with psoriasis.

Topical Therapy

The aims of topical therapy

Local applications may have many aims other than the exposure of the skin to specific pharmacological agents. Such aims include the following:

Cooling. Cooling raises the threshold of itching and so reduces pruritus.

Drying. Drying or astringency is of value in exudative conditions and reduces the risk of secondary bacterial infection of the skin surface.

Hydration. Hydrating the skin may be of value when the stratum corneum is abnormally dry, as in ichthyosis or chapping. The stratum corneum is only pliable and healthy when its water content falls within a certain narrow range. In other circumstances, hydrating the corneum increases its permeability to some pharmacological agents. This type of drug may be incorporated in an occlusive paraffin base which prevents water loss from the skin surface.

Crust removal. The removal of crusts may be important because it allows access of antibiotics to the skin below, for example in impetigo.

Scale removal. Removing scale has the same therapeutic value as removing crusts but it is also of cosmetic importance and increases skin pliability and hence the patient's comfort.

Protection. Visible skin lesions attract the attention of the patient's fingers, even in the absence of pruritus. Rubbing and scratching increase skin damage, promote lichenification and encourage secondary infection. Thick pastes and ointments physically protect the skin from the fingers and hide the lesions from the eyes, lessening the urge to molest.

Drug administration. Specific drug therapy with topical anti-inflammatory agents, antibiotics, etc, brings a drug directly to the target organ where it is wanted and minimizes the exposure of other organs where it is unwanted, thus removing one of the chief drawbacks of systemic drug administration. Such treatment necessitates incorporating the active drug in a suitable vehicle or base. The vehicle must be suitably designed for the carriage and release of the drug and must also be compatible with the other aims and requirements of topical therapy in each particular clinical situation.

Vehicles (bases) for topical therapy

The ideal vehicle or base for topical therapy should not be irritating or sensitizing. It should not react with the stratum corneum or the active agent and should allow the release of the agent into the skin. It should be stable at room temperature, have a long shelf-life and must not tolerate the growth of micro-organisms within it during storage. Its colour and consistency must be physically and cosmetically acceptable to the patient.

Lotions

Lotions are liquid vehicles which may or may not be volatile. A lotion may be aqueous or alcoholic, or it may contain other volatile components. Evaporation of the vehicle promotes cooling and rapidly increases the concentration of active drug. Lotions with an oily base are called linaments, for example oily calamine lotion.

Shake lotions

Shake lotions contain an inert powder in aqueous suspension. Evaporation of the water promotes cooling and leaves a protective deposit of powder, for example calamine lotion.

Creams

Creams are emulsions of either water in oil (oily creams) or oil in water (vanishing creams). An emulsifying agent is needed to keep the system stable. In an emulsion the active agent is dispersed between the oil and water phases according to its partition coefficient. The advantages of such emulsions include miscibility with surface exudation, ease of removal and patient acceptability. Oil-in-water emulsions do not feel greasy and do not retard heat loss. A preservative must be incorporated to prevent microbial growth.

Gels

A gel is a non-greasy, single-phase semisolid with a high viscosity incorporating a single polymer. It is 'clean' and easy to apply and remove, especially in the scalp.

Ointments

Ointments are semisolid and anhydrous, and feel greasy. Ointments may be either hydrophylic or hydrophobic. A hydrophylic ointment is soluble in water and usually contains polyethylene glycols of varying molecular weight which allow the viscosity to be controlled and are solvent, emollient and lubricant. Hydrophobic ointments are not miscible with water and are paraffin based. Mixing hard and soft paraffins controls stiffness and greasiness. Hydrophobic ointments are more protective and have the advantage of preventing heat loss when this is desirable and of hydrating the stratum corneum. Drugs are suspended rather than dissolved in a hydrophobic ointment.

Pastes

Pastes contain a high proportion of powder, such as starch or zinc oxide, in an ointment base. Pastes can be made very stiff, allowing application of a drug to precisely defined lesions, for example in the use of dithranol in psoriasis. They may also play an important protective role. Lassar's paste contains 24% zinc oxide, 24% starch, 2% salicylic acid with 50% soft white paraffin.

Dusting powders

Dusting powders contain zinc oxide, starch or purified talc and are useful as drying agents, absorbers of heat, or occasionally as vehicles for drugs. They are useful in moist body folds.

Soaps

Soaps have a useful defatting action in the seborrhoea of acne vulgaris. A soap medicated with an antiseptic, such as Cidal (U.K.), Dial® or Palmolive Gold® (U.S.A.), may have a place in the treatment and prevention of furunculosis. Simple Soap (U.K.) is free of perfume and other additives and may be useful in perfume-sensitive individuals.

Detergents

These are of value as shampoos. Shampoo containing 1% cetrimide has a useful antiseptic action. Detergent shampoos medicated with tar have a place in the treatment of pityriasis capitis and scalp psoriasis.

Metals

Zinc oxide or starch powders are used very widely, chiefly as inert substances to alter the consistency of lotions, creams, pastes and ointments. Calamine is basic zinc carbonate or zinc oxide coloured with ferric oxide, to give a more natural colour. Titanium dioxide is sometimes added to applications to make them more acceptable cosmetically, and also acts as a sunscreen. Aluminium acetate solution (BPC) 5% in water (Burow's solution) is a mildly astringent solution used as a compress for the oozing stage of various dermatoses.

Medicated dressings

These are of several types. Salicylic acid in a concentration up to 40% may be incorporated into plasters which are cut to shape and applied to plantar warts for 24–48 hours at a time. Bland zinc ointments or ointments containing tar or iodoquinolines can be incorporated into bandages which can be left on areas of lichenified eczema for several days at a time (see p. 92). A proprietary steroid-medicated, translucent, adhesive tape containing flurandrenolone (Haelan Tape, U.K.; Cordran Tape®, U.S.A) is useful in chronic localized inflammatory skin disease which is resistant to conventional therapy and may be used in eczema, psoriasis, lichen planus and discoid lupus erythematosus.

Sunscreens

These may be physical barriers intended to reflect or scatter ultraviolet light. Titanium dioxide or zinc oxide in finely ground forms can be used, incorporated in an appropriate base. Ultraviolet absorbers are of variable efficacy. *para*-Aminobenzoic acid and its derivatives, benzophenones, cinnamates and others are used.

Specific drugs used topically

Antibacterial antibiotics can be used in the topical treatment of skin disease. Where time and resources permit, topical antibiotic therapy should be guided, like its systemic counterpart, by bacteriological culture. Penicillins and streptomycin are *never* used topically because of their sensitizing potential. All those listed below are used, but they can all occasionally sensitize the skin. Neomycin is probably the most sensitizing, and tetracycline the least.

Chlortetracycline

Chlortetracycline is a bacteriostatic antibiotic that is active against most strains of *Streptococcus pyogenes*, although many strains of *Staphylococcus aureus* are resistant. It also has some activity against Gram-negative organisms.

Neomycin and framycetin

These are virtually identical and are very valuable antibiotics for topical use because they are not used systemically and are active against most strains of *Staphylococcus aureus*. They have no activity against *Streptococcus pyogenes*. When used for long periods on eczematous skin they have a considerable predilection to sensitize. They should not be used on ulcers or large erosions, since absorption may lead to nerve deafness or renal damage.

Bacitracin and gramicidin

These are two valuable antibiotics which are not used systemically. *Streptococcus pyogenes* is always sensitive to both, as are some strains of *Staphylococcus aureus*. Either bacitracin or gramicidin is used in combination with neomycin. This combination is of particular value in treating impetigo and infected dermatitis where both *Streptococcus pyogenes* and *Staphylococcus aureus* may be present.

Fusidic acid

This antibiotic is very active against Gram-positive cocci and has been widely used topically. Used systemically, it is a valuable agent in serious systemic staphylococcal infections such as osteomyelitis and postinfluenzal pneumonia. The topical use of fusidic acid should therefore be restricted so as not to encourage the emergence of bacterial resistance.

Gentamicin

Gentamicin is active against *Staphylococcus aureus* and *Pseudomonas aeruginosa*. Like neomycin, it is inactive against *Streptococcus pyogenes*. It is used systemically and considerations similar to those for fusidic acid apply.

Polymyxin

Polymyxin is not used systemically and has a useful range of activity against Gram-negative organisms. It is used in combination with neomycin or bacitracin.

Mupirocin (Bactroban, U.K.)

This is a valuable new topical antibiotic with a wide range of activity against Gram-positive and Gram-negative organisms. It is particularly valuable in resistant superficial staphylococcal infections or carriage, although resistance to it is emerging.

Sulphonamides

Sulphonamides are not used topically on the skin because of their sensitizing potential. Sodium sulphacetamide (Albucid, U.K.) is used in the eye and, incorporated in ethanol (15%), is useful for sterilizing the subungual space in onycholysis.

Antihistamines

Antihistamines should not be used topically bacause of their sensitizing potential. They have no antihistaminic action when applied topically and allay itching by virtue of their local anaesthetic potential.

Local anaesthetics

Local anaesthetics of the procaine series (e.g. amethocaine and benzocaine) should not be used because of the risk of sensitization. Lignocaine (Xylocaine, U.K.) virtually never sensitizes and has a limited role in anogenital pruritis.

Antiseptics

Potassium permanganate is an extremely useful non-sensitizing astringent and wide-spectrum antiseptic. It is used in a dilute aqueous solution of between 1:4000 and 1:16 000 for a few minutes daily as a wet compress or by immersion of the affected part. Povidone iodine in aqueous solution (Betadine, U.K.) is equally valuable. Other antiseptics include benzalkonium chloride 0.1% and chlorhexidine gluconate 1% (Hibitane, U.K.). Iodoquinolines (Chinoform, Clioquinol, Chlorquinaldol) are useful wide-spectrum agents but occasionally sensitize. Sodium hypochlorite solution (Eusol) is now known to be toxic to tissue cells and is little used. Aluminium acetate 5% aqueous (Burow's solution) is also useful.

Corticosteroids

Topical corticosteroids have a central role in the treatment of non-infective inflammatory skin disorders, particularly dermatitis, psoriasis, lichen planus and discoid lupus erythematosus. They suppress rather than cure disease and relapse or even rebound exacerbation may follow withdrawal. They aggravate and change the morphology of cutaneous infections and also worsen acne, rosacea and perioral dermatitis. They should never be applied to ulceration.

They vary widely in potency and the choice of preparation should depend on the disease to be treated, the site and the likely duration of therapy. Thus, dermatitis may respond to mild preparations whereas lichen planus or discoid lupus erythematosus call for potent ones. The younger the patient, the milder should be the product chosen. The skin of the face (Fig. 4.2), neck, flexures (Fig. 4.3) and inner thighs (Fig. 4.3) is more easily damaged than that of the scalp, back or palms. The British National Formulary recognizes four groups (Table 4.1) and classifies every product listed (see Appendix III).

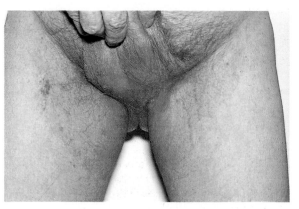

Fig. 4.3 Misuse of strong corticosteroid creams in the flexures leads to striae formation, for example at 90° to the inguinal creases.

Local side effects depend on site, duration and intensity of treatment. Bacterial and fungal infections may spread and assume puzzling forms (see tinea incognito, p. 66). Epidermal and dermal atrophy lead to obvious skin thinning, striae, redness, telangiectasiae, purpura and easy tearing. Local hypertrichosis may occur and pigmentation may be modified. Widespread exposure to potent preparations leads to absorption and therefore the hazards of systemic therapy, especially pituitary-adrenal suppression in the short term and Cushingoid features in the longer term (Fig. 4.4). Death has followed abrupt withdrawal of prolonged whole-body application of large quantities of the most potent preparations. Mothers of atopic children may have facial changes due to unintentional contamination of the skin of the cheeks by the fingers after applying creams to the child.

Dilution of topical corticosteroids

Prescriptions requiring the pharmacist to dilute creams should be avoided. Ointments can be safely diluted in soft white paraffin (mineral oil) when large quantities are needed, for example in generalized exfoliative dermatitis, so that the whole body can be treated twice or thrice daily (which could require 500 g per week). Thus 25 g clobetasol propionate 0.05% (Dermovate, U.K.) can be mixed with 225 g white paraffin to give 250 g of 1:10 ointment.

Antifungal agents

Basic dyes such as 1% aqueous gentian violet lotion are highly effective against fungal infections but tend to be messy and ruin linen. Potassium permanganate and

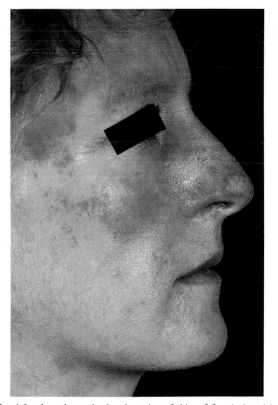

Fig. 4.2 Atrophy and telangiectasiae of skin of face induced by potent topical corticosteroid usage.

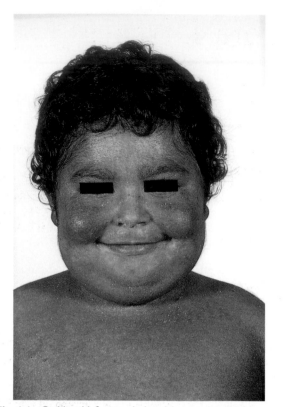

Fig. 4.4 Cushingoid features induced in a young child by prolonged gross exposure to potent topical corticosteroid.

Table 4.1 Potency classification of topical corticosteroids.

Group	Potency	Examples	Maximum dose (per week)
1	Very potent	Clobetasol propionate 0.05% Halcinonide 0.1%	15–25 g
2	Potent	Betamethasone valerate 0.1% Beclomethasone dipropionate 0.025% Difluocortolone valerate 0.1% Fluocinolone acetonide 0.025% Triamcinolone acetonide 0.1%	40–50 g
3	Moderately potent	Clobetasone butyrate 0.05% Flurandrenalone 0.05% Fluocortolone hexanoate 0.1%	70–100 g
4	Mild	Hydrocortisone 1% and 2.5% Alclometasone dipropionate 0.05%	150 g (adults), 60 g (children), 20 g (babies)

iodoquinolines are very useful. Clotrimazole and miconazole nitrate are of particular value, being active against dermatophytes, *Candida* species, tinea versicolor and some bacteria. Another imidazole, tioconazole in undecylenic acid as a solution (Trosyl, U.K.), may prove useful in resistant nail infections with dermatophytes and *Candida*. Griseofulvin is non-active topically.

Hydroquinone

This substance poisons melanocytes and is used as a depigmenting agent. Preparations containing less than 2% hydroquinone may be sold in the United Kingdom without prescription (Ambi, Esoterica, Symba, Ultra Glow). Higher concentrations (5–10%) may be prescribed in melasma, chloasma and rarely on hyper-pigmented patches in vitiligo. Depigmentation may be patchy and chronic overdosage can lead to ochronosis. Monobenzyl ether of hydroquinone should never be used as it may cause widespread metastatic depigmentation.

Many other substances are used topically in dermatological practice and to avoid repetition are mentioned in the relevant Chapters, for example coal tar preparations in psoriasis (Chapter 12) and 5-fluorouracil in actinic keratoses (Chapter 15).

— 5

The Skin and Systemic Disease

In this Chapter a number of systemic disorders and pregnancy are discussed where cutaneous manifestations are important (and of diagnostic value). Infections and neoplastic disease are described elsewhere.

Pregnancy

Pregnant women may need reassurance on a number of minor changes and occasionally treatment of dramatic dermatoses. Spider naevi may enlarge or appear de novo sometimes together with palmar erythema, changes promptly reversed after the birth. Pruritus is common in late pregnancy, especially on the belly. Only rarely is it due to intrahepatic cholestasis. Increasing pigmentation, especially of the face (chloasma), areolae, nipples and anogenital area and mid-line of the abdoment (linea nigra), is usual, as are abdominal striae distensae. The latter may leave permanent unsightly marks. Moles enlarge or may appear in pregnancy, remaining unchanged after birth.

Vaginal candidosis may be a problem and genital wart infections may be particularly exuberant. Psoriasis tends to improve but to relapse and even rebound in the postpartum months. Normal hair loss diminishes only to increase 2–4 months postpartum. When loss is severe, frank alopecia is seen, a form of telogen alopecia (see Chapter 22).

The Rashes of Pregnancy

Several mysterious itching and papular, erythematous or urticarial eruptions are not uncommon. Best delineated is herpes gestationis (better called pemphigoid gestationis since herpes viruses are *not* involved). This is a rare, intensely pruritic, erythematous and blistering eruption which may recur in successive pregnancies, and occasionally is slow to settle afterwards. The mouth is not involved and pathological features are of pemphigoid (see p. 155). There is an association with autoimmune thyroid disease.

Pruritus

Generalized itching may be an important symptom of systemic disease. If no dermatosis is evident and scabies can be excluded, important causes include renal failure, liver disease, hyperthyroidism and malignant disease, especially lymphoma and polycythaemia vera. In addition, anxiety and depression can both cause pruritus.

Dermatological Complications of Diabetes Mellitus

Candidosis. Candidosis is common in presenting or badly controlled diabetes. Recurrent balanoposthitis may be a presenting feature in the adult male, vulvovaginitis in presenting late diabetes of the female.

Staphyloderma. Staphyloderma is common and 'boils' may be a presenting feature; localized infections easily ulcerate, especially on the leg.

Arterial disease. Small vessel disease causes 'diabetic dermopathy', a characteristic pattern of pigmentation and scarring on the shins. Large vessel atheroma may lead to ulceration or gangrene on the feet of elderly diabetics.

Neuropathy. Neuropathic ulceration on pressure points on the feet, characteristically painless, is well recognized in long-standing diabetes. Typically the ulcers are small but deeply perforating, sometimes down to the bone.

Xanthomata. Small multiple pink–yellow eruptive xanthomata may be secondary to the hyperlipidaemia of uncontrolled diabetes (see p. 32).

Necrobiosis lipoidica. Necrobiosis lipoidica (Fig. 5.1) is a rare complication usually seen in adolescent or young diabetics, sometimes well controlled. Typically a solitary patch of indurated erythema spreads very slowly, becoming whitish–yellow and atrophic centrally.

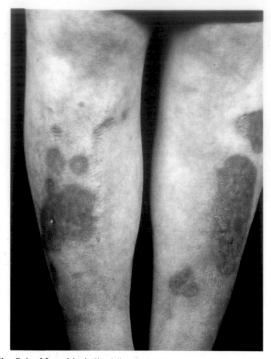

Fig. 5.1   Necrobiosis lipoidica diabeticorum on shins.

Lesions may be multiple and are almost always on the anterior shins. The disease persists indefinitely.

Granuloma annulare. An uncommon disseminated form of this disease may complicate diabetes (see p. 35).

Thyroid Disease and the Skin

The cool dry skin of gross myxoedema is characteristic. There may be diffuse loss of scalp hair and eyebrows. In contrast, frank thyrotoxicosis presents a warm moist soft skin. Sweating may be frequent. Diffuse scalp (but not eyebrow) hair loss may occur. Clubbing is a feature of thyroid acropachy.

Pretibial myxoedema. This is a rare disease, which is usually associated with worsening exophthalmos and clubbing after a thyroidectomy. Smooth hard irregular deposits of a mucopolysaccharide material under the skin of the shins produce red–brown or skin-coloured plaques and nodules which persist indefinitely.

Parathyroid Disease

Primary hyperparathyroidism does not cause skin lesions, although occasionally calcific keratopathy or subcutaneous lumps on the face due to bone cysts present to the dermatologist.

Accidental (surgical) parathyroidectomy with hypo-calcaemia may provoke generalized pustular psoriasis, affects the nails and can cause eczematous eruptions. Idopathic hypoparathyroidism of childhood has characteristic nail changes and may be associated with mucocutaneous candidosis.

Suprarenal Disease

Suprarenal insufficiency (Addison's disease) causes hyperpigmentation, especially on the face and sites of pressure and friction and in the buccal mucosa when blue–black macules are typical. Conversely, vitiligo may occur as an additional autoimmune disorder.

In overactivity (Cushing's syndrome), truncofacial obesity, 'buffalo hump', a plethoric rounded face, hirsutism, acne and striae are found.

Liver Disease

The jaundice and pruritus of acute liver disease are well known. Hepatitis B may have a prodrome of fever, arthralgia and urticaria. In portal cirrhosis, spider naevi, palmar erythema and leuconychia may develop. Later, hyperpigmentation, clubbing and Dupuytren's contracture may appear. In men, body hair may be sparse and gynaecomastia can develop. When portal hypertension worsens, dilated superficial veins over the trunk probably represent collateral portal–systemic connections. Biliary cirrhosis may be associated with xanthomatosis and possibly lichen planus.

Xanthomatosis

The appearance of xanthomata in the skin generally indicates a disorder of lipid metabolism. Six main types of hyperlipidaemia are now recognized (Table 5.1). The disorder may be primary and genetically induced, or secondary to other disease.

Table 5.1 Classification of hyperlipidaemia.

	Cholesterol	Triglycerides	Chylomicrons	LDL	VLDL	HDL
Type I	↑	↑	↑	↓	↓	↓
Type IIA	↑	N	N	↑	N	
Type IIB	↑	↑	N	↑	↑	↓
Type III	↑	↑		↓	↑	↓
Type IV	N	↑	↓	N	↑	↓
Type V	↑	↑	↑	↓	↑	↓

Lipid metabolism

Absorbed dietary lipids and cholesterol are bound by apolipoproteins (which are components of plasma lipoproteins) to form chylomicrons which are taken up by the liver very rapidly. Specialized apolipoproteins (VLDLs) carry triglycerides from the liver and are degraded to low density lipoproteins (LDLs) by the loss of triglycerides. LDL is the major carrier of cholesterol. Tissue cells have a genetically controlled LDL receptor which binds LDLs and regulates cholesterol transfer into the cell. Reverse cholesterol transport back to the liver (and excretion as esters in bile) is achieved by high density lipoproteins (HDLs) which thus prevent cholesterol accumulation.

Clinical patterns of cutaneous xanthoma

Tuberose xanthoma

Tuberose xanthomata (Fig. 5.2) are firm and sometimes tender papules, nodules or plaques, yellow or orange in colour, sometimes with an erythematous

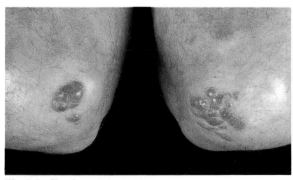

Fig. 5.2 Xanthoma tuberosum.

halo, seen on the extensor points of the elbows, knees and sometimes buttocks. They are seen in Type IIa and III hyperlipidaemia (Table 5.1).

Tendon xanthoma

Tendon xanthomata are firm colourless subcutaneous nodules attached to tendons and usually found at the back of the heel or on the knuckles of the hand. Small lesions are felt most easily on movement of the tendons. They are characteristic of LDL elevation in Type II disorder.

Eruptive xanthoma

Eruptive xanthomata are pin-head or larger yellow papules which are profuse and appear suddenly on the buttocks, shoulder and other extensor surfaces and over the face or oral mucosae. They signify hypertriglyceridaemia (Types I, III and IV).

Plane xanthoma

Plane xanthomata are orange–yellow macules or hardly palpable plaques which may be widespread but which typically affect the palmar creases (Type III disorders). A generalized form may be associated with the monoclonal gammopathy of myeloma or lymphoma.

Xanthelasma palpebrarum

These firm, flat yellow nodules or plaques are seen around the eyes, especially about the inner canthus. Blood lipids are often normal but Type II disorders may be present.

Pathology of xanthomata

Masses of lipid materials are present in cells within the dermis, particularly around capillaries.

Genetic Hyperlipidaemia

Only the two important and common syndromes with cutaneous features are described.

Familial hypercholesterolaemia

This is a common autosomal dominant condition now known to be due to abnormalities of the gene regulating the LDL receptor. The gene has now been cloned and localized on chrommosome 19. Eight mutant alleles have been identified with varying effects on LDL binding and transport into the cell.

The common heterozygote has about 50% LDL binding capacity. Patients present in early adult life with premature chronic heart disease and often tuberose and tendon xanthomata, xanthelasma and corneal arcus senilis. Serum LDL is increased.

The homozygous disease is very rare with almost total inability to bind LDL. It presents with xanthomata in early childhood with gross LDL elevation in the blood, followed by heart disease which is usually fatal by adolescence.

Treatment

The heterozygous disease can be improved by a diet low in cholesterol and saturated fats, and high in polyunsaturated fats. The anion exchange resin, cholestyramine, further lowers serum cholesterol, and nicotinic acid may reduce cholesterol synthesis. Ileal bypass operations help some patients.

Homozygous disease is amenable only to plasma exchange, portocaval shunt or liver transplantation.

Familial (endogenous) hypertriglyceridaemia

This disorder is also common and an autosomal dominant trait. LDL is normal but VLDL is increased. The disease is seen in obese adults, typically with diabetes and hypertension. Eruptive xanthomata are sometimes seen.

Secondary hyperlipidaemia

The important common causes are summarized in Table 5.2.

Table 5.2 Secondary hyperlipidaemia.

Features				Cause
Cholesterol	↑			Biliary cirrhosis
Cholesterol	↑	LDL	↑	Hypothyroidism, nephrotic syndrome
Triglyceride	↑	VLDL	↑	Alcoholism, diabetes, renal failure
Triglyceride	↑	HDL	↑	Oral contraceptives

Nutritional Dermatoses

Vitamin C deficiency. Purpura is the classical sign of 'scurvy' with swollen, bleeding gums. Alcoholics and vagrants are more likely to have bilateral indurated ('woody') oedema of the lower legs with purpura and much haemosiderotic staining.

Nicotinic acid deficiency (pellagra). A scaly dermatitis of backs of hands, fingers and neck is associated with diarrhoea, depression and dementia in gross deficiency (four D's).

Protein energy malnutrition. This term encompasses kwashiorkor, famine oedema, marasmus and cachexia. The classical childhood syndrome of kwashiorkor follows abrupt weaning and is characterized by an exfoliating rash, oedema, fine discoloured hair and hepatomegaly. The child is apathetic or irritable.

Acrodermatitis enteropathica of Danbolt. This is a rare disease of infants. Failure to thrive is associated with a red scaly rash around orifices, diarrhoea and absent hair. It is due to a failure of zinc absorption and can be fatal if not treated with zinc.

Dermatoses Secondary to Gastrointestinal Disease

Dermatitis herpetiformis. Dermatitis herpetiformis is secondary to gluten enteropathy. It is described in Chapter 18.

Pyoderma gangrenosum. This is an uncommon but dramatic complication of ulcerative colitis or Crohn's disease. Small areas of inflammation swell, soften, spread and ulcerate with an alarming speed. Neither infection nor frank vasculitis is present. High dose prednisolone therapy is needed to arrest the process (Fig. 5.3).

Carcinoid syndrome. This presents as recurrent brief dramatic episodes of bright flushing of the face, neck and upper chest. Eventually a chronic plethora may develop. The skin changes may be accompanied by asthma, abdominal pain and diarrhoea. The symptoms and signs are due to release of peptides from a carcinoid tumour in the appendix or small intestine.

Crohn's disease. Perianal abscesses and fistulae are common. Sinus formation may involve the abdominal

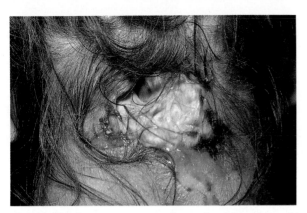

Fig. 5.3 Pyoderma gangrenosum of nape of neck in a 38-year-old woman with Crohn's disease.

wall or groin. The mouth and lips may be affected, with chronic swelling of the lips and a corrugated appearance of the oral mucosa with linear ulcers in the troughs of the corrugations. Erythema nodosum and pyoderma gangrenosum (see above) occur occasionally.

Ulcerative colitis. A variety of changes very similar to those of Crohn's disease may occur.

Dermatoses Secondary to Pancreatic Disease

Panniculitis. Rarely pancreatitis may lead to multiple areas of fat necrosis with inflammation presenting as tender subcutaneous lumps, sometimes tethered to skin. The histology is characteristic.

Cutaneous haemorrhage. In acute pancreatitis, haemorrhage from the pancreas may spread to the body wall leading to 'bruising' of the left flank (Grey Turner's sign) or umbilicus (Cullen's sign).

Thrombophlebitis migrans. Multiple areas of superficial thrombophlebitis may complicate carcinoma of the pancreas.

Haemochromatosis. This disorder of iron absorption and accumulation involves the liver, pancreas (bronze diabetes) and skin whose 'bronze' colour is due to a mixture of melanin and iron pigments.

Glucagonoma syndrome. This presents in women in late middle-life as a distinctive 'necrolytic migratory erythema' in association with weight loss, anaemia, diarrhoea and glossitis. Marginated, eroded and crusted skin lesions particularly involve the anogenital area. Hyperglucagonaemia is associated with a malignant islet cell tumour of the pancreas.

Granulomas of Unknown Origin

Sarcoidosis

This is a fairly common chronic multisystem disease of unknown cause in which epithelioid cell granulomata develop, particularly in lung, skin, lymph glands, eye, bone or central nervous system. It is common in black people of West African origin. The important manifestations are as follows.

Erythema nodosum. This is a presenting feature in 15% of cases, occurring particularly in spring and in young female adults of 20–40 years. Attacks last for 3–20 weeks and may recur. There may be associated flitting arthralgia and hilar adenopathy, often bilateral. This type of sarcoidosis is usually not progressive and carries a good prognosis.

Nodules and plaques. Red–brown papules, nodules and plaques of varying sizes may affect the skin or subcutaneous tissues. The face, nose, ears and neck are common sites (Fig. 5.4). In white skin, lesions are dull red, later becoming brown.

Transient maculopapular eruptions. These may herald the onset of parotid enlargement or uveitis and are probably due to circulating immune complexes. They tend to heal in a few weeks.

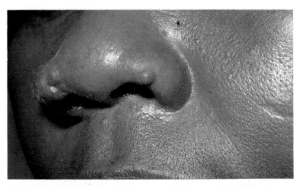

Fig. 5.4 Nodules of cutaneous sarcoid on nose of a black woman.

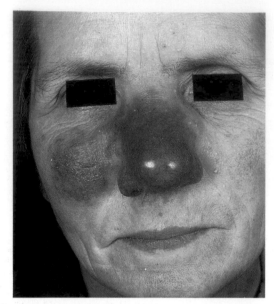

Fig. 5.5 Lupus pernio in sarcoidosis.

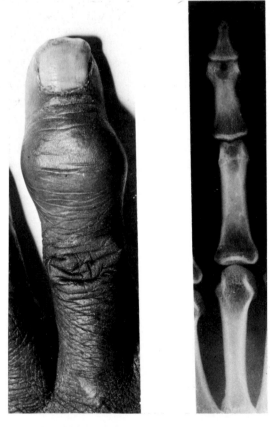

Fig. 5.6 Sarcoidal dactylitis; swelling of finger and radiographic translucencies.

Lupus pernio. This is a striking blue–red infiltration of the nose, face, ears or scalp (Fig. 5.5) and is a feature of chronic progressive multisystem disease. It is found in an older age group than erythema nodosum, i.e. over 40 years, and is more common in females.

Dactylitis. Infiltration of the fingers with flexion deformities and underlying bony involvement occurs occasionally. There may be gross nail dystrophy (Fig. 5.6).

Scars. Old scars may 'light up' and become livid when sarcoidosis develops. Keloids may become sarcoidal, for example in the ears.

Ulceration is not seen in sarcoidosis and histologically caseation is absent.

Diagnosis

Histological confirmation by biopsy is essential. The tuberculin test is usually negative, and the Kveim test positive. Sarcoid must be differentiated from tuberculosis, syphilis, leprosy, leishmaniasis and deep mycoses by appropriate investigations.

Treatment

Spontaneous resolution of erythema nodosum can be expected. Topical corticosteroids are of little value; occasionally intralesional injections of facial lesions with triamcinolone are useful. Oral prednisolone may be needed for progressive systemic disease threatening lung or eye function. Methotrexate 0.1 mg/kg once weekly by mouth for 3 months may be of value. Alternatively, hydroxychlorquine (Plaquenil, U.K.) one tablet thrice weekly for 6–9 months can be used.

Granuloma annulare

Granuloma annulare is a common condition in which there is granulomatous infiltrate in the dermis surrounding foci of collagen degeneration (necrobiosis). The cause is unknown. Probably an antigen–antibody reaction is responsible. Commonest in children and young adults, granuloma annulare can occur at any age. There is a rare disseminated adult type, which may be associated with diabetes. The common sites are the extensor prominences of the hands, arms, feet and legs. The lesions are papules or nodules which are skin-coloured, red or red–blue. The lesions often form a ring or a part of a ring (Fig. 5.7). The diagnosis from ringworm is not difficult because granuloma annulare is sited in the dermis and the epidermis is normal, whereas ringworm produces epidermal changes, i.e. scaling, vesiculation or pustulation. Granuloma annulare and rheumatoid nodules are histologically similar but the latter are subcutaneous. The condition has a strong tendency to improve spontaneously but may persist for years. Granuloma annulare can be influenced by local corticosteroids, either ointments or creams, or by intralesional injection.

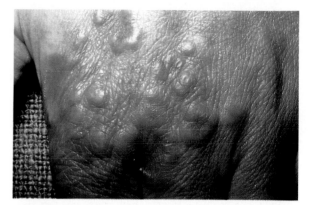

Fig. 5.7 Granuloma annulare on knuckle.

Systemic amyloidosis

Amyloid is a protein-like substance with defined properties. It may be deposited in skin and other tissues. Systemic amyloidosis is due to a plasma cell dyscrasia and is usually associated with myeloma. Characteristic skin and mucosal lesions may be associated with macroglossia, carpal tunnel compression and visceral disease. Waxy, translucent and often haemorrhagic papules and plaques, typically on the eyelids (Fig. 5.8) but also elsewhere, are associated with a striking tendency to cutaneous haemorrhage, spontaneously or on minimal trauma. Death soon follows.

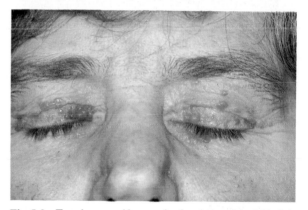

Fig. 5.8 Translucent and haemorrhagic papules of amyloidosis in a woman with myeloma.

6

Cutaneous Manifestations of Malignant Disease

The skin may be involved in systemic malignant disease specifically and non-specifically. Specific involvement means actual neoplastic infiltration of the skin by secondary deposits from an internal carcinoma, such as from the breast, or by deposits of a malignant lymphoma or leukaemia. Morphologically such lesions are likely to be papules, nodules, plaques or ulcers involving mainly the dermis but often with epidermal involvement, as in the case of T-cell lymphoma. The diagnosis is established without difficulty by biopsy.

In contrast, there is no histological evidence of malignant cells in the skin in the non-specific reactions. Clinical experience has demonstrated the importance of a number of cutaneous reactions which are sometimes called 'markers' of malignancy. Their presence calls for further investigation in search of a carcinoma or lymphoma. The mechanisms by which these markers develop are barely understood but immunological factors are thought to play a role in some.

The non-specific markers are best subdivided into three groups, as follows:
- Those almost always associated with malignancy
- Those sometimes associated with malignancy
- Those suggestive of lymphoma

Conditions Almost Always Associated with Malignancy

Paget's disease of the breast

This epidermal disorder of the breast, simulating eczema, is always due to an underlying ductal carcinoma of the breast tissue (see p. 166).

Acanthosis nigricans

This rare but distinctive condition, developing *de novo* in the second half of life, in subjects who are not obese and in the absence of endocrinopathy, indicates an internal malignancy, often a carcinoma in the gastrointestinal tract, especially the stomach. The cutaneous changes may herald the appearance of a detectable tumour or the latter may be well established by the time skin changes are seen.

The cutaneous changes consist of epidermal thickening and hyperpigmentation, particularly in the flexures (Fig. 6.1) and neck. The affected skin may become velvety but patchy wartiness is common. Multiple warty papillomata may be profuse and may involve the lips, mouth and conjunctival margins. The palms and soles may be involved.

Similar but milder changes may be seen in obese adolescents, particularly of dark-skinned ethnic groups such as Arabs and Indians, especially in the axillae and around the neck. Certain endocrinopathies characterized by insulin resistance in children may also be associated with similar changes, sometimes called pseudoacanthosis nigricans and of no sinister significance.

Erythema gyratum repens

This is a very rare but distinctive pattern of erythema

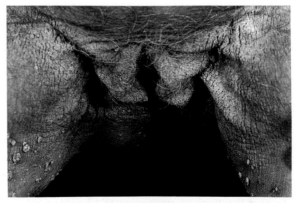

Fig. 6.1 Acanthosis nigricans in groin of a woman with disseminated carcinoma of breast.

in which concentric erythematous rings and wavy patterns are closely packed over the whole body. The patterns change visibly day by day, leaving scaling on the trailing edge of the waves of erythema. The condition may convert to a universal erythroderma. A carcinoma is always present eventually, often of the bronchus.

Necrolytic migratory erythema

This is an equally rare but morphologically and histologically distinctive eruption associated with weight loss, anaemia, diabetes and angular stomatitis. Its presence indicates the existence of a glucagon-secreting tumour, usually malignant, of the α-islet cells of the pancreas (glucagonoma).

Acquired hypertrichosis lanuginosa

This is another very rare syndrome in which widespread fine lanugo hair develops in the absence of virilization. Almost always a tumour is responsible.

Conditions Sometimes Associated with Malignancy

Dermatomyositis

This syndrome is described on p. 147. Cutaneous changes may be absent, as in carcinomatous polymyositis, or the skin changes may predominate or precede myositis by weeks or months. It is the least rare of the 'collagen' diseases in childhood, when it has no malignant implications, but in patients over 40 years, about one-third have or will develop a tumour.

Thrombophlebitis migrans

An uncommon but striking pattern of shifting multiple areas of superficial thrombophlebitis in the legs is sometimes associated with a carcinoma of the pancreas. It may also be a feature of Buerger's disease.

Multicentric reticulohistiocytosis

This is a rare disease of the skin and joints, which usually occurs in women, in which a mutilating and destructive arthritis of peripheral joints is associated with a characteristic eruption of reddish-yellow papules and nodules particularly on the face, shoulders and upper limbs. 'Coral bead' papules around the nail

folds are distinctive. About 25% of patients with multicentric reticulohistiocytosis develop a carcinoma.

Peutz–Jegher syndrome

This genetically determined syndrome features gastrointestinal polyps. Those in the stomach or colon may undergo malignant transformation. Pigmentation of the lips is a constant feature.

Gardner's syndrome

In this rare condition, multiple subcutaneous epidermoid cysts are associated with osseous lesions and polyposis of the colon which can become carcinomatous.

Conditions Suggestive of Malignant Lymphoma

Pigmentation

Marked pigmentation is not uncommon in malignant cachexia. It may be associated with generalized pruritus in Hodgkin's disease. The groins, nipples and axillae are most often involved.

Pruritus

In middle age, intractable generalized itching, in the absence of the well-known causes, may herald a lymphoma, particularly Hodgkin's disease. Pruritus may also be associated with a carcinoma, for example of the stomach. It should be remembered that in old age itching associated with dryness of the skin is common, especially in men.

Acquired ichthyosis

Ichthyosis is usually determined genetically and present from infancy. Appearing for the first time in middle or late life it may have sinister implications of lymphomatous disease. The histological features are non-specific.

Poikiloderma atrophicans vasculare

The combination of atrophy of the skin, patchy pigmentation and telangiectasia is seen in sun-damaged skin and after radiotherapy. Occurring de novo on covered areas it is a feature of lymphomata.

Widespread forms of poikiloderma may develop into T-cell lymphoma. Localized forms may be associated with B-cell lymphoma.

Erythroderma

Universal inflammation of the skin, sometimes called generalized exfoliative dermatitis, has been discussed as a complication of psoriasis (p. 102) and eczema (p. 97) and as a drug-induced phenomenon (p. 198). It may also be associated with a malignant T-cell lymphoma either as a presenting feature or during the course of the illness. In such circumstances, the erythroderma is intractable. Although the histology is non-specific at first, the inflamed skin may eventually become infiltrated with lymphomatous cells. Abnormal T cells (Sezary cells) may be detected in the blood and a leukaemia may develop, often associated with nodular or ulcerated skin lesions.

In all of these conditions modern techniques of cell labelling using monoclonal antibodies, allow earlier recognition of malignant lymphoid cells so that changes which are non-specific on conventional histology may prove to be specific in fact. Nevertheless, repeated skin biopsies at intervals of several months may be needed to establish the diagnosis of T-cell lymphoma.

Arsenic-induced changes

Lastly, although drug-induced changes are described elsewhere, it should be mentioned that cutaneous evidence of previous administration of inorganic arsenic, for example palmar keratoses, raindrop pigmentation, or the presence of intraepidermal (Bowen's) or basal cell carcinomata, implies an increased risk of internal carcinoma, especially of the bronchus.

7

Viral Diseases

Three common exanthemata of children are due to viruses, namely varicella, measles and rubella. These diseases are described in this Chapter as well as the common acute or chronic virus infections which affect predominantly skin or mucous membranes, i.e. herpes simplex and herpes zoster (acute) and molluscum contagiosum and warts (chronic). In addition, several other important but less common viral infections are included. Finally, HIV-related disease is described.

Varicella

Clinical picture

Varicella is a common acute infectious disease caused by a primary infection with the varicella–zoster virus. In children prodromal symptoms of varicella (chickenpox) are unusual. The disease begins with the rash, which may be trivial and easily missed. Itching is variable and more evident in older children. In contrast, in adults, prodromal headache, malaise and back and leg pains may be severe.

The rash is typically centripetal with crops of vesicles at different stages of evolution so that papules, vesicles and crusts are seen. The crusts come away after about 10 days. Lesions may be seen in the buccal mucosa. Skin lesions may leave varioliform (smallpox-like) scars.

Differential diagnosis

Localized lesions may be confused with herpes simplex. In a widespread eruption eczema herpeticum can mimic chickenpox.

Complications

Coccal infection may complicate scratched lesions and worsen the scarring. Pneumonitis may be trivial and unrecognized or, rarely, fulminating and fatal in a few days. Hepatitis and encephalitis are rare.

Treatment

Simple calamine lotion to reduce itching is all that is necessary in a typical childhood case. In adults with very severe disease, pneumonitis, hepatitis or in the immunosuppressed, treatment with intravenous acyclovir or vidarabine may be life-saving.

Measles

Measles (morbilli) is an acute, very infectious disease due to a single-stranded RNA virus, only one strain of which is known. The disease is found worldwide and most susceptible children are infected in the first decade. In the temperate and developed countries biannual epidemics were usual, whereas in the tropics annual epidemics are the rule. In recent years immunization programmes have modified this pattern.

Age of onset

Maternally derived antibody passively protects the child for its first 6 months. In the tropics the disease is not uncommon in the second 6 months, very common in the second year and virtually all children have had the disease by 4 years. In First World countries vaccination has greatly reduced the disease in preschool children but the disease is seen in older children.

Clinical features

Respiratory secretions spread the disease with an incubation period of 10–14 days. Fever and coryza herald the onset. Injected conjunctivae and mild cough follow. At this stage 'Koplik's spots' may be seen as small erythematous macules, sometimes with a white centre, on the buccal mucosa. A day or two later the rash appears on the forehead and neck, with spread to the trunk and limbs over 3–4 days. The exanthema is erythematous and maculopapular, giving way to brownish staining and desquamation as it fades.

In the meantime, cough has usually worsened and respiratory tract complications can occur. The child is characteristically miserable and irritable.

Complications

Tracheitis and tracheobronchitis are usual. Pneumonitis due to various organisms, otitis media, febrile convulsions and encephalitis can all occur.

Measles in the tropics in the very young malnourished child may be devastating. Severe rash, stomatitis, diarrhoea and keratoconjunctivitis are common.

Prevention

Passive immunization with human immunoglobulin is possible within 2–3 days of exposure. Active vaccination with a live attenuated strain of virus is now well established, optimally at 15 months of age. A trivial postvaccination syndrome with slight rash is not uncommon. Antibody responses are excellent.

Rubella

The importance of rubella (German measles) lies not in the mild acquired disease but in its ability to cause serious congenital abnormalities in the babies of women affected in early pregnancy. The disease is worldwide and up to 90% of adults have antibody.

Acquired rubella

Children and adolescents are mainly affected. The incubation period is 2–3 weeks. Typically, mild fever, a sore throat, cervical and occipital lymphadenopathy and a rash characterize the illness. The rash begins on the face, spreading rapidly to the trunk and then the limbs. Pin-head erythematous macules enlarge and may coalesce to produce a generalized flushing. The rash fades in 2–3 days. Milder, fleeting and almost symptomless forms occur, especially in children.

Complications

Arthralgia is common especially in adults, affecting fingers and larger joints. Purpura, thrombocytopenia and neurological sequelae are rare.

Differential diagnosis

Several other viruses may produce an indistinguishable illness, especially in children. Drug eruptions may also be rubella-like.

Laboratory diagnosis

Since the other viruses are not teratogenic, precise diagnosis is crucial in the pregnant woman. Fortunately, accurate and quick serological tests are now available.

Congenital rubella

Cataracts, cardiac defects and deafness are the best known features but thrombocytopenic purpura, hepatitis, bone disease, microcephaly and retardation may all occur. Symptomless babies tend to be of low birthweight and other defects may not become apparent for months or years. The greatest dangers follow rubella in the first 2 months of pregnancy but there are serious hazards up to 4 months. After birth affected infants excrete virus for months.

Prevention

Highly effective vaccines containing attenuated live virus are now available and should be offered to girls between 11 and 14 years who are antibody-negative and to certain groups of adult women, for example teachers, nursery staff, etc, who are at special risk. Postpartum vaccination of women found to be non-immune during pregnancy is also recommended.

Immunoglobulin (1–3 g) can be given within 10 days of exposure to rubella to a non-immune woman in the first 4 months of gestation who is likely to continue pregnancy even if infected. It may reduce the incidence of congenital defects.

Herpes Zoster

Herpes zoster, or shingles, is an acute, painful, self-limiting disease characterized by a unilateral and segmental eruption confined to one or more sensory dermatomes (Fig. 7.1). It is due to the varicella–zoster virus and is a second clinical manifestation of infection which has remained latent in the tissues since an earlier chickenpox infection. Those who have not had chickenpox in childhood, and who yet develop zoster later in life, have had a subclinical attack of varicella when young.

There are many well-authenticated cases of an adult having zoster and children in the same family developing varicella within the next 3 weeks. One attack of shingles confers immunity for many years but second attacks of zoster may occur decades later. Most persons

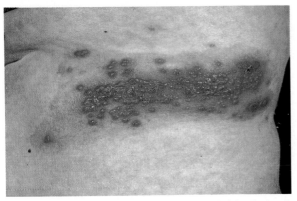

Fig. 7.1 Herpes zoster (shingles) on the lateral abdominal wall. Note the 'clustering' of the papulopustules at the margins.

who develop zoster are otherwise healthy, but there is a higher incidence in those with leukaemia and lymphoma. Zoster has occurred in infants a few months after neonatal infection.

The primary lesion of zoster is almost certainly in the sensory nerve supply of the affected part, but once the virus has entered the sensory neurone it passes peripherally to the skin and centrally to the spinal cord. The vesicles are due to direct action of the virus on the skin. The posterior root ganglion through which the sensory nerve supply passes is acutely inflamed, with round-cell infiltration and haemorrhage. Degenerative changes occur along the posterior nerve root into the root fibres of the posterior columns of the cord, and along the course of the peripheral sensory nerves down to the fine fibrils in the skin at the site of eruption. There are minor cerebrospinal fluid changes in the acute phase.

Zoster affects the skin supplied by all the sensory fibres which pass through the diseased root ganglion. The vesicles are formed in the prickle-cell layer of the epidermis as a result of 'balloon degeneration' of the cells and serous exudation from the corium.

Clinical picture

Zoster affects both sexes. It is seen mainly in the second half of life and is rare in children. Any dermatome may be affected but the thorax is the commonest site. In the aged, involvement of the first division of the trigeminal nerve is particularly common. Zoster of the maxillary division of this nerve is rare and of the mandibular division excessively rare. Disease of the thorax and lumbar segments is easily recognized,

but cervical and sacral segment involvement may be missed because the rash is so localized.

Classically, the eruption is heralded by pain in a segmental distribution for up to a week. Patchy areas of erythema develop and quickly become oedematous. On these areas groups or clusters of papules erupt and rapidly become vesicular (Fig. 7.1). Crusts then form which separate in 14–28 days in the untreated disease. Secondary bacterial infection is unimportant. Enlargement of the draining lymph gland is usual. Sensory disturbances, including pain, paraesthesiae and numbness, persist in varying degrees throughout the attack and postherpetic neuralgia may be a burden to which the aged are particularly liable. Zoster usually leaves scarring and pigmentation in its wake and, if the scalp is involved, cicatricial alopecia is not uncommon.

There are a number of clinical variants. Careful daily examination of the whole skin reveals sparse spattered varicella vesicles in 5% of patients, implying a viraemic phase. In immunosuppressed patients and particularly in patients with Hodgkin's disease undergoing radiotherapy or chemotherapy, the typical eruption may evolve into confluent haemorrhagic and bullous zonal involvement. The affected area may become necrotic (gangrenous zoster) and spread peripherally. A viraemia may lead to fatal varicella pneumonia or encephalitis.

As mentioned above, zoster involves the posterior horn of the spinal cord. Rarely, spread to the anterior horn results in motor involvement and paralysis. Complete paralysis of a limb is rare but usually permanent. Paralysis of other muscles may also occur, for example in the face or abdominal wall.

Mucous membranes may be involved, as in geniculate zoster. In ophthalmic zoster (trigeminal, first division), involvement of the nasociliary branch implicates the conjunctivae.

Differential diagnosis

If the unilateral nature of zoster is borne in mind, diagnosis is rarely difficult. Ophthalmic zoster may cause oedema of both eyelids in the earliest stages, simulating contact dermatitis. Very localized zoster, for example on the genitalia, may mimic herpes simplex but in the latter, pain of the same quality is unusual.

Treatment

If the disease is caught in the first 36 hours of the eruption, application of 40% idoxuridine in dimethyl sulphoxide (Iduridin, U.K.) may be very valuable.

The lotion should be applied at least six times daily or even by continuous wet compress. It should not be used for more than 3 days, because the base is too irritant. It is contraindicated in pregnancy. Alternatively, acyclovir cream (Zovirax, U.K.) applied five times daily for 5 days is less irritant but less effective unless started in the first 12 hours. Once the inflammation is established, however, these treatments are useless. Analgesic tablets may also be necessary. Topical steroids are contraindicated but prednisolone, given orally, is highly effective if started early. It is particularly valuable in the elderly in controlling pain but the evidence that it reduces the incidence or severity of postherpetic neuralgia is unconvincing. So long as there is no contraindication to steroid therapy, a starting dose of 60 mg daily is appropriate. This dose should be continued for 4 days only and then rapidly reduced to zero over 14 days. Oral acyclovir (Zovirax, U.K.) 800 mg five times daily for 7 days is even more effective and can be combined with prednisolone. In immunocompromised subjects intravenous acyclovir is invaluable. Amantadine hydrochloride (Symmetrel, U.K.) 10 ml orally twice daily for 14–28 days is occasionally useful. Vidarabine monohydrate (Vira-A, U.K.) is an expensive and less satisfactory alternative.

Herpes Simplex

This disease is one of the most ubiquitous viral infections of man. In the common recurrent form, localized herpetic eruptions occur which are unrelated to any dermatome but have the same morphology, though a shorter time course, than herpes zoster.

Aetiology and pathogenesis

Two types of *Herpes simplex* virus have been identified: Type I and Type II. Type I is usually the cause of infections of the head, neck or upper limbs. Type II is usually sexually transmitted and affects the genitals, lower trunk or thighs. The two types are easily distinguished by their cultural and serological characteristics. Almost the entire adult population has been infected by Type I at some time, although the infection is often subclinical. The vesicles of the clinical infection are found in the prickle cell layer but no 'balloon' degeneration is seen. The viral inclusion bodies are oxyphilic and intranuclear. The virus can be cultured and antibody detected in the serum.

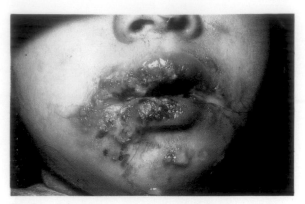

Fig. 7.2   Primary herpes simplex gingivostomatitis.

The clinical picture in primary infections

Primary infections occur in individuals with no specific neutralizing antibodies, recurrent infections in those with such antibodies. Rarely the disease may be congenital, due to birth canal infection. The congenital infection produces bizarre patterns of cutaneous inflammation in the neonate with vesiculation, erosions and even ulceration, and may be complicated by choroidoretinitis or brain involvement. The outcome may be fatal, especially in premature infants. Usually, however, primary herpes simplex infection is seen in infants from about 3 months of age, when the passive maternal antibodies wane, up to about 2 years. Most infections are subclinical.

Primary herpetic gingivostomatitis. This infection is characterized by the sudden onset of painful oral lesions associated with fever, malaise and lymphadenopathy. The gingivae become red and swollen and erosions, blisters and superficial ulcers develop. The whole picture settles spontaneously in 7–14 days (Fig. 7.2).

Primary herpetic vulvovaginitis. This condition is very similar to primary herpetic gingivostomatitis.

Inoculation primary herpes. This is due to direct implantation of the virus into the skin through an abrasion. It may be seen in wrestlers (herpes gladiatorum) and in doctors, dentists and nurses whose fingers encounter infected secretions, particularly from tracheostomy patients. The resulting so-called 'herpetic whitlow' is extremely painful and only slowly becomes vesicular (Fig. 7.3). Pus does not form.

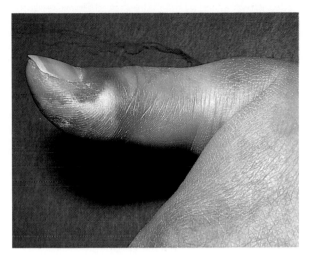

Fig. 7.3 Herpetic whitlow on thumb.

Eczema herpeticum. This is disseminated herpes occurring in a subject with atopic dermatitis (see p. 89). In small children it is alarming and may be fatal in a minority.

The clinical picture in recurrent infections

Sufficient stress, such as prolonged high fever, will facilitate recurrent herpes simplex infection in many adults. Others suffer recurrent attacks, usually in one area, provoked by apparently trivial factors of which the most important are viral coryza (cold sore), minor fevers (fever sore), exposure to strong sunlight or local trauma. The eruption may be preceded for a few hours (or rarely a day or two) by tingling, burning or itching at the site. The erythema is followed by local oedema in which clusters of tiny vesicles, 1–3 mm in diameter, appear. Within 3 days, the vesicles become purulent and crusting follows. Involution takes 5–10 days and occasionally leaves slight scarring, especially after repeated attacks.

Recurrent herpes can occur anywhere but the common sites of Type I infection are the lips and perioral area (herpes labialis). Less commonly, the chin, nose or a cheek is involved, or the hand. Recurrent herpes of the buttock or thighs is usually due to Type II infection and is often preceded by neuralgia for 1–2 days, sometimes radiating down the thigh or into the hip.

Recurrent Type II infections are common on the glans and shaft of the penis, although the site of recurrence often shifts slightly. Attacks are provoked by the trauma of coitus and usually settle in 4 or 5 days but may recur very frequently, sometimes monthly. Herpes simplex may involve the eye, causing keratitis or a dendritic corneal perforation. The Type II virus may cause a chronic cervicitis in women who shed virus in the vaginal secretions.

Complications

Complications are unusual. Secondary bacterial infection is rarely a problem. Erythema multiforme may follow attacks by 5–15 days as an allergic response and may be a serious recurrent problem in some patients. In the immunocompromised patient, viraemia may be complicated by fatal pneumonia or meningoencephalitis.

Treatment

In herpetic whitlow, incision should be avoided. Continuous wet compressing with 40% indoxuridine in dimethyl sulphoxide (Iduridin, U.K.) modifies and shortens the attack. Acyclovir tablets 400 mg five times daily for 5 days are effective if started early. Acyclovir cream is less useful in the finger. Idoxuridine 0.5% eye drops are very useful in herpetic keratitis where steroids must be avoided. In lesions of the lips, face, genitalia and lower trunk, acyclovir cream is now the treatment of choice. The earlier treatment is started, the better will be the response. The cream should be applied every 2–3 hours and can be supplemented by oral acyclovir as above in severe attacks. Long-term prophylactic oral acyclovir (200 mg q.d.s) has a role in serious frequently recurrent disease. In severely immunocompromised patients and in eczema herpeticum in infants, intravenous acyclovir may be lifesaving.

Molluscum Contagiosum

Molluscum contagiosum is a papular eruption of the skin caused by a pox virus which is transmitted either by direct contact or by fomites. Persons of all ages may be affected, but infection is commonest in children. Epidemics may occur in boarding schools and other institutions or among patrons of Turkish baths. It may also be transmitted sexually, when multiple lesions of the lower belly are usually seen. On microscopic examination there is proliferation of the prickle-cell layer with numerous large vacuolated cells with eccentric nuclei, containing closely packed eosinophilic hyaline bodies.

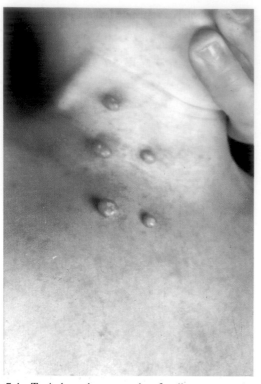

Fig. 7.4 Typical translucent papules of molluscum contagiosum; note the umbilication. These mollusca are unusually large.

Mollusca arise as minute painless papules slowly increasing in size, and varying from 1 to 7 mm in diameter. They may occur anywhere on the body but are usually seen on the upper trunk, axillae, neck and pelvic regions, sometimes in clusters and often distributed asymmetrically. Their appearance is absolutely characteristic, as they form rounded, whitish elevations with an umbilicated centre, and frequently have a glistening, pearly-white appearance (Fig. 7.4). Pultaceous material may be expressed from them. Traumatized lesions may have a surrounding inflammation. Itching is variable.

If left untreated the virus is conveyed on clothes, towels or fingers to other areas, so that groups of mollusca may occur widely. Eventually spontaneous recovery occurs, but the lesions, if untreated, tend to increase in size and number for months.

The mollusca can be easily scooped out with a curette of appropriate size. Cauterization is unnecessary, a dry dressing sufficing. Alternatively, the lesions may be pierced with a spicule of wood which has been dipped in liquefied phenol B.P. (80% phenol w/w in water). Cryotherapy is useful in adults or older children. Occasionally general anaesthesia is needed to deal with a large number of lesions in a very young child.

Warts

Warts, or verrucae, are cutaneous papillomata and may be regarded as localized, circumscribed hypertrophies of the epidermis. Both the skin and mucosae may be affected.

Warts have long been known to be infections but the responsible papova DNA virus was only identified by electron microscopy 35 years ago. Recently, modern molecular hybridization and serological techniques have established the heterogeneity of human papilloma viruses (HPV) and over 45 different viruses have now been identified, which induce cutaneous or mucosal warts. The vast majority of these lesions are benign but dysplasias of the cervix uteri and laryngeal papillomas in adults may evolve into squamous carcinoma. The viruses particularly associated with different clinical lesions are summarized in Table 7.1.

Immunology

Circulating antibodies and markers of cell-mediated responses appear when warts are treated successfully or disappear spontaneously. The outlook for disappearance depends on the HPV subtype involved, the virus load and the patient's immune responses. Immunoincompetent or immunosuppressed subjects may suffer from widespread, large and persistent

Table 7.1 Clinical associations of human papilloma viruses.

HPV subtype	Clinical association
1	Palmoplantar warts
2	Verruca vulgaris Mosaic plantar warts
3	Verruca plana
6	Genital warts
7	Butchers' warts
11	Cervix uteri verruca plana Laryngeal papilloma
16	Cervix uteri genital warts

warts, a problem seen at its worst in the recipients of kidney transplants but to a lesser degree in auto-immune diseases, atopy and occasionally sarcoidosis. Infections by HPV-2, -3, -4 and -10 are particularly associated with a compromised immune system.

Clinical picture

There are five main patterns which are described separately. Two or more types of warts may coexist.

Common warts (verruca vulgaris). These papilliferous excrescences usually occur on the hands but may affect the elbows, face, knees and scalp. On the latter area the lesions sometimes resemble cocks' combs. On the hands the lesions, which tend to enlarge peripherally, may extend round the nail folds. Unless cracked or infected they are symptomless (Fig. 7.5). HPV-2 is usually responsible, but the common hand warts of butchers and meat handlers are due to HPV-7.

Plane warts (verruca plana). These are flat-topped, yellowish papules, 1–4 mm in diameter (Fig. 7.6). They occur chiefly on the backs of the hands, both aspects of the wrists and on the face and may itch. They occur mainly in young people and may persist for years. They may be sparse or profuse, especially on the face. In men, they may disseminate widely in the beard area. HPV-3 and to a lesser extent HPV-10 are associated, the former particularly in immunocom-promised patients. Eventually spontaneous resolution is usual, often simultaneously in all the lesions and often heralded by transient itching and inflammation.

Digitate (filiform) warts (verruca digitata or filiformis). These thread-like warts may be 5–10 mm long with a

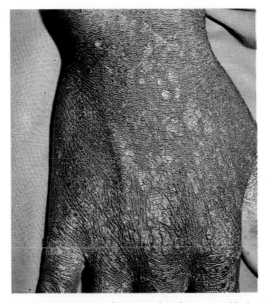

Fig. 7.6 Profuse lesions of verruca plana in a young black man; the backs of hands and dorsal wrists are characteristic sites.

warty top, sometimes dark. They tend to grow on the eyelids and in the axillae, particularly of overweight patients. HPV-2 is generally the culprit.

Plantar warts (verruca plantaris). These warts are most frequently seen in children and adolescents, but when present in adults can persist for years. They are readily contracted, and minor epidemics occur in schools. The lesions are usually isolated and appear as little more than yellowish white, flattened, discrete, tender papules, deeply embedded in hyperkeratotic epider-mis. Tenderness on vertical pressure is usually mini-mal but lateral squeezing elicits marked tenderness, the reverse of the situation in a callosity. In a sponta-neous healing phase multiple black points are embedded in the wart representing thrombosed capil-laries and haemorrhage into the stratum corneum. Occasionally, aggregation of these warts forms a con-fluent hyperkeratotic mosaic-like plaque, especially in chronically hyperhidrotic feet. Single deep lesions are typically associated with HPV-1, but mosaic warts show HPV-2. Multiple punctate palmoplantar warts may be due to HPV-4.

Genital (venereal) warts (condylomata acuminata). These occur in the man on the penile shaft (Fig. 7.7), on the prepuce and occasionally in the pubis. Perianal warts are common and may be associated with rectal

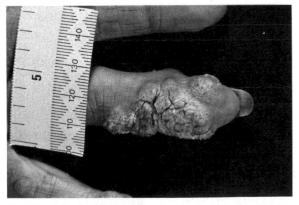

Fig. 7.5 Verruca vulgaris on finger of a patient with psoriasis and on immunosuppressive drug.

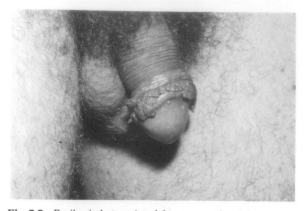

Fig. 7.7 Penile viral warts (condylomata acuminata) in a young man.

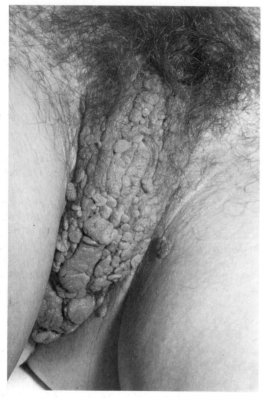

Fig. 7.8 Vulval warts in a young woman.

warts in both sexes if anal intercourse has been practised. Perianal warts in children of either sex and however young should always arouse suspicion of sexual abuse. In women they are found on the vulva (Fig. 7.8), at the introitus, in the perineum or around the anus. There may be vaginal warts and associated cervical lesions. Genital lesions vary from tiny 1–2 mm pink papules, barely warty, to florid cauliflower-like projections. They are encouraged by pregnancy and laryngeal warts may be found in children whose mothers had genital warts at the time of delivery. Persistent pigmented warty papules may occur in either sex which have the histological appearance of intraepidermal carcinoma (Bowenoid papulosis) but usually not the malignant potential. HPV-6, -11, -16 and -18 may be associated with genital lesions. HPV-16 and -18 are of particular importance because of evidence implicating them in premalignant and malignant lesions in both sexes, but particularly in premalignant dysplasia of the cervix uteri.

Epidermodysplasia verruciformis. This is a rare, genetically influenced disease in which myriads of flat plane warts are widely disseminated on the face, trunk and limbs. Multiple HPV viruses are found in each patient, many unique to this disease. Cell-mediated immunity is depressed and malignant transformation to squamous carcinomata is seen eventually in 25% of patients.

Differential diagnosis. Callosity, corn and subungual exostosis must be differentiated.

A *callosity* is an area of epidermal hyperkeratosis in skin subjected to constant pressure. It is due either to inappropriate footwear or to bony deformity in the foot. In the latter situation, cause and effect are usually obvious. A diffuse callosity of the middle of the tread is common in the overweight middle-aged with anterior flat foot.

A *corn* is a small callosity occurring over the dorsal aspect of a deformed toe. A central core of hyperkeratosis may press into the dermis, causing pain or inflammation. Interdigital corns tend to be soft and macerated.

Subungual exostosis (Fig. 7.9) is often mistaken for a verruca. Typically it presents as a hard lump under the free end of a hallux nail, sometimes pushing up the nail. A lateral radiograph reveals an exostosis arising dorsally from the distal phalanx (Fig. 7.10).

Oral warts. HPV-13 and other sub-types have been implicated in verrucous lesions of the oral mucosa. Eventual spontaneous regression is usual.

Treatment

Common warts. Common warts are most easily treated

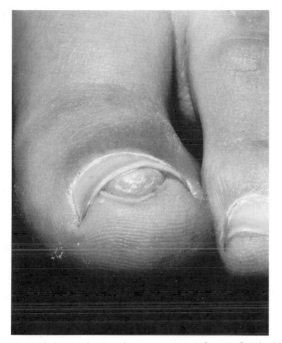

Fig. 7.9 Subungual exostosis on a great toe, often confused with verruca.

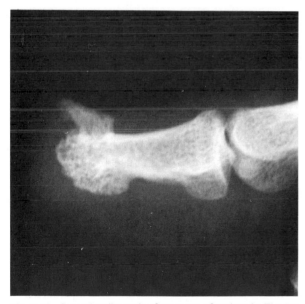

Fig. 7.10 Lateral radiograph of great toe of patient in Fig. 7.9 showing dorsal exostosis.

by cryotherapy using a liquid nitrogen spray. Small numbers of warts in the older child or adult may be curetted out and lightly cauterized under local anaesthesia. If surgery is undertaken for paronychial warts, care must be taken not to damage the nail matrix lest permanent nail deformity ensues. Only the lightest cauterization is advisable for warts at the tip of a digit, since disabling painful scars may otherwise result. Destruction of common warts on the backs of hands by electrical cauterization alone is not advised; it is much more painful than cryotherapy and leaves cosmetically unpleasant scarring. If, for any reason, the above modalities cannot be used or have failed, a lotion containing salicylic acid and lactic acid, 17% of each (Salactol and Duofilm, U.K. and U.S.A.) can be painted on the warts daily, allowed to dry and covered with an adhesive dressing. Other chemical approaches of less value include the daily application of 25% benzalkonium (Callusolve, U.K.) or 10% gluteraldehyde lotion (Glutarol, U.K.). A gel containing salicylic and lactic acids and copper acetate (Cuplex, U.K.) may be useful.

Digitate (filiform) warts. These should be curetted or snipped off and their bases lightly coagulated with electrocautery. Cryotherapy is also easy and effective.

Genital warts. Venereal warts may be approached in several ways. Careful painting of the lesions with 15–25% podophyllin (derived from podophyllum resin) in tincture of benzoin, liquid paraffin or spirit is often rapidly effective. The podophyllin must be applied by the doctor or a nurse after the surrounding skin has been protected with soft paraffin, and any excess mopped up. A gauze dressing is then applied to prevent spread and the application left on for 8–12 hours before being thoroughly washed off by the patient. If necessary, the treatment is repeated two or three times at weekly intervals. Podophyllin solutions are unstable and can be dangerous if used for very extensive vulval and introital warts in the pregnant woman because enhanced absorption may lead to severe neurotoxicity. Podophyllin is also teratogenic and mutagenic. More limited genital warts can be treated by weekly application of 90% trichloroacetic acid by the skilled operator, and liquid nitrogen is useful for small spattered warts on the shaft of the penis. Occasionally excision, curettage and cautery under general anaesthesia are necessary for gross vegetating anogenital warts. Treatment by carbon dioxide laser is also effective. Other venereal infections, possibly transmitted at the same time, should be sought and sexual partners should be examined and treated if success is to be expected. In particular the female sexual partner of men with genital warts should be examined gynaecologically, and cervical cytology and infection checked.

Plantar warts. Single, painful, tender plantar warts which are disabling to the patient or which prevent a child from swimming are best curetted out under local anaesthesia. After the overlying hyperkeratosis has been pared away the wart is defined by blunt dissection and scooped out in one piece. After light electrocautery of the sides of the wound, a firm pressure dressing will control bleeding and need not be changed for 5 days. Relief of symptoms is usually instantaneous and healing uneventful in 2 or 3 weeks. The patient can walk normally from the second day. In skilled hands the cure rate is 80%.

In multiple plantar warts this approach is neither feasible nor worthwhile, and daily soaking of the affected skin in 5% formaldehyde solution is best, prescribed as a 1 in 8 dilution of formalin to give 4.5% formaldehyde in water. After 15 minutes, the foot is rinsed in plain water and dried. Dressings should not be applied. Only the affected skin should be exposed and the toe clefts may have to be protected with a smear of soft paraffin. The warts should be pared once a week using a corn plane. Three or four weeks of such treatment will produce cure in at least one-half of patients.

The various lotions mentioned above for common warts may have to be tried in plantar warts. Mosaic warts in the adult are particularly resistant to treatment, and may persist for years. Adhesive plasters impregnated with 30% or 40% salicylic acid may be successful in their treatment; the plaster should be left on for 48-hour periods, alternating with 24-hour periods of rest. Sodden keratin must be regularly removed with a pumice stone or by sandpapering. Liquid nitrogen may also be useful for small or superficial plantar warts. Usually several modalities have to be used in mosaic warts, changing the treatment every 3–4 weeks. Formalin solution B.P., 20% in ung. Merck and retinoic acid gel (Retin A, U.K.), may be tried or 5% salicylic acid in emulsifying ointment B.P.

If plantar warts are symptomless or becoming less tender on lateral squeezing there is much to be said for doing nothing, since more than 50% will disappear spontaneously in a few weeks. This is particularly so in very young children, in whom the above procedures are difficult or impossible. In the author's view it is only rarely justifiable to use general anaesthesia to deal with plantar warts surgically, and surgical excision and suture should be avoided.

Resistant warts. Vaccination may eventually be feasible. Immunostimulation is being explored. Retinoids can influence wart proliferation but the effect is temporary. Intralesional bleomycin injection is highly effective but may cause severe prolonged pain. Systemic and intralesional interferon are also under valuation.

Other Viral Diseases

Hand, foot and mouth disease

This is a not uncommon infectious disease due usually to the enterovirus Coxsackie A16. Minor epidemics are common, the disease spreading rapidly amongst children and to adults within their families. After a 4–6-day incubation period an oropharyngeal enanthema appears. Transient vesicles give way to superficial ulcers, usually a few millimetres in diameter, which heal within a week. In two-thirds of patients a characteristic exanthema follows the oral lesions by a day or so; rather sparse, 3–7 mm superficial elongated vesiculopustules on an erythematous base are seen on the hands and feet and occasionally elsewhere. Like the mucosal lesions they heal within a week. These mucocutaneous manifestations are accompanied in about 10% of patients by cervical lymphadenitis, coryza, diarrhoea, nausea or transient malaise. The virus can be cultured from the oral or cutaneous lesions to confirm the diagnosis directly, or its presence can be inferred from rising serological titres in serial blood specimens. No treatment is available.

Differential diagnosis is from erythema multiforme. The foot and mouth disease of cattle is a separate disease due to a virus which rarely affects man. A number of other Coxsackie and echo viruses can cause exanthemata of various sorts.

Pityriasis rosea

This is a common disease, possibly viral, characterized by a centripetal rash which lasts for several weeks. It is seen mainly between the ages of 15 and 40 years. Second attacks are rare.

The first sign is a single erythematous oval or circular macule up to 3–4 cm in diameter. This is the 'herald patch' and it appears more often on the trunk than the limbs. The patch may become slightly scaly

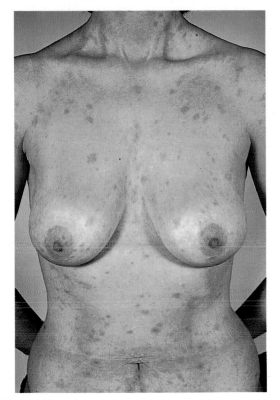

Fig. 7.11 Pityriasis rosea.

and may be 'ringed'. Itching is slight or absent. Within 4–14 days, an exanthema follows in a centripetal distribution confined to the trunk, neck and the proximal parts of the limbs. The eruption is symmetrical and often particularly profuse about the shoulder girdle, including the axillae, and the pelvic girdle (Fig. 7.11).

There are two components: the first, and the more common, is characterized by lesions which have been described as 'medallions' and the second by small maculopapules. Occasionally mixed varieties occur. A 'medallion' is an oval patch which, when fully developed, has a slightly raised peripheral zone, somewhat rose-coloured, with the colour of its outermost edge merging with the normal skin. The inner part of the peripheral zone shows fine scales which tend to be triangular in shape, the apices pointing inwards. The centre of the medallion is smooth, fawn-coloured and soft to the touch. Full evolution from a rosy macule to the complete lesion, which is often some 2 cm in its longest diameter, takes 10–14 days. The long diameters of the lesions on the back run downwards and outwards, producing an inverted Christmas tree pattern.

The lesions of the maculopapular component are irregularly rounded, rose-pink, slightly elevated and covered after a few days with a fine scale.

The rash may take up to 2 weeks to develop fully. As it does so the fine scaling becomes more marked, often forming a 'collarette' around the margin of individual lesions, with its edge facing the centre. The eruption then slowly fades away, having run a total course of 4–8 weeks.

Itching is variable and can be trivial or severe. Fierce attacks are rare but they may cause intolerable itching for a week or more. Minor malaise is not uncommon, especially in young women. Giant urticated and purpuric variants of pityriasis rosea are occasionally seen.

Differential diagnosis is important. The herald patch is often misdiagnosed as tinea. The fully developed eruption must be distinguished from seborrhoeic dermatitis, guttate psoriasis, drug eruptions and secondary syphilis.

The condition is almost uninfluenced by treatment and has to run its course. Oral antihistamines may allay itching, and weak or medium corticosteroid creams may be of limited value.

Orf

Orf is a virus disease of sheep and goats. In man it occurs only among those who handle these animals or their carcasses. The lesions are found most commonly on the fingers, hands and wrists. They begin as red papules, soon become vesicles, and eventually turn into pustules; sometimes the lesions are umbilicated. There are no constitutional symptoms, and the lesions disappear of their own accord in a few weeks.

Erythema infectiosum

'Slapped cheek' or fifth disease is a fairly uncommon contagious disease of children from 2–12 years now known to be due to parvovirus B19. Minor outbreaks have often been recognized in family practice. After an incubation period of 5–10 days, a characteristic bright erythematous exanthema appears on the face (Fig. 7.12), especially of younger children, giving the 'slapped cheek' appearance. This fades in a few days but the erythema may spread on the limbs, where there may be a characteristic lacy network of erythema which can last up to 3 weeks. Constitutional disturbance is trivial. Viral antibody can now be detected reliably, but this is not yet a routine procedure.

Parvovirus B19 infection in a pregnant woman may

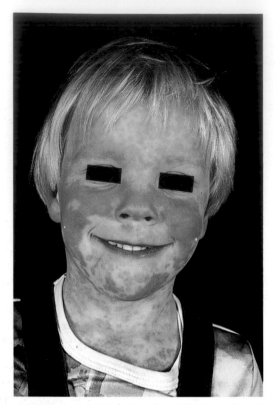

Fig. 7.12 'Slapped cheek' erythema in a child with erythema infectiosum (fifth disease).

cause fetal damage. An acute polyarthritis may also be associated in adults.

Gianotti Crosti syndrome

Gianotti Crosti syndrome (papular acrodermatitis of childhood) is a rare but distinctive syndrome, reported mainly from Italy and France. It affects children aged 2–6 years. Over a few days a profuse papular eruption develops in a centrifugal distribution on the limbs, which lasts a few weeks. There may be slight malaise, lymphadenopathy, splenomegaly and occasionally hepatomegaly. Minor abnormalities of liver function tests occur. The syndrome may be a manifestation of a primary infection with hepatitis B virus, but other viruses such as Epstein–Barr, Coxsackie B and cytomegalovirus can be causative.

Hepatitis B

Apart from papular acrodermatitis in childhood, infection in adults may cause a serum-sickness-like prodrome with purpura, urticaria or vasculitis. Polyarteritis nodosa is rare but serious. A mixed cryoglobulinaemia has been described with purpura, arthropathy, renal involvement and necrotizing vasculitis.

Roseola infantum

This is a transient exanthema of toddlers, also called exanthema subitum or sixth disease. Fever, malaise and lymphadenopathy last 2–3 days, followed by a transient rubella-like rash. Neurological complications may occur. Human herpes virus-6 has recently been identified as the causal agent.

Human immunodeficiency virus (HIV) disease (Table 7.2)

More than one virus is now thought to be implicated. Acquired immunodeficiency syndrome (AIDS) burst upon the world in 1981 as an epidemic of *Pneumocystis carinii* pneumonia or Kaposi's sarcoma in previously healthy young men in New York and California. Very soon male homosexuals, drug addicts and haemophiliacs were recognized as special risk groups, suggesting hepatitis-B-like bloodborne spread. Subsequent isolation of LAV/HTLV-III virus, the development of antibody detection methods and the increasing incidence of the disease are now well known. HIV-related syndromes are defined as follows.

Table 7.2   A working classification of HIV infection.

GROUP I	Acute; associated with seroconversion (Mononucleosis-like syndrome)
GROUP II	Latent; no symptoms or signs
GROUP III	Persistent generalized lymphadenopathy (PGL)
GROUP IV	(a) AIDS-related complex (ARC)
	(b) ARC with neurological disease
	(c) Secondary infectious disease:
	1. AIDS; one or more of 12 specified diseases, e.g. Pneumocystis Carinii Pneumonitis.
	2. ARC; with one or more of 6 other specified diseases, e.g. Hairy Leukoplakia
	(d) With secondary cancers, e.g. Kaposi's sarcoma
	(e) With miscellaneous manifestations, e.g. Thrombocytopenia

AIDS. AIDS is reliably diagnosed opportunistic protozoal, fungal, viral or bacterial infection or certain types of cancer in the absence of other cause and in the presence of HIV antibody in the serum.

AIDS-related complex (ARC). Two clinical manifestations (fatigue, night sweats, lymphadenopathy, weight loss, fever, diarrhoea, oral candidosis) and two laboratory abnormalities (decreased T-helper cell count, hyperglobulinaemia, anergy) and presence of HIV antibody are required for diagnosis.

Persistent generalized lymphadenopathy (PGL). Lymphadenopathy of at least 3 months' duration involving two or more extrainguinal sites in the absence of other causes and the presence of HIV antibody constitutes PGL.

In a few patients, a transient mononucleosis-like illness with fever, rash and lymphadenopathy has been described in association with primary infection and seroconversion.

Mucocutaneous manifestations. Kaposi's sarcoma is common in homosexuals with AIDS, but rare in other groups at risk. The classical involvement of the lower limbs in elderly men is not seen. Instead a widespread papular and nodular eruption is disseminated on the trunk, limbs and face. Nodules may show linear patterning in skin creases. Lesions may be morphologically atypical, mimicking dermatofibroma, granuloma pyogenicum or malignant melanoma. Partial regression of individual lesions is common. The face and particularly the tip of the nose are frequently involved (Fig. 7.13), as is the buccal mucosa of palate or gums. The penis is another common site. Kaposi's sarcoma is rarely the cause of death, which is more likely to be due to opportunistic infection. Epithelioid haemangioma-like lesions, mimicking Kaposi's sarcoma, may be due to the recently described Cat–Scratch Disease bacillus, a Gram-negative rod demonstrable with the

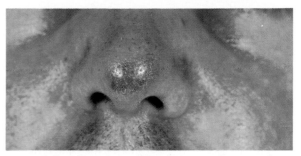

Fig. 7.13 Kaposi's sarcoma of face in a young homosexual man with HIV infection (AIDS).

Warthin–Starry stain. Antibiotics may be effective in treating this infection.

Oral candidosis is universal in AIDS and common in ARC. Patchy palatal involvement, angular stomatitis and glossitis are variants. So-called 'hairy' leukoplakia' of the margins of the tongue is due to proliferation of Epstein–Barr and HPV viruses in the epithelium. Recurrent gingivitis is almost universal and dental abscesses are common. Rarely, severe aphthous ulceration of the mouth is seen. Oral warts may be found.

Seborrheic dermatitis is common and may be severe and extensive, perhaps due to opportunistic cutaneous flora. Spattered nummular eczema is seen. Widespread folliculitis is common, sometimes axillary and pustular or acneiform on the trunk or thighs. Pruritis' may be severe and disproportionate to the physical signs. Pathogenic cocci are usually absent but skin scrapings reveal profuse pityrosporum yeasts. Acquired xeroderma is not uncommon and there is an increased incidence of herpes simplex, zoster and mollusca infections as well as tinea, impetigo or cellulitis. Other interesting features which have been described include premature greying of hair, rapid ageing, diffuse hair loss and an immune-complex mediated cutaneous vasculitis. Patients with HIV-related disease are particularly likely to develop hypersensitivity rashes if treated with co-trimoxazole.

—8—
Bacterial Diseases

Normal skin is inhabited by a large population of micro-organisms, especially in its warm, moist folds. Some are resident but usually non-pathogenic, such as *Staphylococcus albus* or *diphtheroides*. Others are transients which neither multiply nor persist. Pathogenic *Staphylococcus aureus* is carried by up to 20% of people, usually in the nostrils, axillae or perineum. *Streptococcus pyogenes* is usually pathogenic, as are the mycobacteria of tuberculosis, leprosy, etc, and the spirochaetes of syphilis and Lyme disease.

Staphylococcal Infections

Staphylococcus aureus may cause primary epidermal, follicular or ulcerated (ecthymatous) infections or may secondarily infect dermatitis, ulcers, etc.

Impetigo

In the United Kingdom impetigo is usually due to *S. aureus* alone, but a proportion of cases are due to *Streptococcus pyogenes* alone or a combination of these two organisms. Streptococcal participation is important because in tropical and subtropical climates some strains cause nephritis. Impetigo is more common in children than in adults. It may occur in the healthy but is often secondary to a discharging middle-ear infection, nasal vestibulitis, atopic dermatitis, scabies or pediculosis. Poor hygiene, high humidity and squalid social conditions encourage spread. It is very contagious and spreads easily in the family, school or beyond.

Impetigo begins in the subcorneal region of the epidermis and produces erythema and vesicles or bullae in neonates and the very old. The vesicular type ruptures readily and produces honey-coloured crusts. These lesions may be circinate and resemble ringworm (Fig. 8.1), but spread is much more rapid. The bullous type ruptures less readily. The flaccid bullae are clear at first and later purulent. Impetigo is usually asymmetrical and tends to affect the exposed parts, especially the face, the ears and the hands, but may be widespread on the scalp, limbs or trunk. A typical presentation is

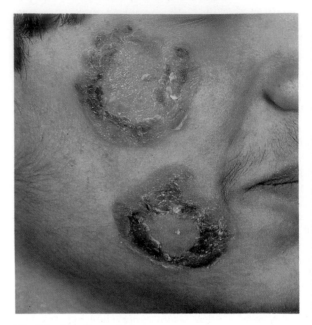

Fig. 8.1 Impetigo contagiosa.

in a small child with a mass of lesions, becoming confluent, around the mouth and nose with crusted nares. Itching is modest and the child may be surprisingly little distressed.

Treatment

If localized, impetigo should be treated with neomycin or framycetin and gramicidin (Graneodin, U.K.; Soframycin, U.K.), neomycin and bacitracin (Cicatrin, U.K.), fusidic acid ointment (Fucidin, U.K.) or chlortetracycline ointment, applied to all lesions and in the nostrils six times daily. Crusts should be wiped away daily. Widespread infections or those secondary to underlying disease should be treated orally for 7 days with flucloxacillin or erythromycin if available, but co-trimoxazole or tetracycline can be used if necessary. Where nephritogenic streptococci are a hazard, penicillin V should be given orally for 10 days, even in apparently trivial infections. In deprived Third World conditions, 1% aqueous gentian violet or brilliant green can be used as antiseptic paints.

Ecthyma

In the debilitated, diabetic, immunodepressed or immunosuppressed, impetigo or folliculitis may ulcerate to produce multiple shallow or occasionally deep round ulcers (Fig. 8.2). Staphylococci will easily be cultured. This is ecthyma and in the Unitied Kingdom is seen mainly in drug addicts, vagrants, poorly controlled diabetes and HIV disease. The appropriate antibiotics should be given orally and topically.

Folliculitis, boils and carbuncles

Staphylococcus aureus folliculitis is common in chronic dermatitis or after treatment of dermatitis or psoriasis with corticosteroid ointments, especially under polyethylene occlusion or in hospital with its hazards of cross-infection. A spattered eruption of 1–5-mm pustules is seen with a halo of erythema, obviously folli-cular and often with a hair emerging from the centre of the pustule, for example on the legs. Shaving-area infections (sycosis barbae) are now rare and the diagnosis in this area is more likely to be pseudofolliculitis due to ingrowing hairs, especially in black men. Severe staphylococcal folliculitis occasionally complicates wax removal of hair from women's legs in salons with poor hygienic practices.

Gross infection of multiple adjacent follicles produces a *boil*. Boils of the head and neck may be due to nasal carriage of cocci, boils of the trunk or thighs to axillary or perianal carriage. Other predisposing factors are obesity, hyperhidrosis, friction, maceration and diabetes mellitus. Multiple adjacent boils may coalesce to form a *carbuncle*. Central necrosis may lead to severe ulceration.

Management of boils

Predisposing factors should be sought and removed where possible. The sensitivities of the *S. aureus* should be identified and swabs for culture should be taken from nostrils, ears, axillae, umbilicus and anus as well as the boil itself. Twice daily baths or showers, vigorous use of soap, fingernail hygiene and frequent washing of clothes are all important. Cetrimide 1% solution (Cetavlon, U.K.), chlorhexidine (e.g. Hibitane cream, U.K.), and povidone iodine preparations (Betadine, U.K.) are all useful. An appropriate antibiotic cream may help to deal with follicular spread around a boil. Often vigorous oral therapy is needed with flucloxacillin, erythromycin or fusidic acid in full dosage for 14 days.

Staphylococcal 'scalded skin' syndrome

This is usually due to phage type 71 staphylococcal infection. It presents as an acute toxic illness in infants, with bright erythema and shedding of layers of outer epidermis, resembling the effects of a severe hot water scald (Fig. 8.3). The mucosae are not affected. It is a serious disease but has an excellent prognosis if treated promptly with flucloxacillin or erythromycin orally. Drug reactions may induce a similar cutaneous picture in adults but with mucosal ulceration, and are often fatal.

Streptococcal Infections

Erysipelas

Erysipelas is an acute, dermal, streptococcal infection

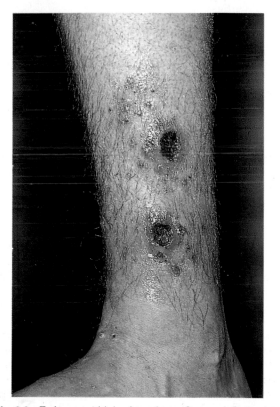

Fig. 8.2 Ecthyma; multiple ulcers due to *S.aureus* infection in a debilitated patient.

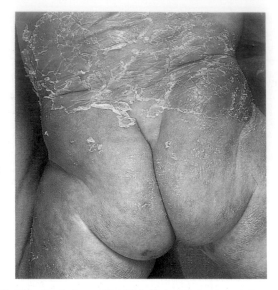

Fig. 8.3   Staphylococcal 'scalded skin' syndrome in an infant.

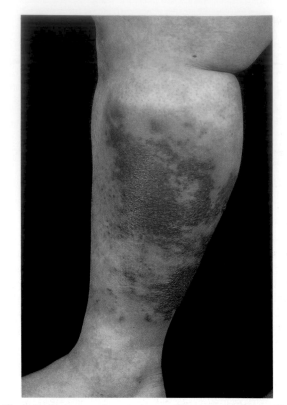

Fig. 8.4   Streptococcal erysipelas on a leg may be complicated by haemorrhagic blistering.

which presents with localized erythema, swelling and tenderness. The margin of the zone of inflammation is usually well defined, and often palpable. The attack is typically heralded by malaise, fever, flu-like symptoms and pain in the affected area, which is almost always the face or one leg, less often an arm. The tenderness, pain and toxicity are crucial in differentiating the episode from urticaria or angio-oedema. On the face, the portal of entry of *Streptococcus pyogenes* may be a fissure in the retroauricular fold, at an outer canthus or at the nostrils or corners of the mouth. In the leg, toe-cleft fissures secondary to tinea or bacterial intertrigo are important. In a limb, a streak of lymphangitis and tender proximal lymphadenopathy may develop. Oedema may be complicated by haemorrhagic bullae (Fig. 8.4). Facial erysipelas may be unilateral or bilateral. Associated eyelid oedema may invite confusion with allergic contact dermatitis, but itching is absent. Untreated attacks subside spontaneously over 2–3 weeks but in the debilitated, streptococcal septicaemia is a serious hazard. Recurrent attacks may lead to lymphatic damage and irreversible oedema.

Cellulitis

Cellulitis is similar to erysipelas but deeper. The area is dark red and often grossly oedematous, tender and painful.

Treatment

Topical therapy is ineffective. *Streptococcus pyogenes* is always sensitive to benzyl penicillin (G) and phenoxymethyl penicillin (V), but these penicillins are not well absorbed orally and tissue concentrations may prove inadequate. Therefore, flucloxacillin or amoxycillin in full dosage is the treatment of choice, continued for 10–14 days. Erythromycin is also almost always effective. In very severe attacks, additional initial treatment with penicillin G 1 megaunit intramuscularly 12-hourly for three or four doses is valuable, if penicillin hypersensitivity can be excluded with certainty. Erysipelas and cellulitis are often recurrent and a history of two or more episodes at one site is a strong indication for long-term (at least 3 years) prophylaxis with penicillin V 250 mg thrice daily or erythromycin 250 mg twice daily or co-trimoxazole, one tablet twice daily. Attention should also be paid to intertrigo in toe clefts, behind an ear or at the angle of the mouth.

Infected fissures

In dermatitis and less often in psoriasis, fissures may develop which become infected with *Streptococcus* pyogenes, painful and purulent. *Staphylococcus aureus* may also be present. Common sites are below the earlobes in children, the hands in chronic dermatitis, the natal cleft and toe clefts.

Miscellanous Infections

Erysipeloid

Erysipeloid is an infection with *Erysipelothrix insidiosa* (formerly *E. rhusiopathiae*). It occurs in those who handle raw meat and fish, and often follows a prick or scratch from a bone. A dull or purplish-red, slowly spreading cellulitis, without constitutional symptoms, results. The erythema tends to spread down one finger and up another. The adjacent joints may also be affected. The treatment is penicillin V 500 mg q.d.s or oxytetracycline 500 mg q.d.s for 7 days.

Erythrasma

In the United Kingdom this infection causes a dry, pale, red–brown, pityriasiform flexural eruption in the axillae (Fig. 8.5), groins or abdominal or submammary folds. In hot countries it may be much more widespread. The lesions, which are macular, fluoresce coral-red under Wood's light due to porphyrin production by the causative diphtheroid, *Corynebacterium minutissimum*. Topical imidazole creams (e.g. Canesten, U.K.) are effective as is erythromycin orally, 250 mg four times daily for 7 days.

Keratolysis plantare

This condition, also known as pitted keratolysis, is a common condition in young unhygienic adults with hyperhidrotic malodorous feet, often macerated by unsuitable occlusive footwear. A well-defined irregular keratolysis produces pitted erosions and extremely shallow areas of confluent brown, slightly depressed discoloration of the heel or sole under the metatarsal heads (Fig. 8.6). The palms are rarely involved. The causative organism is *Micrococcus sedentarius*, but corynebacteria may also be responsible. Treatment calls for better hygiene, less occlusion, use of neomycin or clindamycin topically, 40% formalin ointment, or twice daily soaks with 1:4000 potassium permanganate or 4.5% formaldehyde solution for 10–15 minutes.

Anthrax

Anthrax, due to infection with *Bacillus anthracis*, is primarily a disease of animals. It occurs in those handling imported, contaminated hides, wool and hair, for example tannery workers, dockers, and also those who use bonemeal as a fertilizer. The lesion usually begins on an exposed part, such as hands, arms, face or neck. A papule forms on the site of an abrasion and becomes

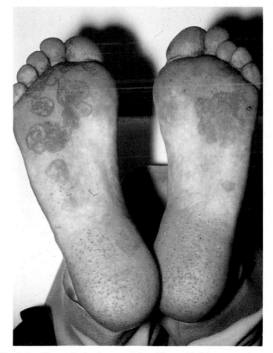

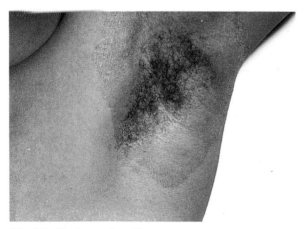

Fig. 8.5 Erythrasma in axilla.

Fig. 8.6 Keratolysis plantare (pitted keratolysis).

surrounded by deep erythema. Bullae or vesicles form and become haemorrhagic. There is gross local oedema, lymphadenopathy and also fever. The diagnosis is confirmed by finding large Gram-positive bacilli in the blister fluid and later by culture. Treatment is with penicillin G, one million units q.d.s. by intramuscular injection or tetracycline, intravenously at first for 3 days, later by mouth (2 g per day for 14 days). Pulmonary and abdominal infections also occur.

Lyme disease

Named after a place in Connecticut, U.S.A., this disease is now known to be a zoonosis, caused by a spirochaete, *Borrelia bergdorferi*, transmitted by the bite of a tick, *Ixodes ricinus*. Its cutaneous manifestation has long been known as *erythema chronicum migrans*, a slowly spreading annular, indurated erythematous plaque, usually on a limb. Weeks or months later neurological or cardiac disease may follow. In the U.S.A., arthritis and cardiac problems are predominant; in Europe, skin and neurological disease are more common. A late skin manifestation, *acrodermatitis chronica atrophicans*, is seen in Sweden and Germany. Diagnosis depends upon the detection of antibody to *Borrelia bergdorferi* in serum and cerebrospinal fluid. The disease responds to high dose penicillin or tetracycline for 10 days.

Mycobacterial Diseases

Tuberculosis of the skin

Common at the beginning of the century, tuberculosis (Table 8.1) is now rare in advanced countries. The pasteurization of milk, the establishment of tuberculosis-free herds, improvements in standards of living and the development of effective treatment have almost eliminated the disease. However, it is still found in the United Kingdom, usually in immigrants of Asian origin, and is still a very common Third World problem.

Lupus vulgaris

This is the commonest type of mycobacterial infection (Fig. 8.7). It arises as a postprimary infection where resistance to the infection is high. It usually begins in childhood and the head and neck (including the nose and inside of the mouth) are common sites, although the shoulders or limbs are occasionally involved. The lesions are red–brown painless nodules which look like apple jelly when pressed with a glass spatula or slide. The nodules heal in the centre and scar, while fresh nodules are formed peripherally, leading to slow spread. On the face, cartilage or even bone may be involved. In neglected disease in the past, the nose, ear, eye and eventually much of the face could be destroyed, causing hideous deformities. On the scalp a cicatricial alopecia was common but is now very rare. In black or brown skin, secondary pigmentary disturbance is usual. Differential diagnosis includes Bowen's disease, morphoeic basal cell carcinoma and discoid lupus erythematosus. Biopsy establishes the diagnosis but it is only rarely possible to culture the organism from biopsy material. Rarely, lupus vulgaris may reactivate after decades of inactivity. Squamous carcinoma may supervene on lupus scarring (Fig. 8.8) and long-term supervision is mandatory.

Table 8.1 Cutaneous manifestations of tuberculosis.

Lupus vulgaris

Warty tuberculosis

Scrofuloderma

Tuberculous ulceration

The tuberculides:

   Erythema nodosum

   Erythema induratum

   Papulonecrotic tuberculide

   Lichen scrofulosorum

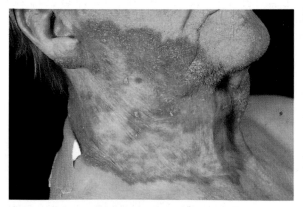

Fig. 8.7 Lupus vulgaris on the neck of an elderly man, untreated for decades.

Warty tuberculosis

Warty tuberculosis (tuberculosis verrucosa cutis) is inoculation tuberculosis in people who are already partly immune from a previous infection. It is found on the hands and wrists of butchers, pathologists and postmortem workers, and on the legs and buttocks of children. It looks like an ill-formed wart or keratotic plaque sitting on an area of cold erythema. It is now very rare in northern Europe or North America but is common in the Third World.

Other tuberculous manifestations

Scrofuloderma

This is the result of involvement of skin over a tuberculous lymph gland or infected bone or joint. A dull red nodule soon ulcerates. Fistulae, scarring and granulations may develop.

Acute tuberculous ulceration

This occurs in debilitated patients with advanced pulmonary, intestinal or urogenital tuberculosis. It is now rare. One or more shallow ulcers with blue–red undermined edges are seen in the skin. The mouth or anus may be involved. *Mycobacterium tuberculosis* is easily demonstrated in the discharge.

Tuberculides

In addition to the above there are four conditions which may be tuberculous manifestations but in which it is rare to detect mycobacteria in the affected skin (Table 8.1). Erythema nodosum is best known; all are now rare in Europe. They are probably due to blood-borne dissemination often from an occult focus, in a patient with high immunity.

Erythema nodosum. This immunological reaction is described in Chapter 16. Other causes are much commoner.

Papulonecrotic tuberculide. This is a rare disseminated profuse papular and necrotic cutaneous reaction to *M. tuberculosis*.

Lichen scrofulosorum. This is an eruption of minute, often lichenoid or follicular, papules.

Bazin's disease (erythema induratum). This consists of indolent nodules on the calves of adolescent girls and young women. The nodules may ulcerate. Differential diagnosis is from nodular vasculitis and, occasionally, perniotic ulceration.

Diagnosis

Biopsy is essential for histopathology and culture, although the latter is rarely positive in lupus vulgaris or the tuberculides. Tuberculin tests (1:10 000 initially) should be performed plus a chest radiograph.

Treatment

Combined treatment with three drugs (rifampicin, isoniazid and ethambutol) for 8 weeks can be followed by treatment with two drugs for a year or more according to response. Pyrazinamide and streptomycin are also available as alternatives if necessary.

Atypical mycobacterial infections

Bacille Calmette–Guerin (BCG) infections

Persistent local reactions may follow BCG vaccination. Small local abscesses and ulcers may be associated with regional lymphadenitis. Oral isoniazid is curative.

Mycobacterium marinum

Inoculation into the skin may follow an abrasion in a swimming pool, and lead to a prolonged dermal granu-

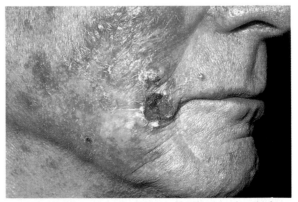

Fig. 8.8 Squamous carcinoma supervening on chronic lupus vulgaris scarring.

loma, for instance on the nose (swimming pool granuloma). Keeping tropical fish tanks (where the fish themselves may be infected) may lead to inoculation on the hand and sometimes a sporotrichosis-like spread with multiple dermal and subcutaneous nodules along the arm (fish tank granuloma). Biopsy for histopathology and low temperature (28–31°C) culture on a special medium confirm the diagnosis. Co-trimoxazole and tetracycline are the most useful drugs, but may have to be given for several weeks.

Mycobacterium ulcerans

Spreading ulceration of the skin occurs in tropical zones due to inoculation from vegetation. The organism can be cultured at 28–31°C. Rifampicin is the treatment of choice.

Other atypical mycobacteria

Immunosuppressed patients, such as those with HIV disease or leukaemia, may develop cutaneous or even disseminated systemic infections with various organisms, for example *Mycobacterium intracellulare*.

Sexually Transmitted Bacterial Diseases

Gonorrhoea

Gonococcal disease is almost entirely non-dermatological. Essentially it is an infection of the mucosa of the genitourinary tract caused by *Neisseria gonorrhoeae*, transmitted sexually. Extragenital sites, including the rectum, oropharynx and eyes, may be involved. Children and babies of infected mothers may be infected non-sexually, especially in the conjunctivae.

Gonococcal septicaemia

Pregnant women are especially at risk. Fever and arthritis are sometimes accompanied by characteristic skin lesions which are papulopustular, purpuric or even necrotic. The lesions are sparse and often distal. The gonococcus or its products can be demonstrated in the lesions. The usual mucosal sites, skin lesions, synovial fluid and blood should all be cultured for diagnosis. Treatment is with 500 000 units penicillin G parenterally every 6 hours for 48 hours followed by ampicillin 2 g daily for 8 days. In areas where penicillinase-producing gonococci occur, spectinomycin 2 g

intramuscularly twice daily for 10 days is preferable and can also be chosen in patients known to be allergic to penicillin. Doxycycline and co-trimoxazole are less effective. In pregnancy, spectinomycin or erythromycin are to be preferred and the latter, continued for 2 weeks, deals with commonly coexistent non-specific genital infection.

Syphilis

Untreated syphilis (lues) is an infectious disease of great chronicity due to *Treponema pallidum*, a spirochaete, with distinct primary, secondary and late stages. It is found worldwide. Penicillin is curative and has radically altered the course and prognosis. Transmission is usually sexual but may be congenital or by infusion of infected blood.

Primary syphilis

After an incubation period of about 3 weeks a small painless papule develops which rapidly ulcerates. This chancre is solitary and usually indurated, remaining painless. It may be 1–2 cm in diameter or trivial and easily missed. In heterosexual men the penis is the usual site (Fig. 8.9). In homosexual men it is on the penis, anal canal or mouth, especially the lip. In women the vulva is the commonest site but the cervix, mouth (lip), buttock or finger are occasionally affected. Painless regional lymphadenopathy is usual within a

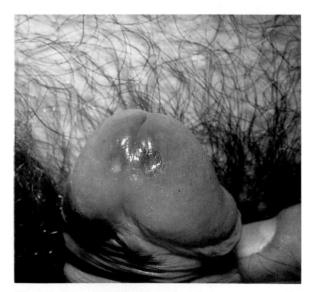

Fig. 8.9   Primary syphilis (chancre) on glans penis.

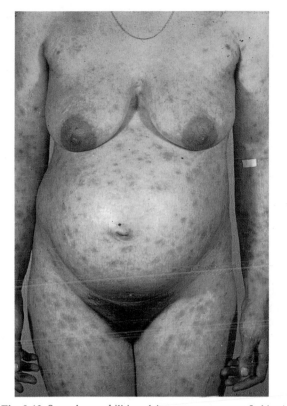

Fig. 8.10 Secondary syphilitic rash in a pregnant woman. Itching is absent or minimal.

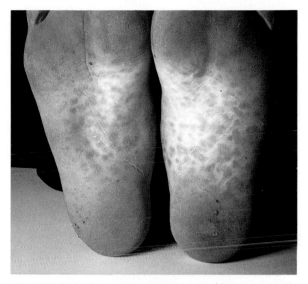

Fig. 8.11 Rash of secondary syphilis on soles of feet.

Table 8.2 Differential diagnosis of secondary syphilis.

Pityriasis rosea
Drug eruptions
Psoriasis
Infectious mononucleosis
Haemorrhoids ⎱ (of condylomata lata) Genital warts ⎰
Aphthous ulceration (of oral lesions)

few days and is bilateral with genital chancres. The spirochaete is demonstrated by dark-field microscopy of wet-mounted material from the chancre.

Secondary syphilis

This stage is characterised by rash, lymphadenopathy and variable malaise. It develops 4–12 weeks after the primary infection. The rash is profuse, symmetrical on the trunk (Fig. 8.10) and limbs and typically involves the palms and soles (Fig. 8.11). It consists of pale pink ('ham-coloured') discrete macules which may become papular or squamous. Itching is *not* a feature. In the tropics pustular and necrotic lesions may occur. In moist flexures confluent plaques may form, called condylomata lata (Fig. 8.12). On the buccal mucosa small grey or white erosions may be seen ('mucous patches') and are sometimes arcuate, producing 'snail-track ulcers'. Differential diagnosis is listed in Table 8.2

Late untreated secondary syphilis is more papulo-squamous and may mimic psoriasis but leaving some scarring in its wake. Patchy 'moth-eaten' alopecia is uncommon.

Lymphadenopathy is generalized. The malaise is variable but can include fever, lassitude, headache and muscular or joint aching. Rare features are laryngitis, meningism, hepatitis, uveitis and periostitis. All the manifestations of untreated secondary syphilis eventually disappear spontaneously.

Latent syphilis

The patient is asymptomatic but with positive serology and is potentially infectious. Untreated, about 40% will eventually develop late clinical syphilis.

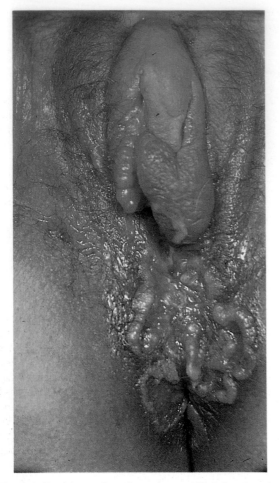

Fig. 8.12 Condylomata lata of secondary syphilis below the vulva. The hyperkeratosis of genital warts is absent.

Late syphilis

Table 8.3 summarizes the main features. Detailed description of visceral disease is outside the scope of this book.

Cutaneous gumma

This is a chronic granulomatous mass showing histologically inflammatory infiltrate including plasma cells and vasculitis including obliterative endarteritis. The clinical lesion is a nodule which enlarges and breaks down to form a 'punched-out' ulcer. It heals very slowly, leaving atrophic scarring. It may be single or multiple; the scalp, face and legs are the common sites.

Table 8.3 Main clinical manifestations of late syphilis.

Skin
  Superficial (nodular) syphilide
  Deep (gummatous) syphilide

Neurosyphilis
  Tabes dorsalis
  General paresis

Cardiovascular
  Aortitis
  Aortic regurgitation
  Coronary ostial stenosis
  Aortic aneurysm

Mucosae
  Gummata

Eyes
  Uveitis
  Choroidoretinitis
  Optic atrophy

Mucosal gumma

This is seen in the mouth or nose and may cause destruction and perforation of the hard palate or nasal septum. Diffuse involvement of the tongue or buccal mucosa produces swelling and inflammation and later, white superficial patches. This 'leukoplakia' is premalignant with considerable risk of eventual squamous cell carcinoma. Differential diagnoses of gumma and leucoplakia are listed in Table 8.4.

Congenital syphilis

The early and late stages are very different.

Early features. Rash appears 2–12 weeks after birth. It

Table 8.4 Differential diagnosis of gumma and leukoplakia.

Gumma	Leukoplakia
Deep mycosis	Candidosis
Tuberculosis	Lichen planus
Leprosy	White sponge naevus
Sarcoidosis	Hairy leukoplakia
Lymphoma	
Halide eruptions	

is usually papulosquamous but may be bullous. The palms, soles and face are particularly involved. The rash may be confluent or eroded on the face, and heals leaving characteristic linear scars ('rhagades'). Hair and nails may be lost and the child may not thrive. The oral and nasal mucosa are involved early, causing rhinitis ('snuffles'). Differential diagnosis is from cytomegalovirus, rubella or toxoplasma infection. The child is infectious.

Late features. Late features include bilateral interstitial keratitis, symmetrical painless synovitis of the knees (Clutton's joints), eighth nerve deafness, optic atrophy, periostitis ('sabre tibia' and 'Parrot's nodes' in the skull) and sometimes neurosyphilis. Central notching of the upper incisors ('Hutchinson's teeth') and 'saddle' nose are other well-known features.

Serological tests

Non-specific reaginic IgG and IgM and specific antitreponemal antibodies are detectable.

VDRL test. This is non-specific but quantitative and titres reflect activity, which is of great value. It becomes positive in the primary stage, reaching a maximum titre in the secondary stage, and becomes very weakly positive or negative after treatment. It is particularly valuable in diagnosis of reinfection.

TPHA test. This is a specific simple *T. pallidum* haemagglutination test and is used routinely in combination with the VDRL test.

FTA-ABS test. This is specific, employing indirect fluorescence with killed *T. pallidum* as antigen, after group antibodies have been absorbed. It is very sensitive but positivity persists long after treatment so it is of no value in assessing disease activity. The FTA-ABS IgM test is valuable in the diagnosis of congenital syphilis.

TPI test. The *T. pallidum* immobilization test is specific but uses live treponemes and is complex and not practical for routine use.

Biological false-positive tests for syphilis

The reaginic non-specific tests may be transiently positive in various infections such as glandular fever (mononucleosis) mycoplasma pneumonitis, and chronically positive in autoimmune disease, leprosy and drug addicts. The specific tests are always negative.

Treatment

Standard treatment is aqueous procaine penicillin, 600 000 units intramuscularly daily for 10 days. A less satisfactory alternative, where compliance is doubtful, is a single depot intramuscular dose of benzathine penicillin 2.4 megaunits. If allergy to penicillin is suspected, doxycycline 300 mg daily for 21 days is effective. Other tetracyclines and erythromycin are alternatives but less effective. The treatment of complicated, late or congenital disease is beyond the scope of this text.

Non-venereal Treponemal Disease

Yaws

Yaws is a common tropical granulomatous spirochaetal disease occurring mainly in rural children. The first lesion is an enlarging, ulcerating papilloma giving way to secondary disseminated cutaneous papillomata which heal in a few months. In drier climates scaly macular lesions are seen. Hyperkeratotic palmar and plantar lesions may mimic viral warts and may be incapacitating. The periosteum of long bones may be swollen and tender. Late skin lesions may be atrophic and ulcerative or proliferative granulomatous lesions resembling gummata. Cardiovascular and neurological disease do not occur.

Endemic syphilis

This is similar to yaws but often starts around the mouth, being transmitted by drinking vessels, and spreads within the family.

Pinta

This treponematosis is seen only in Central and South America and affects the extremities. Spreading plaques coalesce and eventually leave depigmented scars. Penicillin is used in all three diseases.

Granuloma Inguinale

This less common disease is seen predominantly in poor dark-skinned males and is endemic in parts of

India, the South Pacific and West Indies. It is a slowly progressive ulcerative granulomatous infection of the inguinal and anogenital areas due to *C. granulomatis*. Spreading vegetative ulceration has little tendency to heal and cancer may supervene. Penicillin is ineffective but other antibiotics may be successful.

Chancroid

Chancroid is caused by the bacillus, *Haemophilus ducreyi*. The organism enters an abrasion on the penis or vulva leading to formation of a papule which ulcerates and is painful. Ulcers may be multiple. Usually the inguinal glands enlarge and suppurate (the 'bubo').

Healing is spontaneous but not always before mutilation of the genitalia has occurred.

Gram-stains of exudate and culture confirm the diagnosis. Tetracyclines and sulphonamides are moderately effective treatments.

Lymphogranuloma Venereum

Lymphogranuloma venereum does not affect the skin. It is mainly a lymphatic disease due to certain strains of *Chlamydia trachomatis* causing inguinal or femoral lymphadenopathy and sometimes ulcerative proctitis. It is endemic in the tropics.

9

Fungous Diseases

The fungal infections of man are called mycoses. They can be simply classified as in Table 9.1.

The various forms of tinea are due to multicellular fungi called dermatophytes, which form filaments or hyphae. Pityriasis versicolor and candidosis are caused by unicellular fungi which reproduce by budding and are called yeasts.

Tinea

The 'ringworm' dermatophytes live in the stratum corneum of skin, hair and nail, i.e. the dead keratinized tissues which they can digest, but they cannot invade living tissue. Three genera are recognized, called *Microsporum*, *Trichophyton* and *Epidermophyton* (Table 9.2). Within these genera there are very many species, of which about 30 are known to be pathogenic in humans. The dermatophytes can also be divided according to their sources. Anthropophilic species are restricted to man; zoophilic species are essentially pathogenic for animals but may infect man; geophilic species inhabit the soil and only rarely prove to be human pathogens. Fungi vary in their ability to invade skin, hair or nail and in their capacity to excite an inflammatory reaction in the host. Zoophilic species tend to cause much more inflammation than anthropophilic ones.

In the host tissue, the filamentous hyphae of derma-

Table 9.1 Classification of mycoses.

Superficial (cutaneous)	Tinea (ringworm)
	Candidosis (moniliasis)
	Pityriasis versicolor
Deep (systemic)	Actinomycosis
	Sporotrichosis
	Blastomycosis
	Etc.

Table 9.2 Main species of pathogenic fungi.

Genus	Species	Source	Main site	Wood's light
Microsporum	*M. audouini*	Human	Scalp	Positive
	M. canis	Animal	Scalp	Positive
Trichophyton	*T. rubrum*	Human	Nails, hands, feet, groin	Negative
	T. interdigitale	Human	Feet, groin	Negative
	T. mentagrophytes	Animal	Body	Negative
	T. tonsurans	Human	Scalp	Negative
	T. violaceum	Human	Scalp	Negative
	T. schoenleinii	Human	Scalp	Positive
	T. verrucosum	Animal	Body	Negative
	T. soudanense	Human	Scalp, body	Negative
Epidermophyton	*E. floccosum*	Human	Feet, groin	Negative

tophytes segment into chains of arthrospores which are responsible for spread of infection. On suitable tissue, these spores germinate into more hyphae, spreading along the outer epidermis and invading any hair follicles that are present. Some species have the ability to penetrate the hair shaft within the follicle and spread down against the direction of hair growth until the living tissue of the hair bulb arrests further penetration. In an anagen follicle, the fungus may invade newly formed hair indefinitely, perpetuating the infection until the follicle goes into the telogen, or resting, phase. Subsequent shedding of the telogen hair spontaneously 'cures' the infection in that follicle.

Growth of the hair in an infected follicle passively carries the fungus back to the skin surface. If the infected shaft is weakened, it may break, providing a source of potentially infectious material. In some species the arthrospores are formed outside the hair shaft in the infected follicle: this is called ectothrix infection. In others, the arthrospores form only inside the hair shaft, and these are called endothrix spores. The importance of the distinction between endothrix and ectothrix infections for the clinician is that ectothrix spores are associated with the deposition of a fluorescent chemical on the outside of the hair shaft which can be detected by Wood's light examination. Thus, ectothrix infections are Wood's light positive; endothrix infections are not.

The most important species in the United Kingdom are summarized in Table 9.2. *Trichophyton rubrum* is now predominant, with *T. mentagrophytes* var. *interdigitale* and *Epidermophyton floccosum* in second and third place. Infection is much commoner in males at all sites except the lower leg and ankle. It is convenient to describe the clinical patterns of tinea by site.

Tinea capitis

Tinea capitis (ringworm of the scalp) may be caused by *Microsporum* or *Trichophyton* fungi (Table 9.3). *Microsporum* infections are seen mainly in childhood and are of two types: *M. audouini*, which spreads from child to child and may cause epidemics in schools and other institutions; and *M. canis*, which is acquired from kittens and puppies and spreads within the family. *Trichophyton* infections occur in adults and may be of several types, presenting a variety of clinical pictures.

The common *Microsporum* tinea of the child's scalp commences in one or more areas of the scalp as a small, ovoid, scaly patch which spreads at the periphery and may involve the whole of the hair-bearing area. *Microsporum audouini* infections are now rare in the United

Kingdom. The affected parts are covered with broken-off, lustreless hair stumps 1–2 mm in length. There may also be scaling of the skin and *M. canis* infections are more inflammatory than *M. audouini* ones. Viewed under Wood's light in a dark room, the affected hairs on the scalp fluoresce a brilliant green. Scales should be collected with a scalpel or epilating forceps, wrapped in paper and sent to the mycologist for microscopical examination and culture. In the common *M. canis* infection, fungus can often be grown from inanimate objects, such as school desks or bedding.

Scalp ringworm due to *Trichophyton* fungi often presents a different clinical picture. In endothrix infections such as *T. violaceum* and *T. tonsurans*, the hairs may be broken off at the point of their emergence from the scalp, which gives the appearance of small black-heads on the scalp and the name 'black-dot ringworm'. In *T. mentagrophytes* and *T. verrucosum* infections from animals, the patient may exhibit raised boggy swellings on the scalp, where the follicles ooze sero-pus (Fig. 9.1). The suppuration in the follicles causes the hair to fall out, and the disease is self-curative. Small local areas of permanent baldness with depressed scars, sometimes pitted with sunken follicular orifices, may be left. This severely inflammatory form of tinea capitis is called *kerion*, and suppuration is the consequence of the body's reaction to the fungus and is not due to secondary infection. If abscesses on the scalp are bacteriologically sterile the pus should always be cultured for fungi. Kerion is fairly common in rural areas but rare in cities. A large immigrant population in London from the Indian subcontinent, the Middle East and Africa has resulted in *T. violaceum* infections becoming common. The face beard, trunk and even nails may also be affected. The multiple patches in the affected scalp may show minimal scaling, mimicking

Table 9.3 Patterns of tinea capitis.

Species	Source	Clinical	Wood's light
M. audouini	Other children	Patchy alopecia	Positive
M. canis	Puppies, kittens	More scaling	Positive
T. violaceum	Immigrants in U.K.	'Black dots'	Negative
T. verrucosum	Farm animals	Kerion	Negative
T. schoenleinii	Other humans	Favus	Positive

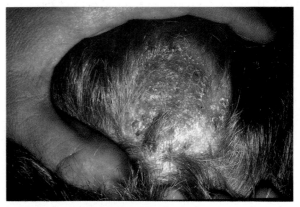

Fig. 9.1 Kerion type of tinea capitis.

seborrhoeic dermatitis or even discoid lupus erythematosus, but sometimes follicular pustules occur.

Favus

This is a distinct form of tinea capitis due to *T. schoenleinii* in which affected hairs do fluoresce a dull grey–green colour. It is rare in northwest Europe. Untreated, favus pursues a chronic course eventually leading to extensive cicatricial alopecia. In the early stages characteristic concave crusts, or scutulae, are seen. Infected hairs do not break easily and long lengths may fluoresce.

Differential diagnosis

Alopecia areata, traumatic (traction) alopecia and various patterns of dermatitis should be considered. If culture reveals *M. audouini*, the source of infection should be sought within the family, friends or school, if necessary enlisting the help of the school medical officer. Large numbers of children can be screened quickly by Wood's light examination. The patient must be kept away from school for at least 3 weeks whilst he and 'positive' contacts are treated. In *M. canis* infections, the family should be examined and infected contacts treated but the child can go to school. The animal source should be identified and treated if possible. The diagnosis of non-fluorescent *Trichophyton* infections can be confirmed by microscopy and culture of scalp scrapings or 'hair-brush' specimens.

Treatment

Tinea capitis cannot be cured by topical fungicides. The antidermatophyte antibiotic, griseofulvin, is given by mouth once daily after the main meal. The daily dose is one 500 mg tablet for adults and 250 mg or 375 mg, as 125 mg tablets or a suspension, for children. Treatment must be continued for at least 2 months and until Wood's light examination is negative in ectothrix infections. In endothrix infections treatment should be continued until the clinical manifestations have disappeared and mycological tests are negative. A topical fungicide can be used in addition.

Tinea corporis

The often ringed lesions of tinea corporis (ringworm of the glabrous skin) give the disease its name. Many different species of fungus may be causative. The erup-

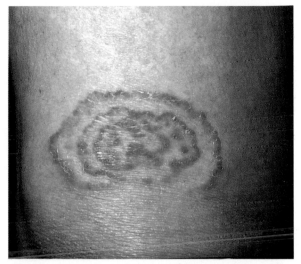

Fig. 9.2 Concentric annular lesions of tinea corporis due to *Microsporum canis*.

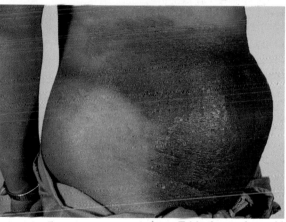

Fig. 9.3 Extensive tinea corporis due to *Trichophyton rubrum* with secondary hyperpigmentation in a Bengali woman.

tion is typically sparse and asymmetrical, with one or more erythematous, scaly, discoid lesions, each sharply defined and spreading slowly centrifugally (Fig. 9.2). In some types there may be marginal vesicles or pustules (Fig. 9.3). Itching is variable. The infection is often of animal origin. If topical corticosteroid creams have been used, the appearance may be atypical with the margins of the ringed lesions losing their continuity and with less scaling.

Treatment

Topical fungicides often suffice for mild infections.

For more serious infections, a 3-week course of griseo-fulvin is curative.

Tinea cruris

The intertriginous inguinal fold is a favourite site of tinea (ringworm of the groin) caused by *E. floccosum, T. mentagrophytes* var. *interdigitale* or *T. rubrum.* The eruption may be due to autoinfection from the feet or to sharing of sports clothing or towels by young men. The first two are seen virtually only in the male but tinea cruris due to *T. rubrum* also occurs in the female, albeit uncommonly. *Epidermophyton floccosum* infections spread only locally on the upper inner thighs to produce a sharply defined 'butterfly' rash more inflamed at its margins. The margin of the rash may be vesicular, pustular or scaly. *T. rubrum* infections often spread much more widely if not treated, extending to the mid-thighs, through the perineum and onto the buttocks (Fig. 9.4), posterior thighs or the lower abdominal wall. The margin is scaly but never vesicular.

Tinea incognito

The natural appearance of tinea cruris is often masked by inappropriate topical steroid therapy which partly suppresses the inflammation and encourages its spread. The distinct margin of the infection is broken up and deeper, inflammatory, 'boil-like' lesions may be seen (Fig. 9.5). The name 'tinea incognito' has been applied to this iatrogenic variant. In chronic lesions, steroid-induced striae may be part of the picture.

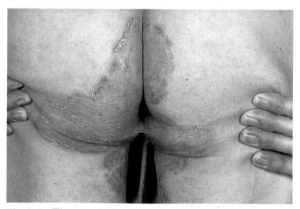

Fig. 9.4   Tinea cruris due to *T.rubrum* spreading to buttocks and posterior thighs.

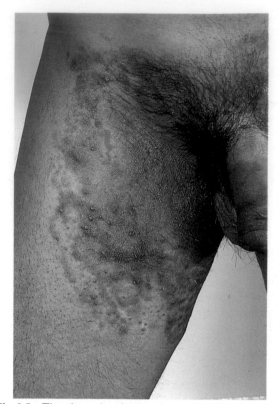

Fig. 9.5   Tinea incognito; tinea cruris treated with topical corticosteroids which have modified the appearance.

Differential diagnosis

Differential diagnosis is from simple eczematous intertrigo, flexural psoriasis and seborrhoeic dermatitis, all of which are more symmetrically distributed above and below the inguinal creases. Candidosis is much commoner in the female and is characteristically vesicular or papulopustular, with outlying 'satellite' lesions. Erythrasma (p. 55) is a more macular, low grade inflammation which flouresces coral-pink under Wood's light. The diagnosis of tinea cruris is confirmed instantly by direct microscopy of unstained scrapings. The causative dermatophyte is identified by culture.

Treatment

The inflamed groin does not tolerate 'strong' local applications and it is easy to induce a secondary contact dermatitis by injudicious topical therapy. Strong topical steroids, if being used, must be withdrawn. If the area is acutely inflamed, 1:8000 potassium permanganate compresses for 10 minutes twice daily for 2 days and then daily for 3 days are invaluable. After this compress, the skin is gently dabbed dry and a cream containing an iodoquinoline antiseptic and a weak corticosteroid (e.g. Vioform-Hydrocortisone, U.K.) applied twice or thrice daily. Later, as the inflammation subsides, an imidazole cream can be substituted, or used from the outset in milder cases. In severe cases and in all *T. rubrum* infections, a 3–4-week course of griseofulvin is indicated.

Tinea pedis

Tinea pedis (ringworm of the feet) is caused by the same three species which cause tinea cruris. It is extremely common in the developed world but rare in those who go barefoot. Those most at risk are young people who share washing, bathing and sports facilities and adults, for example coal miners, who do likewise. Probably the wearing of shoes or boots which compress the lateral toe cleft spaces raises the temperature and humidity in the cleft, encouraging fungal growth. Various bacteria may play a synergistic role in causing symptoms.

Clinical picture

There are three main clinical patterns, all much commoner in males.
- *Intertrigo* occurs especially between the fourth and fifth toes. In minor cases, the webs are itching and scaly. In more severe instances the toe cleft skin in sodden, white, fissured and malodorous and rubs off to leave raw red areas.
- *Vesicular patterns*, usually due to *T. interdigitale*, begin on the sides of toes or on the instep, side or dorsum of the foot. Vesicles, bullae or pustules may be seen. The lesions rupture, dry and leave collarettes of scale. Very acute vesicular tinea is occasionally complicated by secondary allergic vesicular dermatitis (pompholyx) on the remainder of the soles and the palms, the so-called 'id' reaction.
- In the *hyperkeratotic pattern*, diffuse or patchy thickening of the sole is seen. The surface may or may not be reddened but is usually finely exfoliative and the skin creases are accentuated by white scale. This is a chronic pattern almost always due to *T. rubrum*. It is commonly associated with an infection of the toenails. It may slowly spread up the sides of the foot and ankle and to the lower leg.

Differential diagnosis

Differential diagnosis is from endogenous dermatitis, contact dermatitis due to footwear, and psoriasis. Toe cleft intertrigo is sometimes due to candidosis, erythrasma or simple maceration.

Treatment

The mild intertriginous type responds to twice daily application of any efficient topical fungicide. Attention should be paid to foot hygiene and the avoidance of excessively occlusive footwear. Severe intertrigo responds to 1:8000 potassium permanganate compresses and Vioform-Hydrocortisone cream (U.K.) as for acute tinea cruris, followed by resort to other topical fungicides. The same management is appropriate for severe or acute vesicular patterns, although these may be complicated by coccal infection requiring oral erythromycin or flucloxacillin. *Trichophyton rubrum* infections need a 3-month course of griseofulvin. Toenail disease may be incurable.

Tinea barbae

Tinea barbae (ringworm of the beard) is mostly seen in rural areas in farm workers and is acquired from farm animals. *Trichophyton verrucosum* and *T. mentagrophytes* are commonly responsible. Occasionally tinea barbae may be contracted from a cat or dog, when the fungus is *Microsporon canis*, or even from a hedgehog (*T. erinacei*). Human to human spread, for example by *T. rubrum*, is rare. The 'barbers itch' of old was tinea or staphylococcal folliculitis.

The disease commonly attacks localized areas, although it may, of course, spread over the whole of the beard area; the upper lip is seldom affected. In the severe form acquired from farm animals the hair follicles are invaded, and a suppurative condition is set up. The affected area appears as a mass of small boils, at the apex of which a broken-off hair projects through a bead of pus, and is easily pulled out. The picture is thus of kerion. In less severe cases, 'lumpy' swellings may be found, and no pus is visible.

Differential diagnosis

Differential diagnosis is from staphylococcal folliculitis and depends on microscopy of hair and scales, and fungal and bacteriological cultures.

Treatment

Griseofulvin for 3 weeks is indicated. With kerion, loose hairs should be epilated daily. A fungicidal cream can also be used.

Tinea facei

This is infection of the glabrous skin of the face. *Trichophyton rubrum* and *T. mentagrophytes* are the usual causes in the United Kingdom but *Microsporum* species are common worldwide. Erythema, scaling, papules or marginated plaques may be seen but often the inflammation has been suppressed by topical steroid abuse. The patient may complain of itching, burning and sensitivity to light.

Tinea facei may be misdiagnosed as rosacea, seborrhoeic dermatitis, psoriasis, discoid lupus erythematosus or polymorphic light eruption. Microscopy confirms the diagnosis and griseofulvin is rapidly effective.

Tinea manuum

Trichophyton Rubrum is usually responsible for ringworm of the hand. Five clinical patterns are recognized:
- Vesicular discoid patches
- Crescentric exfoliating scaling lesions as seen on the soles
- Discrete red papular and follicular scaly patches on the backs of the hands or wrists
- Erythematous scaly sheets on the backs of the hands, with well-defined margins (Fig. 9.6)
- Hyperkeratotic erythematous finely exfoliative

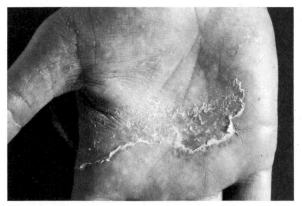

Fig. 9.6 Tinea of hand; note the inflammatory leading edge with a trailing fringe of epidermis.

sheets as on the soles. This pattern is confined to the palmar aspect of the hand and is often unilateral.

Differential diagnosis

Differential diagnosis is from endogenous and contact dermatitis and psoriasis.

Treatment

Griseofulvin is usually indicated. Four weeks suffice for infections of the back of the hand but at least 8 weeks' treatment should be given for hyperkeratotic palmar infections. In addition a topical fungicide should be used.

Follicular tinea of the calves

Often clinicians fail to recognize that certain unusual eruptions on the lower two-thirds of the legs may be due to infection with *T. rubrum*. The infection is usually seen in women.

Usually the lesions are irregularly shaped, unilateral, blue–red patches on which are set indurated follicular papules with some scaling. Occasionally erythema-nodosum-like nodules are seen. The fungus can be demonstrated in the follicles by biopsy.

Treatment

Treatment is by means of griseofulvin and antifungal ointments.

Tinea unguium

Fungal infection of the nails (onychomycosis) is more common in the toenails than the fingernails. *Trichophyton rubrum* is the usual cause in the hands, but *T. interdigitale* and T. rubrum are equally common in the feet. The infection begins at the free end of the nail, often laterally, and gradually extends proximally until the whole nail plate is diseased. The affected nail loses its lustre and becomes brittle and opaque. Its surface becomes roughened and eventually the nail may become grossly thickened or crumble. Subungual hyperkeratosis may develop in the toenails. Paronychia is not a feature. Often the skin of the hands or feet is involved.

Differential diagnosis

Differential diagnosis is from psoriasis and candidosis.

Treatment

In general, toenail infections in the adult due to *T. rubrum* are incurable. Prolonged courses of griseofulvin lasting 4–8 months can cure fingernail infections but, clearly, such therapy should not be undertaken unless the diagnosis has been confirmed by microscopy and culture. Tioconazole lotion (Trosyl, U.K.) painted on the nail plates daily may prove of value.

Candidosis

Candidosis (moniliasis) is an infection of the skin, nails and mucosae, usually caused by the yeast-like fungus, *Candida albicans*, although rarely other *Candida* species are implicated. The yeast is a normal resident of the gastrointestinal and genital mucosae which becomes pathogenic only when an opportunity arises. A number of clinical situations provide such an opportunity and are listed in Table 9.4. The disease is seen at the extremes of life: in the neonate's mouth as thrush, before the normal antagonistic bacterial flora have become established, and in the very old or debilitated. It may also be seen in patients suffering from malnutrition. In extreme situations systemic infection is possible with candidial endocarditis, meningitis or lung infections which may be fatal. Several clinical patterns of candidosis can be seen (Table 9.5).

Table 9.4 Clinical situations favouring candidosis.

Pregnancy	Diabetes mellitus
Oral contraceptives	Hypoparathyroidism
Wide-spectrum antibiotics	Blood dyscrasias
Corticosteroids	HIV infection
Immunosuppressive drugs	

Table 9.5 Clinical patterns of candidosis.

Oral Thrush	Intertrigo
Angular stomatitis	Erosio interdigitalis
Candida granuloma (lips)	Chronic paronychia
Balanoposthitis	Chronic onychia
Vulvovaginitis	Pruritus ani

Thrush

Thrush is oral candidosis which presents as whitish patches on the buccal mucosa. These patches are easily scraped off to reveal an inflamed mucosal surface. The tongue and lips may also be involved. Occasionally oral candidosis can be atrophic or hyperplastic, resembling leukoplakia. Thrush is almost universal in AIDS and related syndromes.

Angular stomatitis and cheilitis

Angular stomatitis involves the skin and mucosae of the corners of the mouth and may be complicated by painful fissuring. It may be the result of sagging of the face in older people with dentures, leading to the formation of an intertriginous fold. In the immunodeficient the whole lip may be involved and granulomatous (candida granuloma).

Balanoposthitis

Balanoposthitis due to *Candida* is a common presenting feature of diabetes in men. Alternatively, it may be caused by candidial vulvovaginitis in the sexual partner.

Vulvovaginitis

Vulvovaginitis is common in pregnancy and diabetes and is a recognized complication of oral contraceptive therapy. It may occur when girls on 'the pill' are being given long-term oral tetracycline for acne vulgaris. The infection causes vulval pruritus, with variable rash and characteristic vaginal discharge. In severe infections the vaginal walls show the features of oral thrush.

Intertrigo

Intertrigo in the submammary (Fig. 9.7), abdominal, anogenital or interdigital folds between the second and third fingers (erosio interdigitalis; Fig. 9.8) is often partly or even wholly due to *C. albicans* in the presence of predisposing factors. The eruption is moist and erythematous, with a well-defined margin which is often scaly or pustular. Outlying, 'satellite' papulopustules may be seen. Occasionally pruritus ani is caused in the absence of obvious intertrigo.

Chronic paronychia

Chronic paronychia is discussed in Chapter 22.

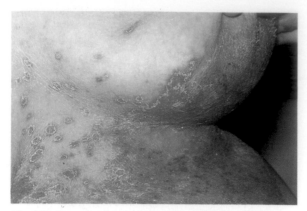

Fig. 9.7 Intertrigo due predominantly to *Candida albicans*.

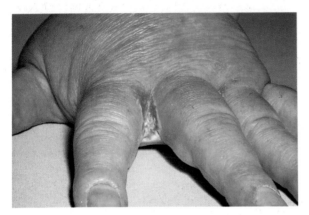

Fig. 9.8 Erosio interdigitalis; in the hand this is almost always due to *Candida albicans*, not tinea.

Onychia

Candidial infection of the nail plate is seen particularly in hypoparathyroidism and in certain rare states of immune deficiency. The nail plate may be grossly disorganized.

Differential diagnosis

Differential diagnosis of candidial infections is from tinea, seborrhoeic dermatitis, flexural psoriasis, pyoderma and contact dermatitis. The diagnosis is con-firmed by microscopy of skin or mucosal scrapings which reveals small oval budding yeasts which may grow into filaments. Culture is less valuable, since it may yield harmless commensals.

Treatment

Underlying predisposing factors should be dealt with as far as possible. A number of preparations are available which are very active against *C. albicans*, for example the antibiotics nystatin and amphotericin B, the iodoquinolines (chinoform, clioquinol, chlorquinaldol) and the various imidazole creams. Gentian violet, 0.5% or 1% in water, is also effective. Nystatin and amphotericin are available as lozenges for the treatment of oral lesions and as pessaries for vaginal treatment. All are available as creams or ointments for treatment of the skin. Nystatin tablets, one twice daily, are effective in the gastrointestinal tract and are occasionally useful for candidial pruritus ani or where recurrent genital infection in the female is thought to originate from the lower bowel. Nystatin is not absorbed from the gut. In the rare systemic infections and in resistant or persistent mucocutaneous candidosis, oral ketoconazole is indicated. Amphotericin B is also effective in such circumstances but has to be given intravenously. Griseofulvin is not active against *Candida* species.

Pityriasis Versicolor

Pityriasis versicolor (tinea versicolor) is caused by *Malassezia furfur* which is the mycelial phase of *Pityrosporum orbiculare*, a yeast which is a component of normal skin flora. The mycelium of *M. furfur* attacks only the stratum corneum and on microscopical examination is seen to consist of short rod-like or bent pieces of fine mycelium, between which lie grape-like clusters of round or oval spores. The malady is slightly contagious but the disease is usually autogenous. In temperate climates it is most common in young adults, uncommon in children and rare in old age. It affects both sexes equally. In the tropics it is rife, affecting up to 40% of the population in some countries. Systemic and topical steroid therapy predispose to this infection, as does Cushing's syndrome.

On white skin the first sign is the appearance of irregular fawn or brownish, slightly scaling macules which coalesce to form irregular figures. Large areas of skin may be involved but the neck, shoulders, upper trunk and upper arms are the usual sites (Fig. 9.9). The

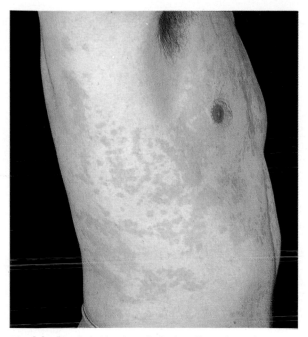

Fig. 9.9 Pityriasis (tinea) versicolor in a Caucasian male.

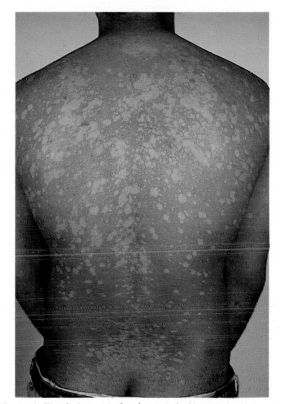

Fig. 9.10 Pityriasis versicolor in a dark-skinned man showing hypopigmentation.

patches have well-defined borders and usually develop in summer. Often the appearance is like a map, with continents and islands painted on the skin in light-brown pigment. In coloured persons and sunburned Caucasians, depigmentation of the infected skin may occur and the infected areas resemble the patches of leukoderma seen in vitiligo (Fig. 9.10). Examination of the patient under Wood's light shows faint orange, gold or buff fluorescence in the affected areas.

It may be difficult to differentiate between tinea versicolor and vitiligo but close examination almost always reveals slight inflammation and fine scaling, which are absent in vitiligo. Usually, it is easy to demonstrate the mycelium and spores in scrapings.

Treatment

Six daily applications of 2.5% selenium sulphide suspension (Selsun, U.K.) are usually curative. The suspension should be applied to the whole body including the wetted scalp, and washed off after 30 minutes. In addition, an imidazole cream can be applied twice daily for 10 days to the affected areas. Griseofulvin is of no value in the treatment of tinea versicolor, but occasionally, ketoconazole 200 mg daily for 5 days only is justifiable and highly effective. When

pigmentation is disturbed the patient must be warned that this will take much longer to settle.

The Deep Mycoses

Actinomycosis

Actinomycosis is an infective granuloma characterized by the formation and spread of nodules, which ulcerate and discharge a typical pus. The disease occurs on the skin, but may commence in other tissues; it may spread by metastasis to any part of the body. It is caused by *Actinomyces*, usually *A. israelii*. *Actinomyces* are anaerobic fungi which often live saprophytically in the mouth and gastrointestinal tract of animals and man; under certain conditions the organisms become pathogenic. The incubation period is unknown, but possibly varies from a few days to several weeks. Adults are more frequently affected than children and men more than women.

Signs and symptoms

The face, neck, chest and abdomen are the most commonly affected parts. The lesions are relatively painless. In Europe, a solitary abscess of dental origin on the cheek is one of the commoner presentations. Infection may occur through an abrasion in the skin, but happens much more often through the mucous membrane of the mouth, from which the disease spreads to the skin. Lesions on the knuckles caused by punching someone in the mouth have been described.

The disease commences with the appearance of a subcutaneous nodule which enlarges, suppurates, forms an abscess and then bursts, discharging a pus which contains greenish-grey or sulphur-coloured granules. These granules consist of small colonies of *Actinomyces*. In rare instances, as one nodule enlarges another forms in close apposition to it, and the clinical picture thus obtained is of a mass of nodules surrounding an ulcerated area. The nodules are frequently 2–3 cm in diameter and are hard on palpation. The disease spreads inwards and may involve bone, leading to sinus formation.

The disease must be differentiated from the other infective granulomata. The clinical diagnosis should be confirmed by microscopical and cultural examination of the pus, which has to be searched carefully for the granules. Precipitating antibodies can be sought by serological methods.

Treatment

High dose long-term penicillin is the treatment of choice. In severe cases, high doses are given parenterally for 14 days, then lower oral doses for months. Wide surgical excision of infected tissue is also advised. In penicillin-sensitive patients, tetracycline 4 g daily for 6 weeks or erythromycin can be used.

Chromoblastomycosis

This is a chronic, slowly progressive fungal infection of the tropics, seen only rarely in northern Europe. It is caused by geophilic *Phialophora* and *Cladosporum* species and may spread metastatically. It is characterized clinically by the development of warty nodules on the skin, usually on the feet, legs or buttocks. Large plaques and tumours may form. Differential diagnosis is from other infective granulomata. The diagnosis is confirmed by histological and cultural examination of biopsy material.

Treatment

Localized lesions may be excised or destroyed by cryotherapy, cauterization or diathermy. Therapeutic claims have been made for isoniazid, thiabendazole and 5-fluorocytosine used systemically. The latter is the best, used alone or combined with ketoconazole. Amphotericin B can be infiltrated intralesionally. Some lesions are resistant to all these treatments.

Sporotrichosis

Sporotrichosis is a contagious disease caused by a fungus and characterized by the formation of nodules which may occur not only in the skin, but in almost any organ or tissue in the body. The nodules break down and, on the skin, form comparatively painless ulcers. The disease is rare in Europe but occurs sporadically in the Americas, Africa and elsewhere where temperature and humidity are high. It is very rare in arid zones. Sporotrichosis is caused by *Sporotrichum schenckii*, which may be contracted from plants and vegetables, but particularly from timber after minor skin abrasions, for example in miners. The fungus is easily cultivated in Sabouraud's medium.

Clinical picture

The patient complains of 'ulceration of the skin'. On examination small nodules are found, which appear to lie in the subcutaneous tissues. These enlarge, become red and form small abscesses which burst causing indolent ulcers, irregular in outline, with undermined and inflamed edges. The disease tends to spread by the lymphatics, and a significant feature is the development of a series of ulcers extending from a primary sore, which often develops at the site of a minor injury, up a limb in the line of the lymphatic drainage (Fig. 9.11). Rarely, sporotrichosis disseminates via the bloodstream and not by the lymphatics; this is usually fatal. Occasionally only one chronic sore, with no metastases, develops. It is usually on an ear exposed to injury, and may take various forms, especially that of an ulcer surrounded by warty proliferations. Involvement of mucosae, eye, organs and bones is not uncommon.

Differential diagnosis

The disease must be distinguished from tuberculosis, syphilitic and venous ulceration. The so-called 'fish-tank granuloma' due to atypical mycobacteria, espe-

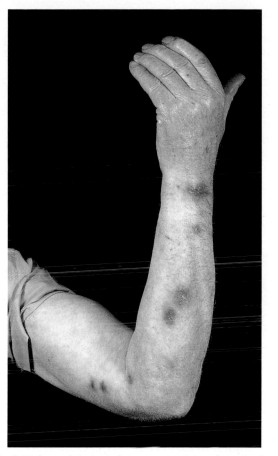

Fig. 9.11 Sporotrichosis; inflammatory nodules along the lymphatic chain in an arm.

cially *M. marinum*, may spread in a sporotrichoid manner on the arm (p. 58). The diagnosis is made by histology and culture of biopsy material.

Treatment

The prognosis is good if the disease is treated energetically. Potassium iodide should be given orally in full dosage for several weeks. The disease may respond to intravenous amphotericin B or oral ketoconazole. Thermotherapy with prolonged daily hot compresses, amphotericin B or 5-fluorocytosine intralesionally have also been used.

Maduramycosis

Maduramycosis (Madura foot) is a chronic granuloma-tous condition which usually affects the lower extremities, generally the foot but occasionally the hand and arm. The disease is endemic in the tropical regions of Asia, Africa and America. It is found mainly amongst the bare-footed population of country districts and is an exogenous infection. It is caused by one of several different fungi and actinomycetes including *Madurella* and *Nocardia* species. These fungi produce, in the diseased tissue, granules composed of hyphae and spores.

The fungi become lodged in small abrasions of the skin. Several months after the inoculation of the fungus, small hard nodules arise in the subcutaneous tissues. Ulceration occurs and a typical oily fluid which contains the granules is exuded. Other nodules form at the periphery, and in time the whole of the foot becomes involved. Necrosis of the bones occurs, and the foot is honeycombed with fistulae. The disease is not usually painful.

The tumour areas consist of granulation and fibrous tissue with abscess cavities and fistulae. The granules are found in the fluid in these cavities. There are three varieties of granules: white or yellow, brown or black, and red. They are 1–2 mm in diameter and irregular in shape and form. The presence of these granules confirms the diagnosis. The fasciae, muscles, tendons and bones are destroyed by the invasion of the fungus.

The prognosis depends on the causative organism. In resistant cases death occurs from cachexia or secondary infection.

Treatment

In early cases the nodules may be excised, but in the later stages amputation at some distance from the foot may be indicated. In general, chemotherapy is unsatisfactory. Nocardial infections (which have been said to account for 50% of cases in most districts) may respond to sulphonamides such as dapsone or co-trimoxazole in full dosage for several months. Rifampicin 450 mg daily for four weeks may be of value.

Subcutaneous phycomycosis

This is a subcutaneous eosinophilic granuloma due to *Basidiobolus meristosporus*, a fungus of the class Phycomycetes. The disease is usually seen in male children in the tropics but cases have been reported in England. It presents as firm, irregular, subcutaneous tumours, usually on the buttocks or thighs. Symptoms are minimal. Potassium iodide by mouth is the treatment of choice after the diagnosis has been established on biopsy material.

Blastomycosis

This chronic granulomatous and suppurative disease is caused by *Blastomyces dermatitidis*. Long thought to be confined in North America it is now known to be widespread in Africa. Primary disease is usually in the lungs but the disseminated disease may cause papular, nodular or ulcerative skin lesions which spread relentlessly. Amphotericin B intravenously is the treatment of choice. Miconazole intravenously or oral ketoconazole may be useful.

Coccidioidomycosis

This is a respiratory fungal infection caused by *Coccidioides immitis*. It is seen mainly in desert areas of the United States and South America. The skin may be involved in hypersensitivity reactions to the infection such as erythema nodosum, erythema multiforme or generalized morbilliform rashes. Disseminated infection can affect the skin but is rare. Amphotericin B intravenously is the usual treatment.

— 10 —
Parasitic Infections and Insect Bites

The important parasitic infections of the skin are listed in Table 10.1.

Scabies

Scabies is a common chronic, contagious, itching disease due to *Sarcoptes scabiei hominis*, a barely visible mite which can live only on human skin (Fig. 10.1).

Biology of the mite

The fertilized female burrows into the skin surface creating an intracorneal tunnel in which she deposits three eggs per day and numerous faecal pellets which contain the allergen which initiates the immune reaction responsible for symptoms. At approximately 3-day intervals, eggs hatch to produce larvae which moult, yielding nymphs. Further moults produce mature adult mites and the 15-day life-cycle begins again.

A rapid build-up of mite numbers is unnoticed by the host until the primary immune response induces itching after about 6 weeks. Thereafter scratching rapidly reduces the female mite population to 12 or fewer. Transmission is by direct human contact,

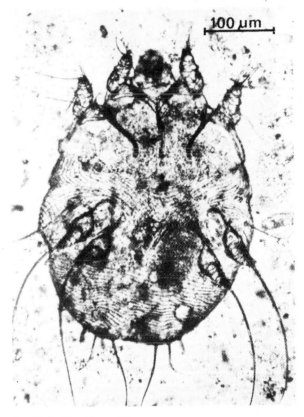

Fig. 10.1 *Sarcoptes scabiei.*

probably usually hand to hand, whether in a familial, childish or sexual setting.

Clinical picture

The patient is typically a young adult of either sex complaining of an intensely itching rash which,

Table 10.1 Parasite infections of human skin.

Disease	Cause
Scabies	*Sarcoptes scabei hominis*
Animal scabies	Animal and bird mites including Cheyletiella
Pediculosis capitis	*Pediculus humanus* var. *capitis*
Pediculosis corporis	*Pediculus humanus* var. *corporis*
Pediculosis pubis	*Pthirus pubis*

incorrectly treated, may last for many months. Itching is localized at first, often about the hands and wrists, but later becomes widespread, especially affecting the penis and scrotum, the umbilical rim, elbows and nipples in the female. It is worse in the evening and in bed or whenever the skin is warmed.

The intensity of the rash depends on the immune response and the extent of eczematization or secondary coccal infection. Typically, small papules, pustules, crusts and excoriations are seen on the hands (Fig. 10.2), wrists and elbows, with a variable erythematous papular and sometimes urticated rash elsewhere on the trunk and limbs. Excoriated papules or even nodules on the scrotum or the shaft or glans of the penis are characteristic. Closer lens inspection of the hands, wrists and sides of the feet usually reveals a few burrows, black–grey sinuous lines up to 10 mm long (Fig. 10.3).

There are many clinical variations. In the tropics, the disease is more widespread and papular, and burrows may be difficult to find. Very clean patients may have few lesions. Topical steroids may mask inflammation. Numerous lesions of palms, soles and head may be seen in infants and atopic eczema may be imitated. Very chronic infections may reveal only a few itching nodules, often genital or pelvic with burrows hard to find. Diminished immune response results in scabies which is less itching and more scaly; atypical patterns are seen in old age, alcoholics, the immuno-suppressed and in Down's syndrome. Very rarely, a total absence of immune response leads to a mite-saturated generalized exfoliative and crusted derma-titis (Norwegian scabies). The admission of such a patient to hospital may lead to infection of many staff, other patients and visitors.

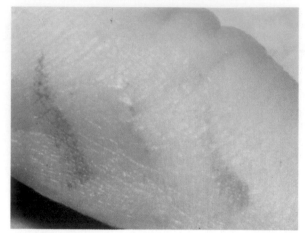

Fig. 10.3 Close-up view of a scabetic burrow on a finger (between marker pen lines).

Diagnosis

In any patient with widespread itching, scabies should be considered. Eliciting the history of an itching 'contact' perhaps months earlier, strengthens suspicion. The finding of a burrow clinches the diagnosis. With practice, the mite can be lifted out of the swelling at the end of the burrow, sticking to the point of a needle, and placed on a microscope slide. Alternatively, scraping a burrow after moistening the skin with liquid paraffin (mineral oil) may reveal larvae, nymphs, eggs and faecal pellets on microscopy.

Treatment

No systemic agent is available but several effective topical scabicides are available.

Lindane. Lindane (gammabenzene hexachloride) 1% cream (Lorexane, U.K.) or 1% lotion (Quellada, U.K.) is very effective. The preparation should be applied meticulously to the whole body below the neck leaving no areas untreated and left on for 24 hours. During this period any part of the body which has to be washed, for example the hands, must be retreated.

Although Lindane has proved to be extremely safe and well tolerated by the skin, it is absorbed and is possibly rarely toxic so is probably best avoided in infants, pregnant women and very thin individuals.

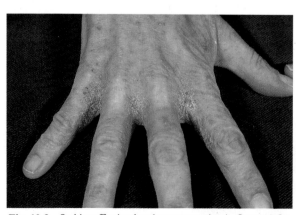

Fig. 10.2 Scabies affecting hands; note crusting in finger clefts.

Malathion. Malathion is available as aqueous liquid 0.5% (Derbac-M, U.K.). Alcoholic preparations have an unpleasant smell and should be avoided. It should be used exactly as lindane. It is safe in infants, where the whole body, including the head and neck, should be treated.

Crotamiton. Crotamiton 10% ointment or lotion (Eurax, U.K.) is a weak scabicide but is non-toxic and non-irritant and can safely be used in infancy and pregnancy. It should be applied daily for a minimum of 7 days and ideally 10 days to ensure cure.

Benzyl benzoate. Benzyl benzoate 25% emulsion (Ascabiol, U.K.) is fairly effective but now rarely used. If applied for more than 2 days it is likely to induce dermatitis and is badly tolerated by infants.

Monosulfiram. Monosulfiram, 25% alcoholic solution, is effective but irritant.

Sulphur. 10% sulphur can be incorporated into an ointment base (e.g. ung. Merck) and applied daily for 3 days. It is potentially irritant.

Whichever agent is chosen, attention to detail and patient compliance are important. It is useful to give the patient an instruction sheet. Those with whom the patient has been in physical contact may have or be incubating the disease and should be treated, i.e. the whole household, children's playmates and sexual partners in adults.

Although 24 hours' treatment with the best scabicides kills all the acari, larvae and eggs, the secondary eruption may take 2–3 weeks to settle completely, during which time crotamiton cream or ointment is the safest application, used daily. Occasionally, even after efficient treatment, intensely itching nodules may persist (postscabetic nodules) due to a dermal hypersensitivity reaction. These respond slowly to a strong topical steroid cream.

True reinfection is possible but uncommon, perhaps because an immediate immune response provokes scratching and burrow destruction.

Animal Scabies

Dogs, cats, rabbits, chickens and birds have their own mites which may cause an itching papular urticaria in exposed humans. Dogs may suffer from sarcoptic mange. Dogs and cats may also be host to another species of non-burrowing mite, *Cheyletiella*. Forage and grain stores may be infested. The distribution of the papules depends upon the particular exposure. The finger webs are usually spared. Arms and neck may be involved but clothing can be penetrated to affect the trunk.

Bird mites may originate from a domestic budgerigar, from air-bricks in a bedroom or from nests in eaves near an open window. Pigeon mites have caused minor epidemics of papular urticaria in long-stay or geriatric hospitals or homes. Thorough cleaning and spraying of windowsills may be necessary to prevent pigeons landing on them.

In all of these mite infestations, examination of appropriate brushings (collected in a plastic bag) by an entomologist will clinch the source of the problem.

Pediculosis

Pediculosis is an infection of the hairy skin or clothing with lice which are wingless, blood-sucking insects. *Pediculus humanus* var. *corporis* lives in clothing and only goes onto the body to feed. *Pediculus humanus* var. *capitis* (Fig. 10.4) and *Pthirus pubis* live in the head and hairy body skin, respectively, and lay their eggs (nits) on the hair.

Pediculosis corporis

In Europe, pediculosis corporis is seen only in tramps (hobos, bums), vagrants and 'down-and-outs', whether alienated, psychopathic, alcoholic or drug-addicted. In

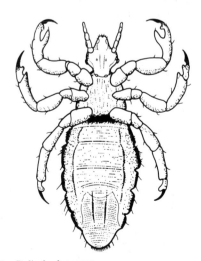

Fig. 10.4 *Pediculus humanus.*

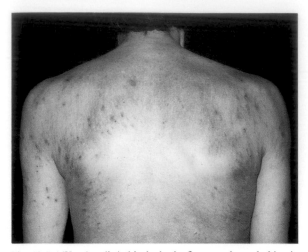

Fig. 10.5 'Vagabond's itch'; the back of a man whose clothing is infested with lice.

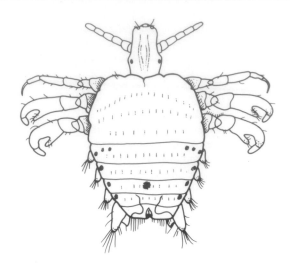

Fig. 10.6 Female pubic ('crab') louse.

times of war and upheaval it may be rife in armies, prison, concentration and refugee camps. The patient is usually dirty, unkempt and malodorous and complains of itching. The skin reveals excoriations, erosions, haemorrhagic crusts and pigmentation, especially on the back (Fig. 10.5). The lice are easily seen crawling in the seams of clothing and underclothing, but not on the patient.

Treatment

Autoclaving of all the patient's clothes is the best treatment. In the United Kingdom most local authorities maintain 'cleansing centres' which offer this service but psychopathic or alcoholic vagrants may not cooperate. Men living in hostels for the homeless may quickly become reinfested. When autoclaving is not available, the clothing should be dusted with 10% dicophane powder B.P.C. or 0.6% gammabenzene hexachloride (lindane) powder (Insect and Louse Powder, ICI, U.K.).

Pediculosis pubis

Crab louse infection ('crabs') is caused by *Pthirus pubis* whose claw-like legs account for its name (Fig. 10.6). Like *P. humanus* var. *capitis* it lives on the body, laying its eggs on hair. Usually it is sexually transmitted and affects the pubis but other body areas are vulnerable, such as the trunk, thighs, axillae and scalp margins. Occasionally the eyelashes may be infected in children but rarely in adults. After mating, the female louse lays 30–36 eggs over her 30-day lifespan, attaching them firmly to a hair proximally. The eggs are brown and shiny and the resultant 'nit' grows out with the hair. Minute nymphs hatch in a week. The empty nit is white and opaque.

Typically, an adult presents with pubic itching. The nits can be seen clearly on the pubic hair and the lice on the adjacent skin. Blue–grey purpura and black excreta may also be visible. The body hair should always be examined widely to determine the extent of the infestation.

Other sexually transmitted disease is common, so appropriate history and examination must not be omitted. The spouse or other sexual partners must be examined where feasible. However, fomite transmission via clothing or bed-linen can occur.

Treatment

Malathion 0.5% aqueous lotion (Derbac M, U.K.) should be applied widely to hairy areas and washed off after 24 hours; this treatment should be repeated in 7 days. Lindane or permethrin 1% cream or lotion can be used in the same way. Alternatively, shaving of the body will quickly cure the disease and this procedure is favoured in Africa and the East. The aqueous malathion lotion can be painted on the eyelashes if necessary. In a young child this is best achieved during sleep.

Pediculosis capitis

Pediculosis capitis is now uncommon in many parts of the United Kingdom but is extremely common world-

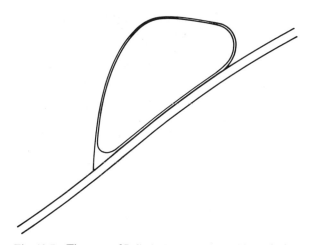

Fig. 10.7   The ovum of *Pediculus humanus* var. *capitis* attached to a scalp hair.

wide. In northern Europe it is as common in the clean as in the dirty and in the wealthy as in the poor, but may be epidemic in refugee camps, armies or in any gross social upheaval. The lice may be difficult to find but nits are plentiful and their distance from the scalp indicates the duration of the infection. They are easily seen, about 0.8 mm long and are cemented to hair (unlike dandruff, which can be slid off) (Fig. 10.7). Occasionally, coarse hair lacquer mimicks nits. Transmission is from head to head when in close proximity so that the head louse may have two or more hosts on any day. The disease is not only transmitted in schools: long-term infections in adults may provide a reservoir and can be detected only by contact tracing. Where there is neglect or lack of hygiene infestation may be gross and the head 'crawling with lice'. Secondary impetigo is common, accompanied by marked cervical lymphadenopathy. Heavily infested children may look pale due to lack of sleep.

Treatment

Malathion aqueous lotion 0.5% (Derbac M, U.K.) should be rubbed into the head and hair and washed off after 12 hours. The treatment should be repeated in 7 days and nits combed out with a metal nit comb. If malathion is not available, carbaryl 0.5% lotion (Caryl-derm or Clinicide, U.K.) should be applied, allowed to dry and left on for 12 hours, again with a repeat treatment after one week. Malathion has a residual effect for weeks, whereas carbaryl persistence is only for a few days. Lindane 1% is now used less because widespread louse resistance has developed and it is not

ovicidal. A new effective pyrethroid pediculocide, permethrin, is available in some countries.

Pediculosis capitis should never be treated with these drugs in shampoo form. The inevitable dilution reduces efficacy, allows lice to survive treatment and encourages development of drug resistance. Lastly, all contacts should be treated and the source of infection traced if possible. Secondary infection may require removal of crusts, aqueous providone iodine applications and oral erythromycin or flucloxacillin.

Insect Bites

Flea bites

Flea bites produce an urticarial lesion with a central punctum. The reaction is an immunological one so that if two individuals are bitten by the same flea, one may react briskly and the other not at all. Bites are usually on the legs, with decreasing ascending density. Women are more commonly affected because their legs are exposed. New lesions may appear daily and itching is variable but sometimes intense. Cat or dog fleas are usually the culprits (Fig. 10.8) and soon infect floors, carpets, bedding, etc, so that the innocence of a well-groomed pet may be protested. Only flea faeces may be seen on the cat's fur but examination of brushings or 'shakings' from the animal and its resting place (put into a polythene bag) reveals faeces, eggs and larvae with a characteristic 'salt and pepper' appearance. Ideally the fleas should be recognized if management is to be logical, and a friendly entomologist may help. It is pointless blaming the cat or dog—and involving the vet in their cure—if hedgehog, rat, poultry or bird fleas are to blame! In the United Kingdom, the Entomology Department of the Royal Army Medical College in

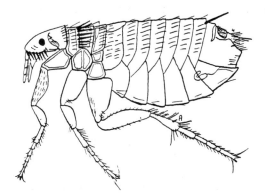

Fig. 10.8   Cat flea.

Millbank, SW1, will inspect brushings (for a fee). Fleas may remain viable for months away from their host.

Treatment

Flea collars on pets are useless. 'New Acclaim Plus' spray or other suitable sprays can be used every 2–3 weeks on the bedding of domestic cats or dogs and around the edges of carpets. If bird fleas are found, spraying under the eaves and under windowsills is useful. Thorough vacuum cleaning of carpets, bedding, etc, is valuable for dog or cat fleas and bedding should be beaten or shaken out of doors.

Bed bug bites

Bed bugs (*Cimex lenticularis*) measure 5 mm by 3 mm (Fig. 10.9) and live in crevices in brickwork, behind peeling wallpaper, in ceilings, floors, occasionally old mattresses and even in old buses and trains. They hide by day but move with agility by night to bite exposed parts, typically producing a linear pattern of urticated papules with a central punctum. Itching is intense. Local Authority help will be needed to disinfect the offending dwelling (and sometimes its neighbours). Where control of the environment is impossible,

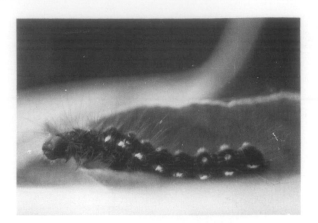

Fig. 10.10 Caterpillar of the brown-tail moth (courtesy of Dr Cicely Blair).

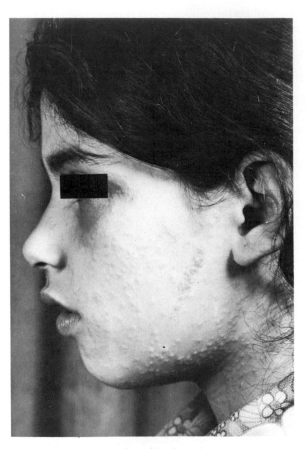

Fig. 10.11 Caterpillar rash; urticated papules on exposed skin.

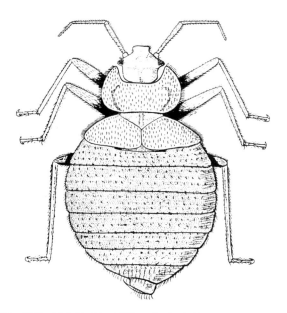

Fig. 10.9   Male 'bed bug' (*Cimex lenticularis*).

prophylactic use of insect repellent gels or sprays on the skin before sleeping is worthwhile.

Other insects

Cockroaches occasionally bite. Blackflies, midges, sandflies and mosquitoes produce minor skin reactions. Horsefly bites may induce a severe inflammatory reaction.

Caterpillar rash

The hairs of the caterpillar of the browntail moth (*Euproctis chrysorrhoea* Linn.) (Fig. 10.10) can cause skin and eye irritation. The resulting rash is papular or vesicular and has a characteristic appearance (Fig. 10.11). It fades in 7–10 days.

— 11 —
Dermatitis

Introduction

Dermatitis (eczema) is a common non-infective inflammatory disorder of the skin. It should be regarded as a 'reaction pattern' and may be provoked by external or internal factors or by a mixture of both. Genetic, immunological, traumatic, chemical and vascular factors may all play a part at different times but there is increasing evidence that immunological events are often central in pathogenesis.

The word eczema ('to flow out') implies an exudative eruption. British authors regard the terms 'dermatitis', 'eczema' and 'eczematous dermatitis' as synonymous. Dermatitis is the term used here. However, in talking to patients, care is necessary since many manual workers think of 'dermatitis' in terms of managerial culpability and litigation. Conversely, the word 'eczema' may frighten the parent of an affected baby and 'dermatitis' may seem less alarming.

Basic clinical features

The symptoms of dermatitis (Table 11.1) are itching and the development of an exuding ('weeping') and, later, crusting or scaling area of inflammation. In acute dermatitis, multiple pin-head to match-head sized papules and then vesicles, uniformly distributed, erupt on a background of erythema and oedema (Fig. 11.1). Exudation may be gross and leads to crusting.

In subacute dermatitis, vesicles and exudation are less marked and thickening and scaling of the skin are

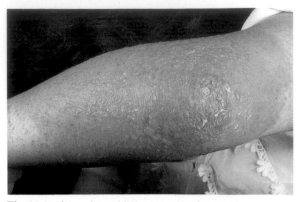

Fig. 11.1   Acute dermatitis (contact) on an arm.

more prominent. Excoriations may be evident and coccal infection is a common complicating factor. Chronic dermatitis takes many weeks to develop and is characterized by skin thickening which is largely the result of an epidermal (perhaps protective) response to constant rubbing and scratching. The skin lines become exaggerated and this stage is called lichenification. Certain types of dermatitis, for example atopic, are particularly likely to become lichenified. On the hands and feet, scaling and fissuring, often painful, are prominent features of chronic dermatitis (Fig. 11.2). Excoriations and sometimes burnished fingernails testify to the pruritus.

Table 11.1 Symptoms and signs of dermatitis.

Symptoms	Signs
Itching	Erythema
Exudation ('weeping')	Oedema
Crusting	Papules
Scaling	Vesicles
	Lichenification
	Fissuring

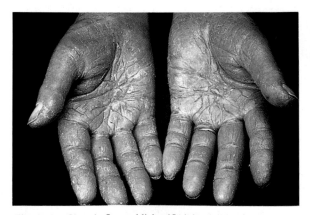

Fig. 11.2   Chronic fissured lichenified dermatitis of palms.

Dermatitis may occur anywhere on the skin, the distribution providing important clues to likely causation. Mucosal surfaces are rarely affected. It has a tendency to spread, particularly if the major provocative factors continue to operate. Spread is initially by local extension but later new areas of dermatitis may develop, sometimes with widespread symmetrical outbreaks, often involving the hands. The mechanisms of spread are obscure. Possibly bloodborne immune complexes or other factors are involved, but sometimes obvious external dissemination of a contact allergen by the fingers is the explanation. Acute and subacute dermatitis may resolve without trace; even chronic dermatitis may do so, but less readily.

Pathology

Dermatitis affects primarily the epidermis and superficial dermis. In the acute stage, extra- and intracellular oedema in the lower epidermis swells and separates the keratinocytes, a process called spongiosis. As the cells are pulled apart, intraepidermal vesicles develop. There is vascular dilatation in the upper dermis, and inflammatory cells congregate and may enter the epidermis. In the subacute stage, epidermal thickening (acanthosis) is added to the spongiosis, and disturbance of epidermal maturation is reflected in parakeratosis (when the keratinocytes of the stratum corneum retain their nuclei and are less tightly bound to each other) and hyperkeratosis; spongiosis eventually becomes subdued. Variable dermal inflammation is present.

Clinical classification of dermatitis

Although an interplay of external and internal factors is at work in every form of dermatitis, it is clinically useful to separate those forms of dermatitis where external factors are predominant (contact dermatitis) from other patterns where internal (endogenous) influences are paramount. The important clinical patterns are listed in Table 11.2.

Irritant Contact Dermatitis

Certain chemicals are capable of causing dermatitis in everyone if applied in sufficient concentration for long enough or repeatedly. Such chemicals are called primary irritants. Some strong primary irritants are capable of causing dermatitis after one exposure. Other, weaker irritants may require prolonged exposure or repeated exposure for weeks or even months

Table 11.2 Classification of dermatitis.

Exogenous	Endogenous
Irritant contact dermatitis	Atopic dermatitis
Allergic contact dermatitis	Seborrhoeic dermatitis (including otitis externa and intertrigo)
	Venous dermatitis of the legs
	Hand dermatitis (including pompholyx)
	Asteatotic dermatitis
	Neurodermatitis (lichen simplex)
	Discoid (nummular) dermatitis
	Generalized exfoliative dermatitis
	Miscellaneous

Table 11.3 Factors in irritant contact dermatitis.

Chemical involved	Additional trauma
Concentration of irritant	Climate
Duration of exposure	Constitutional factors
Site of exposure	

before doing so. Clearly, the development of dermatitis depends on many factors, as follows (Table 11.3).

- The chemical nature of the primary irritant. Acids, alkalis, solvents, mineral oils, surfactants (including soaps) and abrasives are the most obvious examples.
- The concentration of the irritant.
- The duration of exposure, and whether continuous or intermittent.
- The site of exposure. The thick palmar skin has a high threshold of tolerance. Conversely, the face, neck, penis and scrotum are particularly vulnerable. Obviously, it is the hands which are usually exposed in an occupational or domestic setting, but fear of venereal disease in a young man ('the morning after the night before') may lead, for instance, to the application of a strong phenolic

antiseptic to the penis and a consequent acute irritant dermatitis.

- Additional trauma or 'wear and tear'. This applies particularly to the hands in certain industries such as mining and deep sea fishing, and in mothers of very young children and housewives whose hands are constantly in contact with soap, detergent and water.
- Seasonal factors. Intense cold, dry, weather leads to dehydration of the stratum corneum and 'chapping', diminishing barrier resistance. Conversely constant wetting and maceration can be equally damaging.
- Little understood constitutional factors. These seem to influence the threshold of tolerance of primary irritants and may perpetuate irritant dermatitis after the provocative chemical has been avoided. Such factors probably explain the continuation of much 'industrial dermatitis' long after a worker has changed his job or become unemployed.

Clinical features

The hands are much the commonest site. The backs of the hands and the backs and sides of the fingers are most vulnerable, but sufficient chemical insult abetted by trauma may well overcome the resistance of the tougher palmar skin. An acute episode may lead to erythema, oedema, vesiculation and even gross blistering. In chronic forms, scaling, lichenification and fissuring are predominant. In housewives, onset under finger rings is common due to retained soap, etc. Spread to distant sites is very unusual. Other features differentiating irritant from allergic contact dermatitis are listed in Table 11.4. Napkin dermatitis is a special form of irritant reaction described in Chapter 13.

Diagnosis

The history is all important; details of occupational, domestic, sporting or 'hobby' exposures are crucial. Patch testing is valueless and may even be harmful by providing misleading false results.

Management

Prevention may be easier than cure. The wearing of appropriate gloves or other protective clothing by workers and housewives, the organization of industrial processes and assembly lines so as to minimize skin contact with irritants, the provision of adequate acces-

Table 11.4 Differentiation of irritant and allergic contact dermatitis.

Differentiating factor	Irritant	Allergic
Site	Usually hands	Hands, face, elsewhere
Spread	Localized	Tends to disseminate
Eyelid involvement	No	Often
Occupations	Engineering Mining Deep sea fishing Kitchen work	Metal work Rubber work Adhesive work Dye work
Patch testing valuable	No	Yes

sible washing facilities and worker education are all important. So-called barrier creams have little real barrier potential but do enable dirt and chemical soiling to be removed more easily. Bland emollients should be used liberally, especially in 'chapping' weather. Corticosteroid ointments are of limited value but often their use cannot be avoided.

Allergic Contact Dermatitis

Pathogenesis

This is a Type IV (cell-mediated) immunological reaction and cannot develop until the body has become sensitized to a particular agent. Sensitizing chemicals may be complete antigens; others are partial antigens (haptens) which must conjugate with a body protein to form a complete antigen. Clearly, the antigen or hapten must penetrate the stratum corneum and will do so more easily if the epidermis is diseased. Once the agent has penetrated into the epidermis, Langerhans' cells play a key role in taking up the antigen and presenting it to T lymphocytes so that it is carried to regional lymph glands. Sensitization, if it occurs, takes a minimum of 4 or 5 days and results in the production of a clone of sensitized T lymphocytes which reach the skin of the whole body. Subsequent exposure of skin anywhere to the antigen then provokes dermatitis presumably due to the local release of various lymphokines. Possibly immune complexes may also form in certain circumstances and may be responsible for the bloodborne dissemination of allergic contact dermatitis.

Environmental chemicals vary enormously in their capacity to sensitize. For instance, dinitrochlorbenzene (DNCB) will eventually sensitize almost 100% of people, and indeed is used to test ability to mount a 'normal' cell-mediated immune response. Conversely, other chemicals may have almost no capacity to sensitize even after years of exposure.

Clinical features

Any part of the body may be affected but the hands and face are much the commonest sites. The site affected may immediately indicate the likely antigen: thus, dermatitis under the metal studs on the waist of jeans incriminates nickel; dermatitis on one upper outer thigh in a man may be due to matches carried in a trouser pocket or to a wallet (Fig. 11.3). Examples of likely antigens at various body sites are listed in Table 11.5.

Unlike irritant contact dermatitis, allergic contact dermatitis often spreads, especially to the eyelids in both sexes and to the penis in the male. Transfer of allergen by touching is the likely explanation.

The main groups of chemicals responsible are now briefly described.

Metals

Nickel, cobalt and pentavalent chromate are the haptens. Nickel dermatitis is commoner in women because of the use of nickel-containing metal in clothing such as brassière fasteners, suspenders, studs

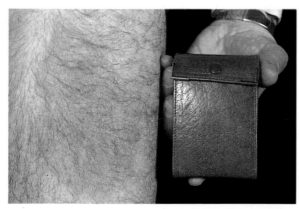

Fig. 11.3 Allergic contact dermatitis of thigh due to a wallet carried in trouser pocket (leather dye).

Table 11.5 Likely sensitizers at various sites.

Sensitizer	Site
Nickel	Earlobe
	Wrist
	Waist (jeans)
Rubber	Hands
	Soles of feet
Nail varnish	Eyelids
	Face
	Neck
Plants	Arms
	Face
Lipstick	Lips
Phosphorous sesquisulphide (matches)	Outer thighs
	Face

Table 11.6 Some environmental sources of cobalt.

Jewellery (with nickel)	Pottery pigments
Cement (with chromate)	Driers in paints
Dental plates	Printing inks
Joint prostheses	

on jeans, hairpins and cheap jewellery, such as earrings, necklaces, bracelets and wristwatch straps. Exposure to nickel may also be occupational. Thus the clerical worker is exposed to metal paper clips, scissors, stapling machines and other office equipment. Cobalt is often added to metal alloys, and nickel and chrome are usually contaminated with cobalt. Cobalt sensitivity is usually associated with nickel sensitivity in women and with chromate sensitivity in men. Various environmental sources of cobalt are listed in Table 11.6. Chromate sensitivity is much commoner in men than in women and is usually occupational in origin. Chromate is often present in cement, causing dermatitis in bricklayers and other workers in the construction industry. Chromate is also used to 'tan' leather, contact with which may sensitize workers in leather goods' manufacture (shoes, bags, belts, etc) or those who wear or use the finished articles (Table 11.7).

Table 11.7   Some industrial sources of chromate.

Cement	Anticorrosives
Antirust coatings	Welding materials
Galvanized metal surfaces	Leather
Primer paints	

Rubber

Unadulterated natural or synthetic rubber is non-sensitizing but many chemical additives are used in the manufacturing processes intended to produce rubber suitable for widely differing purposes. Rubber with properties of heat and friction resistance suitable for tyres would not make ideal surgical gloves or condoms, for instance, where smoothness, softness and pliability are needed. These properties are conferred on rubber by processing which involves many chemicals, mainly antioxidants, accelerators, etc, which are potential sensitizers. Rubber dermatitis may thus be occupational, as in vehicle and tyre manufacture, or due to clothing, for example rubber boots, 'Wellingtons', gloves for wet housework or contraceptive sheaths.

Plastics and resins

Plastic objects in the home rarely cause trouble because the plastic is in the polymerized state. Acrylic monomer occasionally sensitizes dental or orthopaedic surgeons and their nursing assistants because it can penetrate rubber gloves. Light-sensitive acrylates are used in the printing industry and have caused outbreaks of dermatitis.

Epoxy and other resins are used extensively for 'bonding' purposes in industry, as glues in the home and as plastic material for repairing car and boat bodies. Both the resins and the separate 'hardeners' are potentially allergenic. Rarely, spectacle frames and nail varnish cause dermatitis.

Organic dyes

Paraphenylenediamine (PPD) and its many derivatives are well-known sensitizers and may be responsible for dermatitis in hairdressers and their clients (Fig. 11.4), for sensitivity to dye in ladies' stockings, tights or hairnets, or for dermatitis in the photographic industry in workers handling colour developers.

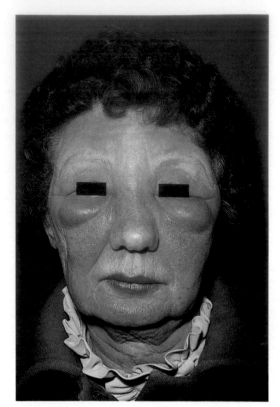

Fig. 11.4   Allergic contact dermatitis due to hair dye (paraphenylenediamine derivative).

Plants

In North America sensitization by poison ivy and poison oak are well known. In the United Kingdom *Primula obconica* is a common household flowering plant; primin (a terpene) in its leaves and stem may easily lead to sensitization. Vesicular or even bullous reactions on the arms are typical of poison ivy and primula eruptions. Chrysanthemums may sensitize, and the gardener and florist are both at risk. 'Tulip fingers'—a contact dermatitis of the fingertips—is well known in Holland and other bulb-growing areas, and is due to an identified allergen in the outer bulb 'skin'. Garlic and other herbs may produce a similar fingertip dermatitis in chefs and cooks (Fig. 11.5). Certain woods, for example teak and African rosewoods, may be an important cause of occupational dermatitis in furniture manufacturing.

Cosmetics

Lipstick, eye and other 'make-up', nail varnish (Fig.

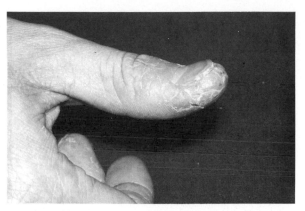

Fig. 11.5 Allergic contact dermatitis of fingertips. See Table 11.12 for likely causes.

11.6), perfumes, body lotions, etc, may all occasionally sensitize by virtue of various chemical ingredients. In recent years, musk ambrette (a synthetic musk), used in male toiletries (e.g. after-shave lotions), emerged as a potent sensitizer and photosensitizer (see Chapter 23) and its use is now strictly controlled.

Medicaments

Both prescribed and freely purchased topical medicaments are a frequent cause of allergic contact dermatitis. Sometimes the drug itself is a sensitizer. Thus, penicillin, streptomycin, chloramphenicol and sulphonamides are never applied to the skin because of their high allergenic potential. Neomycin (and the related framycetin) sensitize but penetrate intact stratum corneum with difficulty and are widely used, but should never be applied for long periods on eczematized or otherwise damaged skin. Local anaesthetics of the procaine series (amethocaine, benzocaine, etc) are potent sensitizers and are found in 'over-the-counter' remedies for insect bites, haemorrhoids, pruritus ani, etc. Lignocaine is not a contact sensitizer.

Ingredients other than the active drug in lotions, creams or ointments may sensitize. Thus lanolin (wool alcohols), hydroxybenzoate preservatives ('parabens'), chlorocresol, cetyl alcohol, ethylenediamine and other ingredients may all be incriminated at times.

Diagnosis

The precise elucidation of the cause of dermatitis and the removal of exposure to a contact sensitizer leading to absolute cure is one of the most satisfying of the

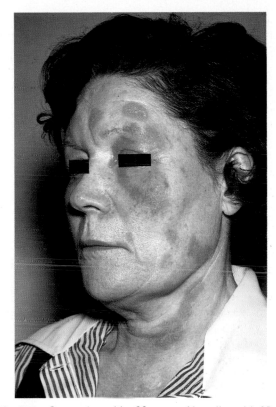

Fig. 11.6 Contact dermatitis of face caused by nail varnish. Note bizarre pattern due to habit of touching face with fingers.

dermatologist's achievements. Clearly, knowledge of common and less common sensitizers is essential. This knowledge, integrated with the occupational, hobby or exposure history and the evident site of onset and distribution of the dermatitis (Fig. 11.7), often leads to a confident clinical diagnosis in which case patch testing is simply confirmatory. In other instances, particularly in hand dermatitis, the clinical diagnosis is less clear. Here, patch testing with 30 or so of the commonest allergens and with other substances to which the patient has been exposed, may be critical in establishing causation.

Patch testing. This involves the controlled application of potential allergens to the unaffected skin. Each patch test is a single immunological experiment. If cell-bound antibody is present a positive test will result; if such antibody is absent a negative result is inevitable. Since such immunological reactions are specific and mutually exclusive, multiple experiments can be carried out simultaneously and it is usual to apply 30 or even more allergens. Internationally

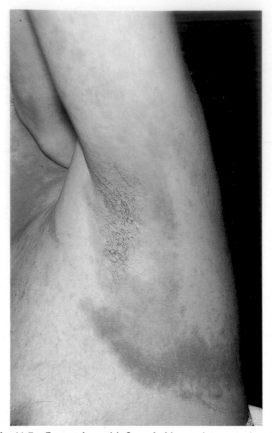

Fig. 11.7 Contact dermatitis from clothing tends to spare the axillary vaults; marginal axillary dermatitis due to a formaldehyde-releasing resin in cloth.

Table 11.8 International battery of contact allergens.

Allergen	Reference number*	Concentration (%)
Potassium dichromate	E0001	0.5
Paraphenylenediamine (PPD)	E0005	0.5
Thiuram mix (rubber additives)	E0023	1
Neomycin sulphate	E0010	20
Cobalt chloride	E0002	1
Benzocaine	E0011	5
Nickel sulphate	E0003	5
Quinoline mix	E0033	6
Colophony	E0017	20
Paraben mix	E0012	15
Black rubber mix	E0024	0.6
Wool alcohols	E0020	30
Mercapto mix (rubber additives)	E0022	2
Epoxy resin	E0021	1
Balsam of Peru	E0008	25
Fragrance mix (perfumes)	E0029	8
Carba mix (rubber additives)	E0026	3
Formaldehyde (aqueous)	E0004	1
Ethylenediamine	E0029	1
Paratertiarybutyl phenol formaldehyde	E0030	1
Quaternium 15 (Dowicil 200)	E0031	1
Primin (synthetic)	E0032	0.01

*Obtainable from Hermal-Chemie Kurt Herrmann, P.O. Box 1228, D-2057 Reinbek/Hamburg, West Germany.

agreed standardized materials are used (Table 11.8).

Each allergen is applied and secured under occlusion for 48 hours. It is suspended or dissolved in an inert, non-sensitizing vehicle, often soft paraffin (mineral oil), and experience must have shown that the concentration used is non-irritant under the conditions of the test, so that confusing non-allergic reactions do not occur. Positive reactions may be delayed, for example with neomycin, so it is usual to read the test sites a second time, a further 48 hours after removal of the patches. A positive test is papulovesicular on an erythematous, oedematous base and itches intensely. Misleading false-positive irritant responses are more likely to be erythematous, bullous or even ulcerative. Sometimes, strongly positive tests are associated with exacerbation of the dermatitis elsewhere.

Management

If the cause can be identified its complete removal alone will cure. Where there is doubt, all suspected agents, for example medicaments, must be withdrawn or avoided. In mild or moderate cases application of a corticosteroid will rapidly suppress the inflammation. Exudative reactions may benefit from preliminary soaks or wet compresses with 1:4000 potassium permanganate for 10 minutes twice daily for 4 or 5 days only. In severe cases, especially with gross facial swelling, oral prednisolone 40 mg daily is highly effective. The dose can be progressively reduced to zero over 7–10 days.

In the latter circumstances patch testing should be delayed until the acute dermatitis has settled. After patch testing the patient and other medical attendants should be notified about proven allergens, particularly

Table 11.9 Some important cross-sensitization hazards.

Topical sensitizer	Related systemic drug
Ethylenediamine	Aminophylline
Balsam of Peru	Benzoin inhalations
Benzocaine	Azo dyes
	Sulphonylureas
Amethocaine	p-Amino salicylic acid
Iodine	Iodide

Table 11.10 Atopy.

Main clinical features	Associated features	Compli-cations	Epipheno-mena
Pruritus			Pallor
Dermatitis	Ichthyosis	Staphyl-oderma	White dermo-graphism
Bronchial asthma	Keratosis pilaris	Herpes simplex (eczema herpeticum)	Serum IgE ↑
Rhinitis	Keratoconus	Viral warts	
Conjuncti-vitis	Caratact (rare)	Mollusca	
Urticaria			

medicaments which will have to be avoided permanently. Clinical notes should be marked boldly (e.g. in red) so that future accidental prescription is avoided. The patient should be given a list of branded names of medicaments known to contain the allergen.

Cross-sensitization

The same or a chemically related drug given orally or parenterally may cause a severe reaction in a patient previously sensitized topically. Some examples are cited in Table 11.9.

Atopic Dermatitis

This is one of the commonest forms of dermatitis worldwide. In Europe, possibly 10–15% of children are atopic. The dermatitis usually begins in childhood, often in infancy, and is relentlessly pruritic. It may be associated later with bronchial asthma, allergic rhinitis or conjunctivitis ('hayfever') and urticaria. Other associated conditions include dry skin (xeroderma), keratosis pilaris (follicular xeroderma), especially on the upper outer arms, a tendency to increased cutaneous vasoconstrictor tone, and eye defects (keratoconus and rarely, juvenile cataract). The predisposition to these disorders is at least partly genetic and is sometimes called the atopic diathesis (Table 11.10).

Pathogenesis

The exact pattern of inheritance is obscure, perhaps Mendelian dominance with variable phenotypic expression. The presence of high levels of serum IgE is a striking feature. Radioallergoabsorbent testing (RAST) reveals that this represents reaginic antibody directed mainly against pollens, cat and dog dander, house dust mite and certain foods. It is easy to believe that Type I hypersensitive reactions, mediated by IgE, explain the hayfever and perhaps partly the asthma and urticaria, but their relevance to the dermatitis is less clear. However, some pollens and house dust mites can also give positive patch tests, and direct contact exacerbation may explain seasonal variations. There are strands of evidence (such as possible abnormal absorption of large molecules in the gut and transient decreased secretory IgA status in early infancy) which could suggest abnormal entry of ingested or inhaled potentially antigenic material into the body, provoking a normal IgE response. A possible deficiency of suppressor T cells could also be relevant, and certainly the peculiar vulnerability of atopic subjects to the *Herpes simplex*, vaccinia and wart viruses suggests a limited defect in cell-mediated immunity, as does the development of dermatitis for the first time after HIV seroconversion in haemophiliacs.

Fascinating recent observations on the transfer of dermatitis and specific allergies (e.g. to food and penicillin) by marrow transplants suggest that the basic abnormality may be due to a bone-marrow derived cell. Where or how the increased cutaneous vasoconstrictor tone fits into this story is utterly obscure. Firm stroking of affected skin produces a white streak of vasoconstriction ('white dermographism') instead of the normal erythematous response. Intradermal injection of acetylcholine analogues induces the same paradoxical response. Presumably the typical pallor of the atopic facies reflects

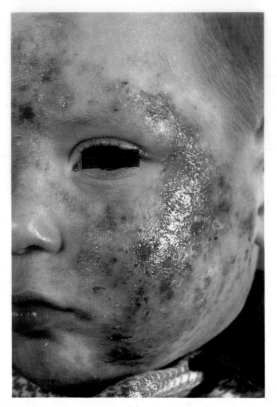

Fig. 11.8   Atopic dermatitis of face in a severe phase.

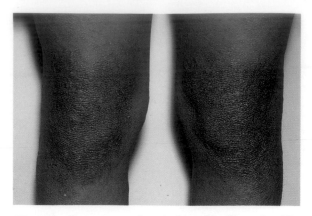

Fig. 11.9   Hyperpigmented atopic dermatitis of knees in a West Indian child.

this phenomenon, which could be due to β-adrenergic receptor blockade. Equally unexplained are the reduced levels of essential fatty acids in the blood of some atopics and the apparent improvement of the skin in some when this is corrected.

Lastly, it is beyond dispute that emotional and psychological factors influence atopic dermatitis but perhaps only by influencing the degree of rubbing and scratching in response to the underlying pruritus. Whatever the fundamental defect, the sequence of events seems to be:

atopic diathesis → pruritus → scratching → dermatitis

It can be demonstrated that dermatitis develops only where the child has access to his skin so that self-trauma is central in the production of skin lesions, albeit that the pruritus comes first.

Clinical picture

The dermatitis typically begins in the third to the sixth month of life as a symmetrically distributed erythematous eruption on the face (Fig. 11.8), trunk or limbs.

Exudation, crusting and scaling may supervene and the child scratches whenever given the opportunity. At 2 years and later, the dermatitis becomes increasingly flexural on the limbs, and lichenification and secondary coccal infection are common. Localized variants may be encountered such as unilateral or bilateral retroauricular (often infected) dermatitis, or lesions about the genitalia in boys. In older children, the disease may remain widespread with lichenification of various patterns becoming an increasing problem.

In the United Kingdom, gross lichenification is a particular problem in black children of Caribbean parentage and may take gross nodular, plaque or profusely disseminated papular forms. In older children, too, the entensor prominences of the limbs may become involved instead of or in addition to the flexural creases. Dermatitis of the great toe and adjacent foot is common in older boys. In black and brown-skinned children, secondary postinflammatory pigmentation adds to the cosmetic defect (Fig. 11.9).

Sports trauma may be important. Chronic hand dermatitis is particularly distressing in schoolchildren. Together with the pallor, rubbed away outer eyebrows and exaggerated infraorbital creases (Morgan–Dennie folds) of the atopic facies, it particularly contributes towards the 'disfigured body image' of the maturing child, which may lead to rejection by schoolmates, so that emotional problems, temper tantrums, aggression and other forms of disturbed behaviour are hardly surprising. Secondary depression is common in severely affected adolescents and sexual problems may stem from genital involvement. In a very small minority, severe atopic dermatitis remains as a permanent life-ruining disability.

At a far younger age, many atopic children soon learn to use their disease to manipulate parents, be it to gain entry to the parental bed or to avoid school, domestic chores, etc, in later years. The consequences of severe atopic dermatitis tend to envelop the whole household. Often both parents attend consultations and, surprisingly often, the mother is a dominating personality. The atopic child is often hyperkinetic, particularly in the consulting room, adding to the wearying of parents, child minders and the physician.

Complications

Coccal infection. Secondary bacterial infection with staphylococci or streptococci is the commonest cause of exacerbations of atopic dermatitis.

Eczema herpeticum. The atopic dermatitis patient has a peculiar vulnerability to the *Herpes simplex* virus which spreads easily on the skin to produce a viral pyoderma. This is not apparently related to immunodeficiency and sometimes may be a primary infection.

Eczema herpeticum is common, usually mild and localized, resolving spontaneously in about 10 days. Frequently it is unrecognized. Rarely it is severe, very widespread and potentially fatal, especially in infants. Recurrent attacks occur.

The eruption is monomorphic, vesicular or pustular, often with umbilicated varioliform lesions occurring in clusters.

Treatment. If the eruption is spreading, very extensive or the patient is toxic, intravenous acyclovir is given in a dosage of 1.5 g/m^2/day for 2–3 days, followed by oral acyclovir (2.4 g/m^2/day in divided doses).

Viral warts and mollusca. Viral warts and mollusca both tend to be more numerous and persistent. Other viral infections of childhood behave normally.

Contact dermatitis. Atopics have no special liability to allergic contact dermatitis but anaphylactic reactions to drugs, especially penicillin and antisera, are a hazard. Their threshold tolerance of primary irritants is reduced and this vulnerability may dog them years after the dermatitis had seemed to disappear. Thus, irritant hand dermatitis may develop in adolescent girls on taking up hairdressing or nursing, or in the newly married housewife or mother of a first child. The hands of engineering apprentices or coal miners may 'break down' soon after starting working life. Nipple dermatitis may be a problem in young women.

Prognosis

Many parents of atopic children become disillusioned by dogmatic medical statements that the disease will disappear by a certain age. It is safer to stick to statistical generalities. In the United Kingdom, 90% of atopic children have cleared up by 15 years, although a small proportion may relapse later (see above). It is established that certain factors worsen prognosis in general and these include a family history of alopecia areata or ichthyosis, onset later than 2 years of age, social and particularly maternal deprivation, and the persistence of a discoid pattern of dermatitis for months or years.

Management

Very mild atopic dermatitis is easy to treat. At the other end of the spectrum of severity, the disease may tax the endurance of parents and physicians to the limit over many years (Table 11.11).

Table 11.11 Essentials of management of atopic dermatitis.

Counselling
Emollients
Hydrocortisone ointment
Medicated bandages
Oral antihistamine
Oral antibiotics (short courses)

At all stages of management time spent with the parents in explanation and the answering of questions will be rewarded. Advice on the avoidance of excessive bathing, overheating the child with clothing or bedding, irritating the skin with rough, especially woollen clothing and keeping the finger and toenails short, smooth and clean is all important. Excessive drying and prolonged wetting of the skin are equally harmful in worsening itching. The parents will soon learn for themselves whether contact with cats, dogs or horses leads to worsening, but may not appreciate the link with house dust (and its mite) from small children rolling on floors and carpets. In mild or moderate disease, five modalities form the mainstay of treatment and can be combined according to need.

- Liberal and frequent use of emollients (but intolerance is common).
- Use of hydrocortisone ointment. Stronger topical

steroids should be prescribed reluctantly and their use quantified.

- Use of zinc or tar ointments and bandages medicated with these substances.
- Topical and systemic antimicrobial agents usually in short courses to discourage emergence of resistant strains of staphylococci.
- Oral antihistamines, especially at night, and often on a long-term basis.

The use of these modalities is described in Chapter 14. Emulsifying ointment B.P., soft white paraffin B.P. or a 50 : 50 mixture of liquid paraffin and soft white paraffin can be tried as emollients. Hydrocortisone (ointment rather than cream) can be used freely, except in babies, but at times short intensive courses of treatment with a Potency I corticosteroid ointment are needed to control intolerable exacerbations, the strength of the steroid then being reduced when control is established.

Occlusive medicated bandages may not be tolerated by day but are useful overnight. Tolerance may easily develop to the sedative antihistamines given at night, and the antihistamine should be changed every 2–3 months. Several preparations that are safe for children are available.

If these methods are not sufficient, dietary manipulation should be considered although its value is controversial. Conflicting evidence has been presented on the value of breast feeding infants with an atopic diathesis. Initially, a simple empirical withdrawal of egg and cow's milk is justifiable, particularly in very young children. The assistance of a dietician is essential if protein, calcium or vitamin deficiencies are to be avoided when dietary restriction is prolonged beyond a few weeks. If egg and milk withdrawal has not helped after 6–8 weeks, the diet should be abandoned. If it seems to help it should be continued for a year (provided that well-balanced nutrition is maintained) and the offending proteins then reintroduced one at a time and cautiously.

In older children, prick testing on the forearm for Type I allergy is rarely valuable. Food allergens may give false-negative prick tests, and a few specific RAST tests are more likely to be informative. Food challenge as a guide to dietary manipulation is not without risk but can be considered in older children and adults. Urticaria will develop within 12 hours of successful challenge but dermatitis may take 3–4 days to develop so foods should be introduced weekly. Nuts, fruits, jams, colourings and flavours have all occasionally been incriminated. The risk of anaphylaxis should not be forgotten. Sodium cromoglycate orally is of no

Table 11.12 Dry fingertip dermatitis.

Occupation	Cause
Dental surgeon	Local anaesthetics
	Acrylates
Dental nurse	Adhesives
Chef	Garlic
Market gardener	Tulip bulb
Bank clerk	Rubber finger stall

proven value. In adolescents and adults, oil of evening primrose (given orally as Efamol) can be tried and is safe. Rarely, in very severe atopic dermatitis, alternate-day prednisolone therapy is justifiable and very effective but is best used after growth has ceased. Occasionally, resort is necessary to PUVA therapy or the use of azathioprine orally in adults.

Seborrhoeic Dermatitis

This name is unfortunate since the patterns of dermatitis so labelled are unrelated to seborrhoea (excessive sebum production), but no better term has gained acceptance. It is a disease of adults and should not be confused with the unrelated 'seborrhoeic dermatitis' of infants (p. 110).

Pathogenesis

Although there is certainly an endogenous, and sometimes obviously genetic, factor, clinical evidence points to an important role for cutaneous flora, particularly the yeast-like *Pityrosporum ovale*. Such evidence includes clinical response to imidazole creams and the emergence of rampant seborrhoeic dermatitis as one of the manifestations of HIV-related disease. Some patients also seem to be especially susceptible to recurrent coccal infections. Curiously, in the United Kingdom severe seborrhoeic dermatitis is much less common than it was 50 years ago, and possibly improved nutrition and hygiene (particularly more frequent shampooing) in the wake of rising standards of living are responsible.

Clinical picture

Two main patterns are seen.
- Dry persistent redness and scaling, not necessarily with much itching, are seen on the face, particularly

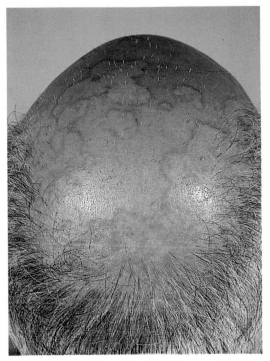

Fig. 11.10 Seborrhoeic dermatitis of scalp in a man. Note the marginated petaloid pattern.

at the sides of the nose, along the eyebrows and in the central forehead, sometimes with chronic blepharitis. Often there is associated redness and scaling of the scalp. In men, the scalp eruption may be strikingly marginated and petaloid (Fig. 11.10), and a similar eruption may be seen in the mid-line of the chest over the sternum and, less often, on the upper central back.

Persistent, moist or even exudative dermatitis occurs in the retroauricular, submammary, axillary and anogenital folds. One or more folds may be involved. There is a strong tendency to coccal colonization or even frank infection, and increased humidity, temperature, sweating and friction encourage secondary infection. This latter type is sometimes called *seborrhoeic intertrigo*.

In either pattern, a 'seborrhoeic' folliculitis can affect the scalp.

Differential diagnosis

In the scalp, flexures, chest and back, psoriasis may clinically 'overlap' and be difficult to distinguish. On the trunk, pityriasis versicolor may have to be excluded by microscopy of scrapings. On the face, atopic or allergic contact dermatitis should be considered.

Treatment

In the scalp, frequent washing with a medicated shampoo containing coal tar extracts or ketoconazole or selenium sulphide is important. For the dry facial and truncal patterns, an imidazole cream should be used first but may have to be combined or alternated with hydrocortisone cream. In the exudative flexural cases, iodoquinolone antiseptics combined with the weaker corticosteroids and a suitable antibiotic such as chlortetracycline are needed. Intermittent treatment may be needed long term and the hazards of contact sensitization by medicaments and corticosteroid overuse should not be forgotten. Oral ketoconazole is invaluable in the persistent seborrhoeic dermatitis of AIDS but should only rarely be used otherwise.

Chronic otitis externa

This pattern of seborrhoeic dermatitis is probably provoked by infective, climatic or chemical factors. Infection derived from the middle ear should be obvious and distinguishable from the spectrum of Gram-positive or Gram-negative secondary bacterial invaders. The entities of 'desert ear' and 'swimming pool ear' testify to the importance of excessive climatic dryness and wetness, respectively. Chemical factors are secondary but may be important in perpetuating the condition. Sensitization by nickel hairpins or by phosphorous sesquisulphide from red-headed matches used to scratch the ear or by the constituents of creams and ointments is not uncommon.

It is convenient to consider pruritus ani and pruritus vulvae here although these conditions may not have an eczematous basis.

Pruritus ani

Pruritus ani is a common symptom. In childhood it is usually due to threadworm infestation. In adult life it almost always affects men. It may be transient or chronic and has many causes. Infective causes include viral warts, candidosis (e.g. after wide-spectrum oral antibiotic therapy), erythrasma and tinea. Perianal infection in children, especially with viral warts, should always raise suspicion of sexual abuse. Bacterial infection also plays a role in seborrhoeic intertrigo (see above). Other forms of dermatitis which may be responsible are contact dermatitis medicamentosa and neurodermatitis. Other skin diseases such as psoriasis and lichen planus may involve the perianal skin and present as pruritus ani. Surgical causes include fistula, fissure in ano, haemorrhoids and skin tags. Any rectal discharge may cause pruritus so that occasionally a carcinoma of the rectum, gonococcal proctitis, rectal incontinence or excessive use of liquid paraffin as a laxative may be responsible.

Notwithstanding this long list of established causes, pruritus ani may occur in the absence of any of them and may persist or be intermittent for decades. Obesity, a tendency to hyperhidrosis in the anogenital area, poor hygiene after defaecation, especially in the hirsute, and imperceptible leakage of rectal mucus onto the perianal skin may each be relevant. When no physical cause of such an intractable symptom can be found, psychogenic explanations are sometimes tempting. It is true that some men with this symptom readily present the anus for examination, an observation which has been cited as evidence of latent or suppressed homosexuality. They may also display a good deal of anxiety in various ways, particularly in a desire for lengthy and frequent consultations. In the author's view, psychogenic factors are often important but psychosexual theories are less convincing.

Whatever the cause, the physical signs vary from slight erythema to excoriation, lichenification and secondary folliculitis. In all cases, examination must be thorough and should include digital rectal examination, proctoscopy and Wood's light examination of the perianal skin. If no treatable surgical or dermatological entity is found, management should include attention to bowel habit and hygiene after defaecation. Cleansing the area gently after defaecation with soap and water rather than toilet paper may be helpful. Hydrocortisone ointment 1% may be useful, as may a preparation combining hydrocortisone with lignocaine (Xyloproct ointment, U.K.).

Pruritus vulvae

This is a common symptom which may present to the general practitioner, gynaecologist or dermatologist. Usually a physical explanation can be found. The important causes are:
- Vaginal discharge, whether trichomonal, candidial or due to Gardnerella or cervicitis
- Urinary incontinence or glycosuria
- Local skin disease such as pediculosis pubis, psoriasis, dermatitis of various types, senile atrophy, lichen sclerosus et atrophicus, epithelial hyperplasia or dysplasia and HPV infection

As in men with pruritus ani, obesity and poor hygiene may increase the liability to intertrigo.

Possibly the replacement of stockings by occlusive tights has also been an aggravating factor in some cases. When no physical cause is apparent, psychosexual explanations have been invoked, particularly in unmarried women, but are hard to establish.

Treatment depends on the cause. In idiopathic cases, weak topical corticosteroid creams such as 1% hydrocortisone cream are useful. Oestrogen cream has a place in the management of senile atrophy.

Venous Dermatitis

Chronic dermatitis is a central feature of the syndrome of chronic venous insufficiency in the legs (fully described in Chapter 16). Several previously used terms for this pattern of dermatitis are unsatisfactory. 'Varicose' implies that varicosities are the cause, which they are not, venous hypertension in deep veins due to previous thrombosis and valvular incompetence being far more important. 'Stasis' and 'hypostatic' are equally to be deplored, since stasis does not occur. 'Gravitational' is equally unsatisfactory since gravity and dependency alone do not cause dermatitis.

Hand Dermatitis

Determining the cause of dermatitis of the hands (and feet) is one of the dermatologist's most difficult problems. Since such dermatitis often begins in an industrial setting, medicolegal problems frequently complicate the matter. In an attempt to create order, some dogmatic statements may provide a frame of reference.
- In pre-pubertal children, hand dermatitis is almost always atopic.
- *Pompholyx* ('bubble') is the name given to a distinctive vesicular pattern of dermatitis seen on the palmar aspects of the hands and, less often, the plantar aspect of the feet. The thick stratum corneum at these sites prevents rupture of vesicles or escape of epidermal oedema, so that a striking uniform sago-grain-like eruption of deep vesicles appears (Fig. 11.11). In its most severe form, these vesicles aggregate to form large bullae so that large areas of stratum corneum are lifted away from the skin, 'de-gloving' the hand in the healing exfoliative phase.

Pompholyx may be an idiopathic phenomenon, typically recurring in adolescents and young adults in spring or summer. In its most minor seasonal

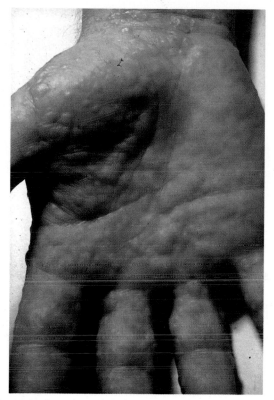

Fig. 11.11 Acute 'pompholyx' dermatitis of palm.

- Nummular (discoid) dermatitis (p. 96) in adults may occur on the back of the hand, knuckle or wrist. The nummular pattern in atopic children is a bad prognostic factor.
- Primary irritant hand dermatitis is common and is described earlier in this Chapter.
- Allergic contact dermatitis of the hands is also common in adults.
- Hyperkeratotic, dry patches of eczema on the thenar or hypothenar eminences, the central palm or sides of fingers are common in adults and usually difficult to attribute if patch tests are negative. The author has the impression that the condition may be stress-related in the middle-aged and elderly.

Differential diagnosis

Psoriasis and tinea must always be considered, especially *T. rubrum* infections. Patch testing is usually necessary.

Treatment

Irritants and potential or known allergens must be avoided. Mild acute or sub-acute summer pompholyx dermatitis may respond to Potency I or II corticosteroid cream or ointment. Gross pompholyx dermatitis with threatened 'de-gloving' calls for prompt oral treatment with prednisolone 30–40 mg administered daily initially, the dose then rapidly being reduced according to response. Weak potassium permanganate compresses reduce the risk of secondary coccal infection, but often it is prudent to give flucloxacillin or erythromycin orally at the same time. Tense blisters can be pricked with a sterile needle and allowed to drain. Only bland local applications are needed at this stage—calamine cream or Lassar's paste. In the later healing dry stage, emulsifying ointment B.P. or soft white paraffin are appropriate, or a corticosteroid ointment if there is persistent activity of the dermatitis.

Chronic lichenified and fissured hand dermatitis calls for corticosteroid ointments, emollients and the use of gloves when contact with irritants is unavoidable. In mild cases a urea-hydrocortisone cream may be useful (Alphaderm or Calmuid–HC, U.K.).

Localized dry hyperkeratotic dermatitis of the fingers, or palms, is notoriously resistant to treatment. Potency I corticosteroid ointment (e.g. Dermovate, U.K.) or occlusive corticosteroid tape (Haelan Tape,

form, a line of itching pin-head papulovesicles develops along the sides of several fingers. When more severe, pain, redness and oedema may precede the outbreak of vesicles so that pompholyx in a big toe may occasionally mimic acute gout at first. Rarely, pompholyx appears to be a hypersensitivity reaction to events elsewhere on the skin. Thus, it can be provoked by a fiercely inflammatory tinea pedis or by continuously provoked allergic contact dermatitis (for instance, by neomycin) around a venous leg ulcer.

Chronic pompholyx in adults is not uncommon, often with variable scaly dermatitis. Usually no cause can be found nor is a cure possible. Some such patients have positive patch tests to nickel, chromate or cobalt and their pompholyx can be worsened by oral administration of these metals. Such evidence raises the possibility that summer pompholyx could be related to inhaled or ingested antigens, for example pollens. It seems clear that chronic vesicular dermatitis of the extremities is multifactorial. Where irritant or allergic provocation at work is evident, the attribution of chronicity between endogenous and external factors may prove contentious.

U.K.) may have to be tried. A steroid salicylic acid ointment mixture can also be useful (Diprosalic ointment, U.K.).

Asteatotic Dermatitis

Sometimes called *eczema cracquelé*, this pattern of dermatitis is seen mainly in the elderly, particularly in winter, and usually on the legs. It consists of slight erythema, fine scaling and very superficial 'crazy pavement' fissuring which combine to produce a very characteristic pattern. Hypothyroidism and chronic diuretic therapy may contribute to its development. It is common in institutions for the elderly.

Treatment

Liberal use of emollients and urea-containing creams, sometimes combined with hydrocortisone, is rapidly effective. Strong corticosteroid ointments should be avoided, as the skin is usually already atrophic due to ageing.

Neurodermatitis

The term 'neurodermatitis' is as confusing as 'seborrhoeic'. In the author's opinion, the term should be reserved for the peculiar, localized lichenification, lichen simplex chronicus. This type of skin disorder is seen mostly in adult women, particularly on the occipital scalp, nape, sides of the neck (Fig. 11.12), high on the ulnar forearm near the elbow, on the volar wrist, on the sides of the lower calves and the sides of the natal cleft. Chronic pruritus ani and pruritus vulvae may lead to localized lesions. Neurodermatitis is remarkably common in both men and women in the Bengali community around the author's hospital in London.

The lesions are sharply defined, raised plaques and often ovoid or elongated. Hyperpigmentation is common and the surface shows exaggerated skin markings. The yellow/brown races are particularly susceptible to this pattern and to lichenification in general. Sometimes, habitual scratching, rubbing and pinching of the skin induce a nodular form of lichenification, a condition sometimes called *nodular prurigo*.

Itching is intermittent and intense, and patients usually admit that they habitually rub the lesions, particularly when agitated. These patients commonly reveal evidence of emotional stresses so that retention of the term 'neurodermatitis' seems justified.

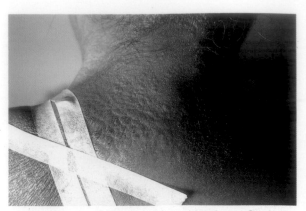

Fig. 11.12 Lichen simplex (neurodermatitis) of nape of neck.

It should be mentioned that the term 'disseminated neurodermatitis' is often used for generalized atopic dermatitis in the United States.

Differential diagnosis

Neurodermatitis has to be differentiated from psoriasis; on the legs hypertrophic lichen planus can cause confusion. Occasionally, warty granulomas (such as verrucous tuberculosis or chromoblastomycosis) will mimic neurodermatitis. A biopsy may be necessary to confirm the diagnosis.

Management

Attention to the skin without consideration of the patient's psychological problems rarely gives more than transient benefit. Nevertheless, impregnated tar or zinc paste bandages can be useful, as is a steroid-medicated tape. Bland pastes help to keep the fingers off the skin. Intralesional triamcinolone injections are less useful than in hypertrophic lichen planus.

Nummular (Discoid) Dermatitis

This is a little understood pattern of endogenous dermatitis in adults characterized by the appearance of multiple well-defined discoid lesions, usually on the limbs but sometimes on the trunk. The lesions tend to recur at the same sites, sometimes over years. Nummular dermatitis is often very symmetrical and the intensity of the dermatitis varies considerably. Sometimes oedema is prominent so that the plaques of dermatitis stand out and may be vesicular. At other times, the lesions are almost flat and scaly. In young adults the cause is rarely apparent but an atopic background is likely in a minority, especially in young women with localized lesions of the nipple and areola. However, in older men (50–75 years), emotional stress often seems to be the precipitating factor and the prognosis is better in this age group.

Differential diagnosis

Distinction from the nummular pattern of atopic dermatitis is perhaps academic. More important, allergic contact dermatitis may take a nummular form on the backs of the hands and wrists, and in localized disease at these sites patch testing should be carried out. Psoriasis and neurodermatitis are unlikely to be confused but the possibility of tinea corporis should never be forgotten.

Treatment

Topical corticosteroids are the mainstay of management. Secondary coccal infection may invite the addition of an iodoquinoline antiseptic or chlortetracycline to the cream or ointment.

Generalized Exfoliative Dermatitis

This is a distinct entity, sometimes called erythroderma, in which the skin becomes universally inflamed, i.e. erythematous, oedematous and scaly but not vesicular. It may be complicated by marked loss of scalp and body hair (reversible), by thickening and deep fissuring of the palms and soles and by gross nail hypertrophy. There may be secondary lymphadenopathy (dermatopathic lymphadenitis). The disease is rare and is usually seen in men in the second half of life. Fortunately it tends to be self-limiting. Generalized exfoliative dermatitis may follow injudicious provocation of a contact dermatitis but usually develops subacutely from an unclassified dermatitis of the head, neck or hands. It may be a sequel of photosensitivity in chronic actinic dermatitis. The potential metabolic sequelae are described on p. 102.

Differential diagnosis

A drug cause of erythroderma must always be excluded. Sulphonamides, sulphonylureas, indomethacin, allopurinol, gold and many other drugs may precipitate it. Psoriatic erythroderma must be differentiated by the history, as must a mysterious entity called *pityriasis rubra pilaris*. Lymphomas and leukaemias may cause or even present as erythroderma and can be recognized by evidence of systemic disease and on skin biopsy.

Management

Admission to hospital is often necessary. Removal of any possible causative factor is the first essential. Prevention of excessive heat loss and replacement of protein and water loss are crucial. A potent corticosteroid ointment well diluted in soft white paraffin (mineral oil) is usually the best topical treatment. Sometimes oral prednisolone, starting with 40 mg daily, is needed to control the disease.

Miscellaneous

Drug eruptions may be eczematous, for example due to methyl dopa. Rarely, metabolic disorders are associated with dermatitis, for example phenylketonuria in infants, Wiskott–Aldrich syndrome, steatorrhoea and Danbolt's acrodermatitis enteropathica. Congenital lymphatic dysplasias may predispose to dermatitis in the lower leg. Polymorphic light eruption is a dermatitis of the exposed parts occurring in spring and summer; the patient may react abnormally to short-wave ultraviolet light and to longer wavelengths. Infection with staphylococci can occasionally provoke a localized pattern of spreading dermatitis of the hand, with a moist, scaly edge which responds rapidly to an appropriate antibiotic. This entity is sometimes called *infective eczematoid dermatitis*.

— 12

Psoriasis, Reiter's Disease and Lichen Planus

Psoriasis

Psoriasis is a very common, chronic, non-infective, inflammatory skin disease characterized by the presence of sharply defined salmon-red plaques with a scaly surface. Psoriasis is found in 2% of the population of northwest Europe and North America, but is less common in the yellow–brown and black races. The sex ratio is equal. Although psoriasis can start in infancy, onset before 4 years is rare and before 8 years uncommon. The peaks of incidence are seen in the second and third decades but the disease may begin at any age, even in senility.

Aetiology and provocative factors

The predisposition to psoriasis is inherited multifactorially. This has been established by population surveys, twin studies and family pedigree analyses. Strong positive correlations of psoriasis with the HLA antigens CW6 and DR7 have been demonstrated. Psoriasis is a polygenic disease, the predisposition depending on the presence of a number of genes whose combined action draws the patient closer to a threshold beyond which provocative environmental factors can precipitate clinical disease (Table 12.1).

Table 12.1 Provocative factors in psoriasis.

Trauma
Infections
Hormonal epochs
Drugs (lithium, chloroquine)
Emotional stress
Sunlight (uncommonly)
Hypocalcaemia (rare)

The provocative factors include trauma, for instance a cat scratch or operational incision; infection, particularly the role of streptococcal pharyngitis in precipitating guttate psoriasis of childhood; and hormonal disturbance, especially childbirth. Less common precipitating factors are sunlight, although it improves the condition in the majority, drugs such as chloroquine and lithium, hypocalcaemia and psychological stress.

Pathogenesis and pathology

Exciting strides in understanding of the pathogenesis of psoriasis have taken place in the last 15 years, the landmarks being the recognition that both the epidermis and dermis are involved and that clinically unaffected skin is abnormal. The active, psoriatic epidermis is hyperkinetic with increased cell production. Production of new cells is increased by a factor of 20–30, leading to an increased epidermal volume, i.e. acanthosis. Epidermal turnover or replacement time is shortened from the normal 30 days to as little as 3 or 4 days. The increased cell production rate is due to an expanded germinative cell population, a much higher than normal proportion of whose cells is actively cycling. Cell cycle times are not much changed. The rate of nail growth is also increased.

At present it is controversial whether the epidermal maturation defect which results in the abnormal scaly stratum corneum, is the result of accelerated epidermopoiesis or whether the latter is compensatory and due to a feedback mechanism, i.e. secondary to maturation fault. Current research using monoclonal antibodies against various keratinocyte components may elucidate these problems. Various abnormalities of arachidonic metabolism have been identified, particularly an excess of leukotriene B4 in psoriatic epidermis, the formation of which is catalysed by lipoxygenase enzymes. Such abnormalities may explain the strong chemotactic attraction of the abnormal epidermis for polymorphonuclear leucocytes which results in microabscess formation in the epidermis, a central feature of the histopathology of psoriasis.

The epidermal changes can be summarized as acanthosis with striking epidermodermal infolding, parakeratosis, i.e. the formation of an abnormal nucleated loose scaly stratum corneum, absence of the stratum granulosum and the presence of polymorphonuclear microabscesses. The equally important dermal changes are capillary hypertrophy in the papillae and a superficial infiltrate of mainly lymphocytes and macrophages. The epidermal changes may be secondary to lymphocyte abnormalities.

Clinical picture

The expression of psoriasis is enormously varied, both in space and time. The disease may be trivial or universal, transient or chronic over decades with every variation between these extremes. The clinical spectrum is complicated by morphological variants and curious locations, but most adult psoriasis is characteristic and easily recognizable.

Discoid psoriasis. The plaque is sharply defined and is palpable. The colour is red with a dull salmon-coloured hue. It is covered by a white scale which is easily detached by scraping, and bleeding points are easily provoked. The scratched scale assumes a silvery colour (Fig. 12.1). The primary papule can grow into a plaque of any size or may coalesce to form 'geographical' patterns. Discoid psoriasis has a predilection for the extensor aspects of the limbs, especially the points of the elbows or knees, the lower back and the scalp, especially at its margins.

Table 12.2 Clinical patterns of psoriasis.

Discoid psoriasis	Rupioid psoriasis
Guttate psoriasis	Pustular psoriasis
Napkin psoriasis	Nail psoriasis
Flexural psoriasis	

There are many variants of this classical picture (Table 12.2). The main ones are briefly described.

Napkin psoriasis. Eruptions spreading from the napkin area in infants may be sharply defined and psoriasiform. The occurrence of this rash in babies of psoriatic families and the occasional later emergence of typical psoriasis support the belief that the eruption is a form of psoriasis (Fig. 12.2).

Guttate psoriasis. Guttate psoriasis is an acute exanthematic papular psoriasis, uniformly distributed on the trunk and limbs and often precipitated by an upper respiratory infection. It is usually seen in children but can occur in adults (Fig. 12.3).

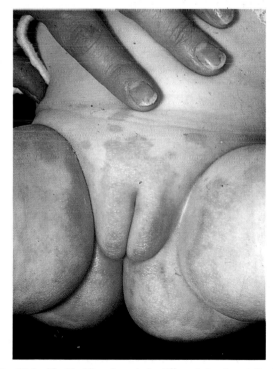

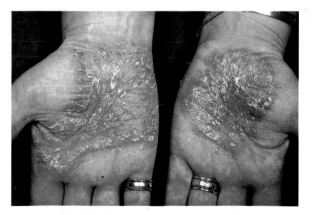

Fig. 12.1 Typical discoid psoriasis but the involvement of the palms in this pattern is unusual.

Fig. 12.2 Napkin (diaper) psoriasis; differentiation from infantile seborrhoeic dermatitis may be difficult.

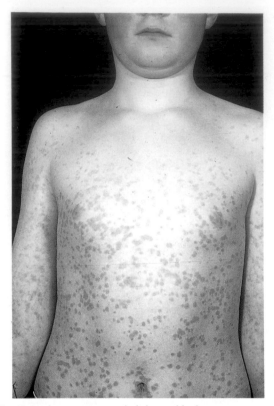

Fig. 12.3   Acute guttate psoriasis in an older boy.

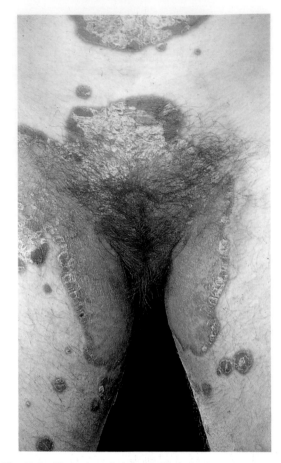

Fig. 12.4   Flexural psoriasis in an elderly woman.

Flexural psoriasis. In some patients, particularly the elderly, psoriasis affects the axillary, submammary and anogenital folds (Fig. 12.4). The scale is rubbed off by intertriginous friction, leaving smooth, glazed but well-defined plaques. Pruritus ani may be the presenting symptom (Fig. 12.5).

Pustular psoriasis. Uncommonly, the epidermal micro-abscesses become exaggerated and macroscopic so that visible yellow pustules are set in the psoriatic skin. Such pustules are sterile. This pattern is seen usually in middle life as an indolent eruption of the palms or soles where the pustules slowly desiccate to leave discrete brown stains in the desquamating stratum corneum. The thenar and hypothenar eminences, heels and insteps are particularly affected (Fig. 12.6). Rarely, pustular psoriasis may be generalized, acute and even fulminant (see Complications).

Rupioid psoriasis This is a variant of pustular psoriasis in which heaped-up, conical, orange–yellow papules form. It is indistinguishable from the 'keratoderma blenorrhagicum' described in some cases of Reiter's syndrome.

Localized patterns

Some of the variants described above have characteristic locations but ordinary discoid psoriasis may also be peculiarly localized. It will not escape recognition if simple rules of diagnosis are remembered. Thus, psoriasis confined to the scalp may be misdiagnosed as dandruff. The important features are the patchy, particularly marginal, involvement and the fact that lesions are palpable as well as visible (Fig. 12.7). Persistent lesions on the shaft or glans of the penis (see Fig. 2.8), on the umbilicus or in the external ear are common in the adult. In children, small patches may be seen in an axilla, inguinal crease, on the belly or even on the face or eyelid. Acral psoriasis may be associated with psoriatic arthritis or Reiter's syndrome (Fig. 12.8).

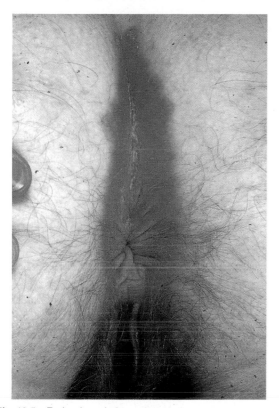

Fig. 12.5   Perianal psoriasis causing pruritus and soreness.

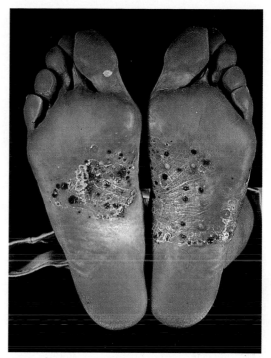

Fig. 12.6   Chronic palmoplantar pustular psoriasis. Ordinary psoriasis is sometimes found elsewhere.

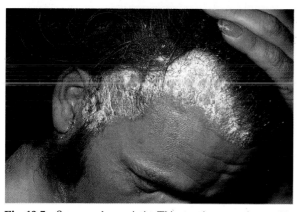

Fig. 12.7   Severe scalp psoriasis. This may be a very intractable pattern.

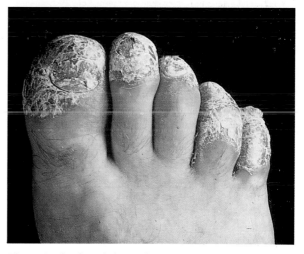

Fig. 12.8   Acral psoriasis associated with distal psoriatic arthritis.

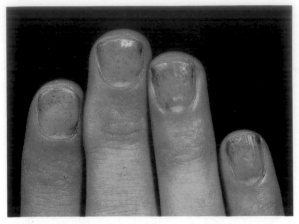

Fig. 12.9 Psoriatic 'pitting' of finger nail plates.

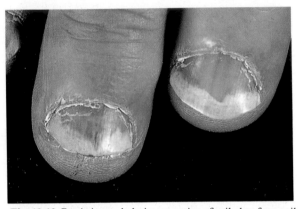

Fig. 12.10 Psoriatic onycholysis; separation of nail plate from nail bed distally.

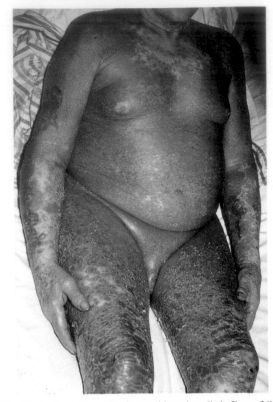

Fig. 12.11 Psoriatic erythroderma; this patient died of heart failure consequent upon the skin disease.

Psoriasis of the nails. Psoriasis affects the nails at some time in up to 50% of patients. It may disturb the matrix or the nail bed (hyponychium). Matrix disease causes pitting (Fig. 12.9) or ridging of the emerging nail plate. Nail bed psoriasis leads to separation of the plate (onycholysis), particularly at the free end laterally (Fig. 12.10), and subungual heaped-up parakeratosis. The latter is particularly common in the toes, whereas pitting is seen more in the fingernails.

Complications

Complications of psoriasis include erythroderma, generalized pustulation and their metabolic sequelae, and polyarthritis. Secondary bacterial infection is rare, but plaques may be colonized by staphylococci which could be a hazard to others, for example in a psoriatic surgeon or nurse.

In erythrodermic or generalized exfoliative psoriasis, the localized plaques are submerged in a universal inflammation of the skin. Involvement of nails, palms and soles is gross and much hair may be lost. The skin is bright red, oedematous and uncomfortable (Fig. 12.11). Exfoliation of scales may be profuse and continuous. This pattern is rare, occurs in adults and may run a subacute or chronic course. It occurs spontaneously but can be precipitated by injudicious topical therapy, drug reactions and corticosteroid withdrawal.

In acute generalized pustular psoriasis, fever, nausea and malaise usher in a fierce skin inflammation which may rapidly become universal. Masses of pinhead sterile pustules erupt, coalesce and desquamate in crops (Fig. 12.12). A leucocytosis is usual. Attacks may be fatal but fortunately this complication is rare.

Metabolic complications of erythroderma

Universal erythrodermic psoriasis may cause serious constitutional disturbance (Table 12.3). Thermo-

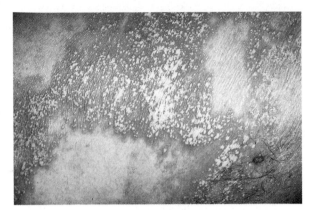

Fig. 12.12 Generalized pustular psoriasis (acute).

Table 12.3 Metabolic complications of universal psoriasis.

Disturbed thermoregulation
Increased water loss
Increased protein loss
Cardiovascular strain
Malabsorption

regulation is disturbed, cutaneous vasodilatation causing excessive heat loss with the danger of hypothermia in a cold environment. Conversely, in high ambient temperatures, hyperthermia is possible because the psoriatic skin is anhidrotic, due to blockage of the sweat ducts in the disordered epidermis. Cutaneous bloodflow is greatly increased, demanding an increased cardiac output. If the cardiovascular system is compromised by disease, cardiac embarrassment and then failure may supervene. Persistent exfoliation represents a protein loss since keratin is a fibrous protein. Hypoalbuminaemia may ensue. Transepidermal insensible water loss is also greatly increased due to the impaired barrier qualities of psoriatic skin, but cutaneous electrolyte loss is not a problem. Other secondary metabolic problems may include malabsorption, hypocalcaemia and folate deficiency, the last partly due to increased utilization.

Psoriatic arthritis

Psoriasis and an inflammatory polyarthritis are seen together more often than chance alone would dictate.

The arthritis is similar to rheumatoid but, in its classical form, has a predilection for the distal interphalangeal joints of the fingers and the small joints of the toes. In the fingers, the distal joint is swollen and tender, and may be fixed in flexion. The adjacent nail is likely to show psoriatic changes. Sausage-like deformity of the toes is characteristic but the lateral deviation of rheumatoid arthritis is absent because the metacarpophalangeal and metatarsophalangeal joints are relatively spared. Rheumatoid subcutaneous nodules are absent. Radiographs reveal an erosive arthropathy (Fig. 12.13). Rarely, in psoriatic arthritis mutilans, joint destruction and bone lysis may be extreme (Fig. 12.14) and can be followed by bony ankylosis, functionally destroying the hands. However, many patients have an arthritis very similar to rheumatoid, but tending to be less symmetrical and with more spinal involvement. The only important differentiating laboratory feature in all of these groups is the absence of serum rheumatoid factors so that the Rose–Waaler and latex fixation tests give negative results. Eye complications associated with arthritis include conjunctivitis and uveitis. There are 'overlap' associations of psoriatic arthritis with ankylosing spondylitis, Reiter's syndrome, ulcerative colitis and Crohn's disease.

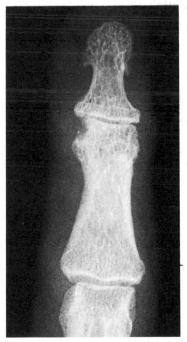

Fig. 12.13 Erosive arthropathy in distal interphalangeal joint of a finger.

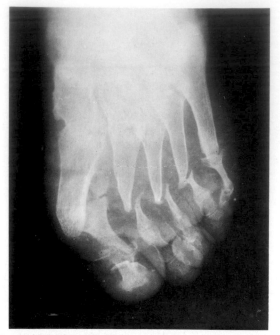

Fig. 12.14 Radiograph of foot showing gross osteolysis of metatarsal heads; psoriatic arthritis mutilans.

Table 12.4 Therapeutic modalities in psoriasis.

Topical	Systemic	Topical and systemic
Coal tar	Methotrexate	PUVA
Dithranol (anthralin)	Hydroxyurea	
Corticosteroids	Etretinate	
Ultraviolet B	Cyclosporin A	
Salicylic acid		
Shampoos		

Management

Psoriasis is a chronic relapsing disease for which the physician can offer suppression but not cure (Table 12.4). The patient therefore needs social and psychological support as well as physical remedies. Attention should always be paid to any accompanying disease, such as arthritis, anaemia or depression, which may critically lower the patient's tolerance of his disability. Its non-infective nature should be stressed. Most psoriasis is treated topically; systemic therapy, which is more hazardous, is reserved for severe and disabling disease.

Topical therapy

Tar, dithranol and corticosteroids are of accepted value. Detergent shampoos, salicylic acid ointments and pastes, and short-wave ultraviolet light (UVB) are adjuncts to treatment.

Tar. Coal and wood tar extracts are often effective, probably by virtue of their weak antimitotic action. Coal tar solution B.P.C. (100 ml to 100 l) can be added to a daily bath, or a coal tar medicated soap can be used. Alcoholic extract of tar (liquor picis carbonis) or crude coal tar can be incorporated into an ointment, for example 2–6% in soft yellow paraffin. Coal tar paste B.P.C. can be used. Cleaner, washable proprietary tar creams are available, for example Alphosyl (U.K.), CarboDome (U.K.) or Zetar® (U.S.A.). For the scalp, coal tar and salicylic acid ointment B.P. is messy but extremely valuable, as is Leeds Pomade (U.K.) which consists of 2% sulphur, 2% salicylic acid, 4% prepared coal tar, 25% emulsifying wax and liquid paraffin to 100%. The head is washed, initially daily, with a proprietary tar-based shampoo, such as Polytar (U.K.) or Zetar® (U.S.A.), or with 50% teepol and 1% glycerine in water. One popular regime, introduced 50 years ago by Goeckermann, is effective in most inpatients over 4–6 weeks and involves a daily application of tar paste which is wiped off the following day with oil and the skin exposed to UVB through a film of residual tar and oil. The paste is then reapplied.

Dithranol. Dihydroxyanthranol (anthralin) is a more potent topical antimitotic but is more difficult to handle because it is an irritant to the unaffected skin. It is therefore incorporated in a concentration of 0.01% increasing to 0.5% in a stiff paste, zinc and salicylic acid paste B.P. (Lassar's paste). Dithranol stains linen permanently so the paste is applied once daily precisely to the lesions and then covered with tube gauze or an orthopaedic stockinette (Fig. 12.15). The following day it is thoroughly removed in a tar bath, the patient exposed to UVB and the procedure repeated; this is the Ingram regime. Dithranol cannot be used on the face, ears, genitalia and flexures, and is highly irritant if introduced accidentally into the eyes. Efficient use of the Ingram regime for inpatients or outpatients attending a day-care centre will clear discoid psoriasis in most patients in about 3 weeks. A residual deep brown staining of the skin (Fig. 12.16) disappears within a month of the termination of

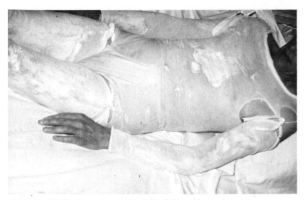

Fig. 12.15 Patient dressed with dithranol (anthralin) paste and covered with tubular gauze dressings.

treatment. The addition of UVB and the tar bath are not crucial. Dithranol is also available in an ointment base (Dithrolan, U.K.) in stable cream formulations (Dithrocream, U.K.; Drithocream, U.S.A.) and in a urea-containing cream (Psoradrate, U.K.). Recent realization that long exposures are unnecessary, as well as inconvenient, has led to a vogue for short-contact dithranol therapy, the preparation being removed 15–60 minutes after application according to strength. Up to 4% dithranol with 0.5% salicylic acid in soft white paraffin (Vaseline) has been tried; 10 minutes may suffice with such high strengths.

Corticosteroids. These are cleaner, non-irritant and much easier to use than tar or dithranol and are the treatment of choice for the face, ears, flexures and genitalia. However, prolonged use of the most potent preparations may destabilize the psoriasis, especially on withdrawal. Such preparations also induce cutaneous atrophy with consequent striae, telangiectasia, skin fragility and purpura. The rate of development and severity of these effects is proportional to the strength, quantities and duration of exposure. The face, flexures and backs of hands are particularly at risk. Widespread application of strong steroids in amounts exceeding 50 g per week may lead to Cushingoid features and hypothalamo–pituitary–adrenal suppression due to systemic absorption. Nevertheless, judiciously used, corticosteroids have a valuable place in therapy. Lotions and gels of betamethasone valerate and fluocinolone acetonide are useful in the scalp. On the body, creams and ointments containing clobetasol propionate (Dermovate, U.K.; Demovate, U.S.A.), betamethasone valerate (Betnovate, U.K.; Diprolene® U.S.A.), etc, can be applied once to thrice daily. For

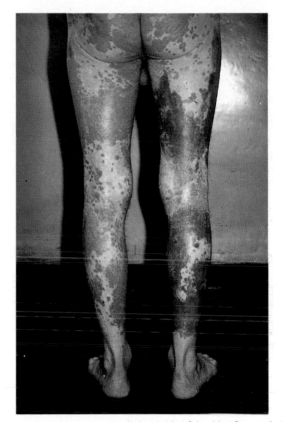

Fig. 12.16 Dithranol (anthralin) staining of the skin after psoriasis has cleared. This disappears in 2–3 weeks.

maintenance treatment, medium strength preparations such as flurandrenolone (Cordran® U.S.A.) and hydrocortisone butyrate (Locoid, U.K.) are applicable.

Systemic treatment

When psoriasis is life-threatening or physically, socially or economically disabling and either resistant to efficient topical therapy or relapses immediately after such treatment, various systemic options are available.

Methotrexate. Methotrexate is the longest established systemic treatment. This folate antagonist is given orally once weekly in a dose of 0.2 mg/kg, increasing if necessary to 0.4 mg/kg. It probably acts by inhibiting epidermal cell mitosis. Similar doses can be administered intramuscularly or intravenously. Response begins at 2–3 weeks and progresses for several weeks.

Before treatment is begun it is essential to establish that renal, hepatic and marrow function are all normal. Alcoholism, liver disease, active infection and a history of peptic ulceration or colitis are contraindications. Maintenance treatment is effective and safe in experienced hands but regular red and white cell and platelet counts are essential. Nausea or headache lasting 24–36 hours are the commonest minor side-effects. The principal long-term hazard is the development of hepatic fibrosis and even cirrhosis. Methotrexate is abortifacient and teratogenic and cannot be used in pregnancy.

Hydroxyurea. Another cytostatic drug of value is hydroxyurea (Hydrea, U.K.). In a dosage of 750–1000 mg daily, it is slower and less potent than methotrexate and should be given a 2-month trial. It has the merit of causing no gastric discomfort and is not hepatotoxic. Marrow function must be watched closely.

Etretinate. This retinoid (available as Tigason, U.K.) has moderate antipsoriatic activity but is particularly useful in severe hand or foot psoriasis and in pustular forms. Taken orally in a dosage of 0.3–1.0 mg/kg daily it is a useful new weapon, especially in conjunction with topical tar or corticosteroid treatment. It can also be combined with hydroxyurea therapy and with PUVA (Re-PUVA). Etretinate is likely to be replaced by its metabolite acetretin which has a much shorter half-life.

Photochemotherapy (PUVA). This is a highly effective form of treatment. It involves the oral administration of 8-methoxypsoralen (P) which is a photoactive coumarin compound of plant origin, followed 2 hours later by whole body exposure to a high potency source of long-wave ultraviolet light (UVA) (Fig. 12.17). The treatment is given three or four times weekly initially and leads to steady clearance of psoriasis, together with the development of a flattering tan. Maintenance treatment is feasible every 14–28 days to keep the psoriasis at bay. The long-term hazards include premature and accelerated ageing of the skin, lentigo development and cutaneous carcinogenesis. The eyes must be protected with UVA-blocking plastic spectacles on the whole of the day of treatment, because of a theoretical hazard of cataract. Immediate side-effects include nausea, pruritus and acute sunburn.

Miscellaneous. Other systemic treatments are only experimental. Various forms of dialysis have been reported to be of benefit. Theoretically, lipoxygenase

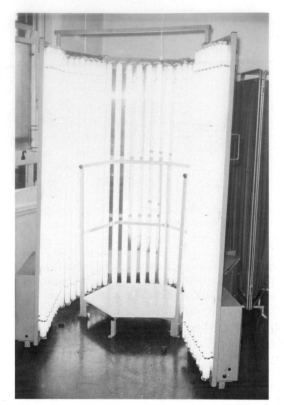

Fig. 12.17 Photochemotherapy (PUVA) unit with vertically arranged UVA-emitting tubes.

inhibitors could be beneficial and indeed benoxaprofen, now withdrawn because of its severe toxicity, was shown to have antipsoriatic efficacy. Rarely, cyclosporin A is used in exceptionally severe and resistant psoriasis.

Reiter's Disease

Definition

This is a disease in which a non-suppurative polyarthritis lasting more than one month follows closely a lower urogenital or enteric infection, particularly in young men carrying the HLA-B27 antigen. Inflammatory eye disease and mucocutaneous manifestations are common.

Pathogenesis

The disease seems to be due to a triggering infection in a genetically predisposed male, usually HLA-B27 positive. Chlamydia trachomatis, ureaplasma, Shigella and other organisms may be responsible.

Clinical features

Mainly young men are affected. A non-gonococcal urethritis or enteric infection is followed by a non-suppurative polyarthritis, usually of the lower limbs. Conjunctivitis occurs early but iritis may occur later. The skin lesions are psoriasiform (keratoderma blennorrhagicum) but erosive lesions may affect the penis (circinate balanitis) or mouth. Rupioid acral lesions are typical and nail involvement may be gross. The skin and joint disease may develop slowly into typical psoriasis and psoriatic arthritis. Rare complications include heart block, aortic incompetence and pericarditis, and various neurological syndromes.

Treatment

There is no specific treatment. The initial infection is treated as usual. Antiinflammatory analgesics and rarely prednisolone are needed for the arthritis. Topical steroids are useful for the skin lesions.

Lichen Planus

Lichen planus is a fairly common subacute or chronic mucocutaneous disorder of adults, characterized by a pruritic papular eruption.

Aetiology

The cause is unknown. An indistinguishable 'lichen-oid' drug eruption can be caused by gold, mepacrine, chloroquine and some beta-blocking agents, suggesting an immunological mechanism. Lichen planus may be a manifestation of graft-versus-host reactions, strengthening this supposition. Whether a single or multiple antigens may be involved in 'idiopathic' lichen planus is not known.

Clinical features

The elemental lesion is a small (2–3 mm) flat-topped papule with a characteristic blue–red (violaceous) hue which develops a fine lacy white pattern on its surface—Wickham's striae. The flexor aspect of the wrist is a typical site but similar lesions may occur elsewhere on the limbs and trunk, particularly on the arms, lower trunk, legs and ankles. The eruption may

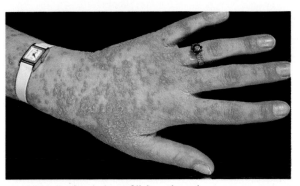

Fig. 12.18 Profuse lesions of lichen planus in a young woman.

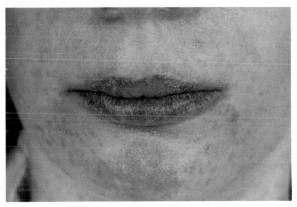

Fig. 12.19 Lichen planus of lips in same patient as Fig. 12.18.

be sparse or profuse (Fig. 12.18) and usually itches, often intensely.

The lesions may enlarge and coalesce to form plaques 1–2 cm in diameter. Sometimes annular patterns are formed. The glans and shaft of the penis are commonly involved (Fig. 2.9).

About 50% of patients develop lesions in the buccal mucosa, tongue or lips (Fig. 12.19). Oral lesions are white, slightly thickened and of lacy pattern with variable erythema. Discomfort may be minimal or intense.

Clinical variants

Many morphological variants may occur. Lesions on the legs are common, usually on the anterior or lateral shins where large (1–3 cm) hypertrophic plaques form. The ankles and insteps are often involved, and palmar or plantar lesions may have a pseudovesicular or pseudopustular appearance. Occasionally, enlarging intractable annular lesions are seen with central atrophy. The scalp is usually spared but, rarely, fulminating lichen planus can sweep through the scalp in a few weeks causing irreversible cicatricial alopecia if not checked. Gold-induced lichen may affect the scalp similarly.

Linear patterns are uncommon and usually seen on a limb. In very active disease, short 'streaks' of papules may be due to trauma (Köbner or isomorphic phenomenon).

In black people an acute profuse centripetal lichen planus may mimic pityriasis rosea in its early stages. Rarely the disease is ulcerative—in the mouth, lips, penis or elsewhere.

The finger nails are involved in about 10% of patients. Mild changes consist of fine ridging and grooving. Sometimes the nail becomes thinned and spoon-shaped. Complete nail destruction with pterygium formation is rare.

Prognosis

The course is variable. Often the disease settles spontaneously in 6–24 months but may recur at intervals. Oral disease, hypertrophic leg lesions and atrophic annular lesions may persist for years or even decades. Generally, resolution is accompanied by a typical macular hyperpigmentation which takes a year or more to resolve. The hyperpigmentation is particularly gross after an attack of centripetal lichen in black patients.

Pathology

The biopsy findings are singular. Histologically there is hyperkeratosis and acanthosis with a prominent stratum granulosum. An intense, mainly lymphocytic infiltrate forms a band in the upper dermis 'hugging' the epidermis which tends to present a jagged ('sawtoothed') epidermodermal junction with destruction of basal keratinocytes, the relics of which may be seen near the junction as amorphous pink 'colloid' bodies.

Differential diagnosis

A typical case is instantly recognizable. Psoriasis may be mimicked at times and hypertrophic leg lesions have to be distinguished from psoriasis and lichen simplex.

In the mouth and lips, candidosis, hairy leukoplakia (viral), white sponge naevus and premalignant dysplasia must be differentiated. Linear lesions have to be distinguished from epidermal linear naevi, lichen striatus and linear morphoea. Solitary annular lesions may mimic 'morphoeic' basal cell carcinoma.

Treatment

Clearly, if a drug is suspected it must be withdrawn. Mild cases are treated with a corticosteroid cream. Oral antihistamines may help the pruritus.

Very pruritic hypertrophic lesions on the shins respond well to intralesional infiltration with triamcinolone hexacetonide (5–10 mg/ml). Very severe generalized attacks and scalp involvement threatening alopecia merit early vigorous oral prednisolone therapy. Usually 40 mg daily initially is appropriate, the dose being progressively reduced. A few patients need long-term maintenance with 5–10 mg prednisolone for years to suppress the disease. Oral and lip lesions are difficult to influence. Use of steroid gels and oral pellets is disappointing.

Neonatal and Childhood Disorders

The main disorders encountered in the skin in early childhood are described. Genetically determined diseases are covered mainly in Chapter 14.

There are three factors, potentially additive, exposing the neonate to toxic hazards from topically applied chemicals of which the physician, nurse and mother should be aware. Firstly, the skin of the neonate is more permeable than in adults, especially so in the premature infant. Secondly, mechanisms of metabolism and detoxification of absorbed chemicals are immature. Thirdly, surface to volume ratio is higher.

The preterm baby

Acrocyanosis and oedema are common. Lanugo hair is prominent. The head is relatively large and the ears very soft.

The post-term baby

The skin is scaly and child's appearance may be marasmic.

Toxic erythema of the newborn

This is a common transient eruption of macular blotches, becoming papular, and sparing the palms and soles. The cause is unknown and it settles in a few days. Rarely, it is pustular.

Cutis marmorata

This mottled, reticular, cyanotic response to cooling is common in infants, and clears on gentle warming.

Miliaria neonatorum

An erythematous micropapular or vesicular eruption due to sweat retention is common in neonates. It responds to commonsense measures.

Milia

'Millet seed' milium cysts are common and can be ignored.

Impetigo neonatorum

Coccal impetigo may easily become bullous in the neonate: hence the old name of 'pemphigus neonatorum'. It responds rapidly to oral flucoxacillin or erythromycin. Staphylococcal 'scalded skin' syndrome is described on p. 53.

Subcutaneous fat necrosis

This is a curious erythematous induration of subcutaneous tissues with well-defined edges due to cold injury or birth trauma. It gets better spontaneously.

Neonatal intertrigo

This mild inflammation is common in the flexural folds of fat babies.

Granuloma gluteale infantum

This uncommon but alarming papulonodular eruption of the napkin area is benign and probably due to an unusual tissue response to a bowel infection, for example with *Candida*.

Acrodermatitis enteropathica

This rare and dramatic vesicular or pustular inflammatory dermatosis of infancy, resembling candidosis, begins around the various orifices, typically in association with diarrhoea and hair loss in a child who is failing to thrive. Malabsorption of zinc appears to be the cause but there may be a genetic factor. Zinc replacement is dramatically effective.

Acropustulosis of infancy

This recently recognized disorder is far from rare in black infants. An itching papulopustular eruption develops on the hands and feet in the first year and may persist for a year or more (Fig. 13.1). The differential diagnosis of pustulosis in infancy is shown in Table 13.1.

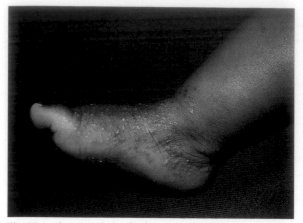

Fig. 13.1   Acropustulosis of infancy—almost always seen in black babies.

Table 13.1   Causes of pustulosis in infancy.

Impetigo	Toxic erythema of newborn
Herpes simplex	Acropustulosis of infancy
Candidosis	Congenital syphilis
Neonatal acne	

Dermatitis in Childhood

Several forms are characteristic of childhood:
- Seborrhoeic dermatitis of infancy
- Napkin dermatitis
- Pityriasis alba
- Juvenile plantar dermatosis
- Atopic dermatitis (described in Chapter 11)

Seborrhoeic dermatitis of infancy

This common eruption begins in the first few weeks of life. It may affect any of the scalp, face, neck, axillae, anogenital and other body folds and areas. In the flexures a bright, moist, shiny, well-marginated erythema with scaling is seen. On the scalp a coarse yellowish crust–scale is seen ('milk crust'). The child is well and itches little, if at all. The condition may persist for months but disappears before the end of the first year. Serum IgE is normal (whereas in atopic dermatitis it is usually raised by 9 months).

Differential diagnosis

Napkin dermatitis spares the anogenital flexures; atopic dermatitis itches, whereas candidosis is more pustular. Psoriasis may be mimicked and some of such children may have a psoriatic diathesis ('napkin psoriasis'—see p. 99).

Treatment

Hydrocortisone 1% cream, particularly in combination with clioquinol 3%, is usually effective. Stronger corticosteroids are rarely needed. Salicylic acid 2% in emulsifying ointment B.P. and mild shampoo will clear the scalp.

Napkin (diaper) dermatitis

This form of primary irritant contact dermatitis is extremely common. Probably 50% of babies are affected sooner or later. It may begin in the early weeks but is uncommon after one year of age. Wetting of the skin is probably the major causative factor leading to mechanical abrasion and increased permeability. Mixing of urine and faeces allows ammonia formation, pH rises and probably allows increased activity of faecal proteases and lipases which compound skin damage.

A bright erythema, occasionally complicated by papules, pustules and even erosions, is seen on the convex prominences of the napkin area, tending to spare the sheltered creases. The penis and scrotum may be affected. In neglected infants the skin may ulcerate. A disseminated non-itching rash may follow, resembling seborrhoeic dermatitis or psoriasis. In black children, hypopigmentation may be striking but is temporary (see Fig. 21.4).

Treatment

Frequent stools, infrequent napkin changes and excessive occlusion by plastic pants may aggravate the condition. Improved sensible hygiene, frequent napkin changes and, in severe cases, nursing without a napkin, are effective. Modern absorbent and the latest superabsorbent napkins make a modest contribution to reduced wetting of the skin and their use is spreading, but they occasionally induce miliaria. Aqueous cream B.P. can be used as a soap substitute but 1% hydrocortisone or chinoform–hydrocortisone may be needed. Rarely, Tri-Adcortyl (U.K.) ointment is needed for a few days only.

Pityriasis alba

This is a minor form of endogenous dermatitis, sometimes atopic, in older children where secondary loss of suntan or true postinflammatory hypopigmentation produces relatively pale areas of slightly scaly ('pityriasiform') skin, particularly on the face and upper arms or trunk. It is very common in black children in the United Kingdom. Vitiligo must be differentiated. Hydrocortisone 1% cream suffices.

Juvenile plantar dermatosis

This puzzling dermatosis has become common in the United Kingdom in the last decade perhaps because of older boys' addiction to 'trainers' as their exclusive footwear. A red, glazed, dry and sometimes superficially fissured dermatitis is seen on the distal part of the sole and weight-bearing area of the toes (Fig. 13.2). Discomfort is variable. The condition is not responsive to steroids and emollients are usually best, together with conversion to less occlusive footwear. It may be very slow to clear. Some of these children are atopic.

Vascular Naevi

These are extremely common.

Naevus simplex ('salmon patch')

Perhaps one-third of all children are born with macular pink areas of erythema on the nape, brow or eyelids. On the brow the patch usually fades and disappears in a few months but nuchal patches often persist.

Naevus flammeus ('port wine stain')

This is a common disorder of superficial dermal capillaries and is now regarded as an ectasia of normal vasculature, perhaps due to local abnormal neural control. Present at birth, it is usually unilateral and on the face but can occur anywhere. It grows only in proportion to the child and does not involute spontaneously. The colour varies from pale pink to deep purple and tends to darken with age. Later in life, angiomatous papules may supervene (Fig. 13.3). Very large lesions are occasionally associated with neurological disorders. Some lesions may be genetic but alcoholism in pregnant women increases the risk of such lesions.

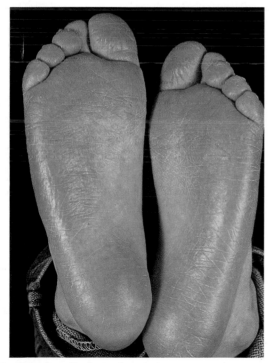

Fig. 13.2 Juvenile plantar dermatosis.

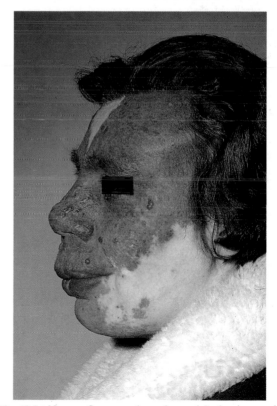

Fig. 13.3 Naevus flammeus (portwine stain) showing angiomatous proliferation in adult life.

The psychological effects of a large facial lesion may be profound. Expert cosmetic camouflage is desirable and in the United Kingdom the British Red Cross Society provides an excellent service. Laser treatment may be helpful in adults.

Sturge–Weber syndrome

A naevus flammeus in the dermatome of the first division of the fifth cranial nerve is associated with ipsilateral vascular malformations in the meninges or brain which may cause epilepsy in infancy and later hemiplegia and mental retardation (Fig. 13.4). Neurological manifestations are likely to occur early or not at all. Glaucoma is a hazard if both eyelids are involved.

Klippel–Trenaunay–Weber syndrome

This rare syndrome usually presents in older girls. An extensive vascular malformation of an arm or leg with arteriovenous aneurysm is associated with a naevus-flammeus-like angioma of the overlying skin. The disease may only present when the orthopaedic consequences of disproportionate overgrowth of the affected limb become apparent. Massive arteriovenous aneurysms may lead to high-output cardiac failure.

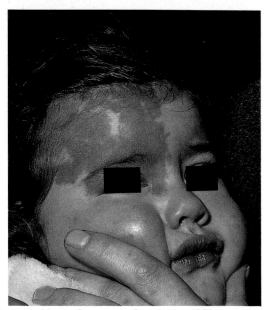

Fig. 13.4 Naevus flammeus in first division of fifth cranial nerve (see Sturge–Weber syndrome).

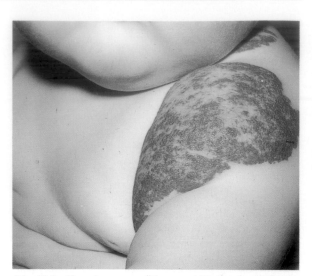

Fig. 13.5 'Strawberry naevus' (cavernous haemangioma) showing early involution.

Strawberry and cavernous haemangioma

The 'strawberry' naevus is usually not present at birth but appears within a few weeks as a rapidly growing vascular papule which reaches full maturity by about 6–9 months. A stationary phase is then followed by slow involution (Fig. 13.5) over several years. Usually single, two or more may occur in a minority of children. Mature naevi vary from 0.5–5 cm or more in diameter and giant lesions are occasionally seen. Those in the napkin area may ulcerate or bleed; large lesions on the eyelid or lip may interfere with binocular vision or with feeding.

Cavernous haemangioma is a similar lesion with a deeper component and may be present at birth. Its outline is less distinct and it may have a blue colour. Most occur on the head or upper trunk. Mixed patterns do occur. Involution is slower and often less complete.

Management should be conservative. A series of photographs demonstrating involution is invaluable in reassuring anxious parents.

Kasabach–Merritt syndrome

This is a rare event in very young infants in which massive haemorrhage complicates a large deep cavernous haemangioma, usually at the root of a limb. Thrombocytopenia due to platelet sequestration in the angioma appears to be the cause. Deep progressive blue–brown swellings due to haemorrhage may press on vital structures. Transfusion and oral prednisolone may be needed.

Eruptive disseminated angiomatosis

In this rare condition, multiple cutaneous cavernous angiomata are associated with multiple similar lesions in internal organs. Arteriovenous shunting may cause cardiac failure. If the child survives, all the lesions may disappear. Prednisolone may be of value.

Blue rubber bleb naevus syndrome

Multiple small cavernous angiomata tend to increase in size and number, may be tender or painful and may be associated with gastrointestinal lesions with a tendency to bleed.

Syndromes with Mental Handicap

Down's syndrome (Trisomy 21)

These children are prone to infections such as scabies, blepharitis, angular stomatitis, gingivitis, otitis externa and tinea. Alopecia and syringomata may develop. Down's syndrome can be diagnosed confidently in utero by ultrasound imaging and confirmed by fetal biopsy early enough to allow termination.

Phenylketonuria

This is a rare autosomal recessive disorder in which a specific enzyme deficiency leads to phenylalanine accumulation and the abnormal excretion of its products in the urine. Untreated children are fair-skinned and are liable to develop eczema and pyogenic infections. The disease is detectable by urine testing at birth and the mental deficiency is preventable by prompt use of a low phenylalanine diet.

Congenital infections

Rubella, toxoplasmosis, cytomegalovirus and syphilis can all lead to mental retardation, neurological damage and various cutaneous signs.

Neurofibromatosis (p. 116), tuberose sclerosis (p. 117) and Sturge–Weber syndrome (p. 112) are described elsewhere.

Miscellaneous Uncommon but Important Disorders

Congenital aplasia cutis

This localized absence of skin and underlying tissues is present at birth and usually affects the scalp. One or more localized areas of weeping granulation or ulceration occur close to the midline of the scalp. Birth injury must be differentiated. Later the scarring alopecia may be misdiagnosed as tinea.

Mastocytosis (urticaria pigmentosa)

In this uncommon sporadic disease, multiple guttate or larger pigmented macules appear on the trunk and limbs of a baby (Fig. 13.6). The mother may have noticed that the lesions are sometimes erythematous and swollen (for instance, after a bath) and then itch. Rarely, frank blistering is seen or larger solitary nodular lesions (mast-cell naevus). The diagnosis is confirmed clinically by inducing urtication in one or two lesions by brisk rubbing. A biopsy reveals abnormal numbers of mast cells in the dermis. Usually the condition disappears before puberty. An adult-onset form of mastocytosis occurs rarely where lesions persist indefinitely and systemic lesions may occur.

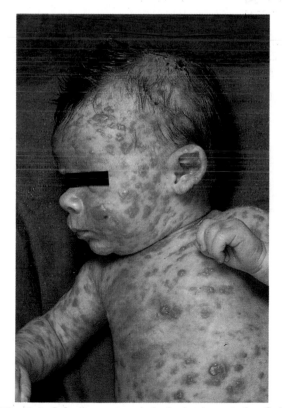

Fig. 13.6 Infantile mastocytosis (urticaria pigmentosa); a florid disseminated example.

Kawasaki disease (mucocutaneous lymph node syndrome)

Common in Japan and increasingly recognized elsewhere this is a self-limiting disease of children under 5 years. It is characterized by fever lasting several days, conjunctival injection, cheilitis, 'strawberry' tongue, a red throat, a macular erythematous exanthema beginning on the palms and soles but becoming widespread, progressing to oedema of the hands and feet and often cervical lymphadenopathy. The peeling of a 'toxic' erythema follows. Cardiac and neurological complications may occur, especially in infant boys. Coronary occlusion can be fatal. The cause is unknown.

Juvenile xanthogranuloma

This is a rare, benign, self-limiting disorder characterized by the appearance of symptomless multiple smooth yellow or reddish-brown papules and nodules, usually on the head, trunk or proximal parts of the limbs. The condition appears in the first year of life and involutes spontaneously. Histologically, there is a dermal infiltrate of foamy histiocytes.

Histiocytosis X (Langerhans' cell histiocytosis)

The disordered Langerhans' cell is now known to be the usual cause of histiocytosis, although rare non-Langerhans'-cell forms, both benign and malignant, do occur.

The disease is rare. It may involve a single organ (usually bone) but more often is a multisystem disease. It affects mainly male children. The commonest features are proptosis (due to retro-orbital proliferation), otitis externa, bony middle-ear lesions leading to mastoid infection, recurrent pneumothorax, hepato-splenomegaly and skin lesions.

Skin lesions are common and superficially resemble seborrhoeic dermatitis of infancy, but erosions and ulceration, especially in the flexures and scalp, should alert the clinician.

Therapy is difficult. Topical steroids and mustine may be valuable. Progressive disease calls for oral prednisolone and chemotherapy. The disease is occasionally self-limiting.

Sebaceous naevus

This relatively common form of epidermal naevus presents at or soon after birth as a barely raised, orange–yellow velvety ovoid plaque, usually 1–2 cm in length, and generally on the scalp. The plaque is hairless and may only attract attention later in childhood as a patch of alopecia. After puberty the plaque gradually gets thicker and becomes elevated.

Biopsy reveals masses of mature sebaceous glands with epidermal hyperplasia. Buds of basaloid cells represent 'abortive' hair follicles.

Various benign or malignant appendageal and epidermal tumours may eventually complicate this naevus. For this reason and to remove the bald defect, complete excision and primary closure in adolescence is the usual practice.

Focal dermal hypoplasia (Goltz's syndrome)

In this rare genetic syndrome, streaky atrophic skin lesions are present at birth. The dermal collagen is grossly hypoplastic so that the dermis appears to be invaded by fat. There may be many associated defects.

Lick dermatitis

A sharply defined peri-oral zone of erythema, pigmentation and scaling is seen in children who habitually moisten the peri-oral skin with the tongue (Fig. 13.7). Some of these children are atopic.

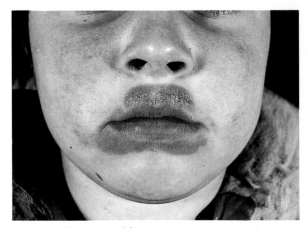

Fig. 13.7   'Lick' dermatitis.

— 14
Genetic Diseases

Introduction

The structure and function of normal skin are determined by the individual's genetic endowment, the *genotype*. Multiple genes are involved in many physical characteristics, for example skin colour. The somatic result of genetic interplay is called the *phenotype*.

Some human disorders are not only influenced by multiple genes, i.e. are *polygenic,* but are multifactorial in the sense that genetic and non-genetic environmental influences determine disease expression. In dermatology, atopic dermatitis and psoriasis are good examples.

In this Chapter the most important *genodermatoses* are briefly described, i.e. those diseases where genotype is all-important and non-genetic influence is absent or minimal.

Genetic definitions

- *Genes* transmit characteristics to the next generation.
- *Chromosomes* are paired and carry large numbers of genes in fixed positions (*loci*).
- *Homozygous* implies that the corresponding loci on a chromosome pair are occupied by identical genes.
- *Heterozygous* implies that the corresponding loci on a chromosome pair are occupied by genes which differ, variant forms of the gene being called *alleles*.
- A *dominant gene* exerts its *full* phenotypic effect even in the heterozygous situation.
- A *recessive gene* exerts its *full* phenotypic effect only in the homozygous situation. There may be very limited phenotypic effects in the heterozygous situation, sometimes very subtle, but which can be detected by special means, so-called *genetic markers*.
- The *expression* of a gene refers to the qualitative or quantitative variations in the resultant phenotype; there may be variable expression.
- The *penetrance* of a gene is a measure of the frequency with which it exerts any phenotypic influence. Thus penetrance can be partial or complete.
- *Autosomal* inheritance depends on genes carried on any chromosome pair except the sex chromosomes, and implies transmission to either sex. However, an environmental factor may determine expression so that *sex-limited* effects are possible. Thus, the male pattern of alopecia often induced by androgen excess in women suggests that common baldness may be controlled by an autosomal gene where phenotypic expression is dependent on androgenic activity.
- *Sex-linked* characteristics depend on genes transmitted on the sex (X and Y) chromosomes.
- A *mutation* occurs when a gene is altered or changed for whatever reason.

The principal features of the three main patterns of inheritance are summarized in Tables 14.1–14.3.

Table 14.1 Characteristics of autosomal dominant inheritance.

Parent affected (unless mutation)
Half of children affected (on average)
Vertical involvement in family pedigree
One abnormal allele causes diseases
Homozygous state may be lethal
No consanguinity of parents expected

Table 14.2 Characteristics of autosomal recessive inheritance.

Parents unaffected
One-quarter (on average) of the children of heterozygous parents affected
Horizontal involvement in family pedigree
Patient must be homozygous for abnormal allele
Increased incidence of consanguinity in parents

Table 14.3 Characteristics of sex-linked recessive inheritance.

Only males affected
Never transmitted from father to son
Mother's brothers often affected
All daughters of an affected man are heterozygote carriers

Histocompatability (HLA) antigens

The imperatives of tissue matching for donation and grouping purposes led to the discovery of antibodies which react with surface markers on white blood cells (HLA antigens). These antigens are controlled by specific loci on a particular chromosome pair. These loci are named A, B, C, D and DR.

HLA antigens have proved to be useful 'markers' of certain diseases, probably because of '*genetic linkage*', i.e. the HLA gene and the disease gene may be neighbours on the same chromosome and are transmitted together. Thus the association of HLA-B27 with ankylosing spondylitis is well known. In dermatology the association of Reiter's disease with B27, psoriasis with C6 and DR7, pemphigus with DR4 and dermatitis herpetiformis with B8 are important examples.

Prenatal diagnosis

Invasive procedures for prenatal diagnosis are ethical only if the fetus is at risk of a disease with severe consequences and if accurate diagnosis is possible at a gestational age at which abortion is available and legal. Such procedures should only be performed after full, careful and skilled counselling. It is now possible to obtain material from the fetus and its amniotic fluid at an early stage of pregnancy, thus allowing termination if genetically determined or other abnormalities are detected and, conversely, removing the need for termination if such defects can be shown to be absent.

Amniocentesis, chorioncentesis and cordocentesis at about 16 weeks provide amniotic fluid and cells for cytogenetic or biochemical examination, as well as for detection of abnormalities of DNA or RNA synthesis or repair. Fetoscopy at about 20 weeks allows fetal tissue biopsy, especially of the skin, and direct visual inspection of the fetus. Ultrasound imaging can detect major physical defects, and often very small defects; in addition it is invaluable for direct guidance of invasive techniques. These techniques, allied to rapid progress in DNA analysis allowing detection of mutations and gene tracking, provide confident diagnoses of an increasing number of genetic disorders. Some of the diseases thus detectable are:

- *By fetal skin biopsy*: epidermolysis bullosa (certain types), ichthyosiform erythrodermas, lamellar ichthyosis and Harlequin fetus, Sjögren–Larsson syndrome, oculocutaneous albinism (tyrosinase-negative), hypohidrotic ectodermal dysplasia
- *By amniocentesis (DNA/RNA studies)*: Down's syndrome, xeroderma pigmentosum, Bloom's syndrome, ataxia–telangiectasia
- *By amniocentesis (biochemical studies)*: certain types of porphyria, Fabry–Anderson disease

Genetic counselling

Advice to prospective parents, pregnant women and their husbands is clearly of crucial importance in certain conditions. Expert counselling calls for detailed genetic understanding, knowledge of the relevant diseases and thorough familiarity with the current capabilities of prenatal diagnosis. It is best left in expert hands in special centres.

Inherited skin diseases

More than a hundred genetically determined diseases, where skin is involved have been described. Only a few of the more common ones are described in this Chapter.

Neurofibromatosis

Two distinct forms are now recognized.

Von Recklinghausen's peripheral neurofibromatosis

This neurocutaneous syndrome is relatively common (1:3000 births). It is inherited as an autosomal dominant trait with variable expression. It is characterized by the almost invariable presence of *café au lait* macules and few or multiple cutaneous neurofibromata.

Cafe au lait spots are light-brown oval pigmented macules with sharply defined borders, usually 2–5 cm in length which appear progressively in childhood. Six or more greater than 2.5 cm in diameter are diagnostic. *Axillary freckling* is common and pathognomonic.

Cutaneous neurofibromata (molluscum fibrosum) are soft, skin-coloured or slightly pink or blue nodules

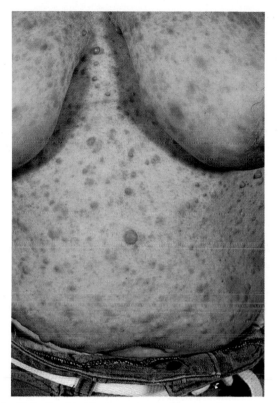

Fig. 14.1   Von Recklinghausen's neurofibromatosis.

with a smooth normal overlying epidermis. They are sessile but may become pedunculated. They vary in size and number. Occasionally they are isolated but usually dozens (and sometimes hundreds) are found (Fig. 14.1). They arise from Schwann cells of the peripheral nerves but have a collagen matrix. They may spread along a large nerve, forming *plexiform neuroma*, or be associated with gross cutaneous overgrowth to produce *elephantiasis neuromatosa*.

Other features include pigmented hamartomas in the iris (Lisch nodules) in 90% of cases and oral lesions. Uncommon features are short stature (in 4%) and scoliosis (in 3%); various endocrine disturbances include acromegaly, Addison's disease, hyperparathyroidism and phaeochromocytoma. Pseudoarthrosis and renal artery stenosis are rare.

Neurological complications (40%) include epilepsy and spinal neurofibromas. Intelligence is low (IQ < 70) in 10%. Malignant sarcomas may eventually develop in 6%.

Bilateral acoustic central neurofibromatosis

This is also an autosomal dominant trait. Typically, bilateral acoustic neuromas develop in patients who have minimal cutaneous manifestations but who do have a marked tendency to other cerebral tumours, particularly meningioma.

Routine investigations of all people affected may not be prudent, but long-term follow-up and immediate investigation of symptoms suggesting neurological or endocrine complications are essential. Genetic counselling is important; 50% of children will be affected. Individual skin lesions which are causing problems can be excised. Recently, genetic prediction has become possible in selected families by DNA analysis using gene tracking.

Tuberose Sclerosis

This syndrome (epiloia, Bourneville's disease) is characterized by hamartomatous development in many organs. Inheritance is autosomal dominant with very variable expression. It is rare.

Clinical features

Epilepsy in infancy or childhood is often the presenting feature. Mental deficiency or secondary dementia of variable degree is common. Ovoid or elongated hypopigmented macules ('ash leaf patches') may be detectable in infancy, especially with the aid of Wood's light. 'Adenoma sebaceum' is an acne-like eruption of angiofibromatous papules of the muzzle (Fig. 14.2) in late childhood or adolescence. Periungual fibromata arise as pink projections from the nail folds (Fig. 14.3). The 'shagreen patch' is an angiofibromatous raised plaque, usually on the lower back. Retinal phakoma is seen as white streaks along fundal vessels. Radiological

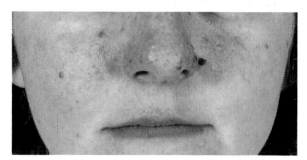

Fig. 14.2   Adenoma sebaceum of tuberose sclerosis.

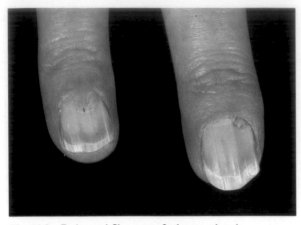

Fig. 14.3   Periungual fibromata of tuberose sclerosis.

investigations may reveal hamartomata in various organs and in bone.

Prognosis is enormously variable. Cauterization of 'adenoma sebaceum' is useful cosmetically. Genetic prediction by gene tracking is sometimes possible.

Connective Tissue Disorders

Ehlers–Danlos syndrome

This term embraces a group of at least 11 inherited disorders of collagen structure and metabolism. The most characteristic features are increased elasticity (but not laxity) of skin and joints, and increased fragility of blood vessels, tending to haemorrhage. The collagen in skin, joints and blood vessel walls is decreased in quantity and abnormal in quality.

Classical Ehlers–Danlos syndrome (Type I) is an autosomal dominant trait. The skin is easily lacerated and heals with scarring which may be blue and spongy. Joints are hypermobile and the facies is distinctive. Easy bruising is a feature.

In the other types severity is variable and different defects, for example haemorrhage, may be prominent. Some types are recessive and possibly X-linked. No treatment is known.

Cutis laxa

This is usually inherited but is rarely acquired. There is profound loss of elastic tissue in the dermis so that skin becomes lax and pendulous. The collagen may also be abnormal. The skin hangs in folds, giving a 'bloodhound' appearance of the face. Emphysema and cardiovascular changes are common. Dominant and recessive types differ in various ways.

Pseudo-xanthoma elasticum

There are four types of this rare but important disease which may show dominant or recessive inheritance. The elastic tissue (and collagen) in the dermis, blood vessels and eye are abnormal and calcium is deposited on the elastica. In its complete form, typical skin lesions are associated with 'angioid streaks' in the retina and various vascular problems. The skin lesions are best seen on the sides of the neck. The skin is loose, lax, wrinkled and yellow ('chicken skin') and contains multiple, often linearly arranged papules, mimicking xanthoma. Vascular involvement may present as hypertension, claudication or angina. Massive haemorrhages may occur in the gut or brain.

The Ichthyoses

This is a group of disorders in which the skin is persistently dry and scaly. The ichthyoses are disorders of stratum corneum formation and desquamation. There are six main types, with differing patterns of inheritance (Table 14.4).

Ichthyosis vulgaris

This common disorder (1:250 births) is inherited as an autosomal dominant trait with high penetrance. It is a disorder of cornification of the epidermis. The granu-

Table 14.4   Classification of ichthyoses.

Type	Inheritance
Ichthyosis vulgaris	Autosomal dominant
X-linked ichthyosis	X-linked
Bullous ichthyosiform erythroderma (epidermolytic hyperkeratosis)	Autosomal dominant
Non-bullous ichthyosiform erythroderma	Autosomal recessive
Lamellar ichthyosis	Autosomal recessive
Refsum's syndrome	Autosomal recessive

lar cell layer is reduced or absent. Onset is between 1 and 4 years. The skin is dry and shows small whitish scales, particularly seen on the extensor limbs and back. Keratosis pilaris and atopy are common associated features. The limb flexures and face are almost always spared but palmar and plantar markings are increased.

X-linked ichthyosis

X-linked ichthyosis is much less common than Ichthyosis vulgaris, at about 1:7000 births. Onset is earlier (sometimes from birth). The scales are more widespread, larger and darker and usually do not spare the flexures. The face, scalp and neck are all involved.

The enzyme steroid sulphatase is deficient in keratinocytes and has also been shown to be reduced in cultured fibroblasts. However, the biochemical defect may be more complicated, as aryl sulphatase is also deficient. For diagnostic purposes, the increased levels of the substrate cholesterol sulphate can be detected easily by serum lipoprotein electrophoresis.

Bullous ichthyosiform erythroderma

This autosomal dominant defect is fortunately rare (1:100 000). The skin is clearly abnormal at birth being odiferous, red, moist and eroded in parts. Over the subsequent few months the erythema lessens to be replaced by large scales which are particularly thick in the flexures. A biopsy reveals vacuolization of the cells in the upper prickle and the thickened granular cell layers with overlying hyperkeratosis, hence the alternative name favoured in the U.S.A. of epidermolytic hyperkeratosis.

Non-bullous ichthyosiform erythroderma

This autosomal recessive disease is equally rare. At birth, the picture is of 'collodion baby'. If this gives way to variable redness and thickening of the skin, fine whitish scales, universal involvement including face and flexures and mild palmar and plantar keratoderma, this diagnosis is very likely. Ectropion may be present. Histologically there is acanthosis but no hyperkeratosis.

Lamellar ichthyosis

This rare autosomal recessive condition is also likely to be present at birth as 'collodion baby' giving way to persistent large dark scales with little or no erythema. Palmoplantar keratoderma is marked.

Refsum's syndrome

This rare autosomal recessive disease is characterized by progressive visual impairment due to retinitis pigmentosa, peripheral neuritis, cataracts, cerebellar ataxia and ichthyosis. It is eventually fatal.

Excess phytanic acid can be demonstrated in the triglyceride fraction of the serum lipids and other tissues. The disease is due to deficiency of a single enzyme involved in hydroxylation of phytanate.

Management of the ichthyoses

Minor forms of ichthyosis demand only regular use of emollients and moisturizing creams. Treatment should always be simple, cheap and cosmetically acceptable. Creams containing urea (e.g. Calmurid, U.K.) may be valuable.

Ichthyosiform erythroderma in the neonate calls for skilled paediatric intensive care. Thermoregulation is grossly disturbed and fluid loss through the skin may be massive. Later in childhood, etretinate and acetretin may have a role in very severe forms but the long-term skeletal effects of the retinoids are causing concern.

Incontinentia Pigmenti

This rare disorder is either autosomal dominant or X-linked, and is fatal in male fetuses, being seen almost exclusively in girls. The first manifestations are cutaneous, lesions evolving through several stages.

Stage 1. Within the first 2 weeks of life a symmetrical eruption of vesicles and pustules appears on the limbs, often with linear or whorled patterning. It lasts for weeks or months. The scalp may be involved, leading to cicatricial alopecia. There is no fever or malaise but there may be early blood eosinophilia.

Stage 2. The vesicles may give way to warty papules most marked distally, i.e. on the dorsa of the hands or feet. Over several months the lesions disappear.

Stage 3. The first two stages always give way to highly characteristic whorled or 'swirling' patterns of macular brown or blue–grey pigmentation on the trunk or limbs. This reaches its peak in the second year and then fades away over many years.

Stage 4. Streaky depigmentation, especially on the calves, may remain in older children and adults as a marker of the disease.

Systemic manifestations

Various neurological sequelae include epilepsy and mental handicap of varying degrees. Eye abnormalities include squint, cataract, optic atrophy and retinal damage. Various dental anomalies are common, including 'peg-teeth' and delayed dentition. Rarely, cardiac and skeletal abnormalities are seen.

The mother and other female family members should be examined for stigmata and genetic counselling is essential.

Focal Dermal Hypoplasia

This rare disorder is seen only in females. Streaky erythematous, linear and sometimes atrophic patches are characteristic. Other features include soft, floppy 'spaniel ears', 'lobster claw' deformities of the limbs and bony changes. Prenatal detection by ultrasound is now possible. The histology of the skin shows absence or hypoplasia of dermal components, and fat herniations into the skin.

Genodermatoses with Photosensitivity

Several genetic syndromes share disabilities of DNA repair mechanisms, rendering the patient sensitive to light or to mutagenic chemicals.

Xeroderma pigmentosum

In this rare but fascinating disease there is a failure of DNA repair mechanisms which are normally constantly vigilant, repairing DNA damage throughout the body, however induced. Ultraviolet light is perhaps the most important damager, so that skin bears the brunt of the disease. Photosensitivity may begin in infancy and striking freckling of exposed skin is seen in early childhood. Carcinogenesis eventually follows and, in severe forms, multiple cutaneous malignancies are seen in childhood and adolescence leading to early death. There may also be deafness and other neurological abnormalities. Depending on the precise error in DNA excision–repletion, several forms are now recognized.

The disease can now be diagnosed prenatally by study of DNA repair in cells obtained by amniocentesis.

Bloom's syndrome

This autosomal recessive syndrome is characterized by facial erythema and telangiectasia, immune abnormalities and a predisposition to malignancy.

Congenital poikiloderma (Rothmund–Thomson syndrome)

This is a rare autosomal recessive disorder characterized by early onset of poikiloderma (atrophy, telangiectasia and pigmentation), especially on the cheeks, sparse eyebrows and lashes, short stature, juvenile cataracts, photosensitivity and sometimes bony, endocrine and dental defects and mental retardation.

Epidermolysis Bullosa

This name encompasses at least 16 genetically distinct congenital blistering skin disorders. These can be simply grouped as in Table 14.5.

Epidermolysis bullosa simplex

The blisters form as a result of cytolysis in the basal epidermal cells. The disease is often mild and localized, for example to the palms and soles, but severe generalized variants occur. The teeth and nails are unaffected. With time, the blistering may improve spontaneously.

Junctional epidermolysis bullosa

Dermoepidermal separation occurs in the lamina

Table 14.5 Main types of epidermolysis bullosa*.

Type	Inheritance
Epidermolysis bullosa simplex	Dominant
Junctional epidermolysis bullosa	Recessive
Epidermolysis bullosa dystrophica	Dominant
Epidermolysis bullosa dystrophica	Recessive

*An acquired type of epidermolysis bullosa in adults is now known to be the result of an autoimmune reaction to Type VII collagen in the dermis.

lucida. Some forms are quickly lethal but less severe variants are now recognized.

Dominant dystrophic epidermolysis bullosa

Clinical severity is variable but scarring may occur, sometimes with milia formation. Nails and mucosae may be affected. Electron microscopy shows separation deep to the basal lamina, with reduced and abnormal anchoring fibrils. In one variant (Pasini type), increased synthesis of sulphated glycosaminoglycan has been demonstrated in cultured fibroblasts.

Recessive dystrophic epidermolysis bullosa

This scarring type is commoner than the dystrophic dominant variety but separation is at the same level. Increased and abnormal collagenase activity has been demonstrated in dermal fibroblasts. Epanutin, which inhibits collagenase synthesis, may be of therapeutic value.

Genodermatoses Involving Vascular Tissue

Hereditary haemorrhagic telangiectasia (Osler's disease)

This is an autosomal dominant disorder. Onset is in adolescence or early adult life and epistaxis may be the presenting symptom. Multiple punctate telangiectases develop on the skin of the head and upper body and on the mucosae of the mouth (Fig. 14.4), nose and eyes, as well as throughout the gastrointestinal tract. Pulmonary arteriovenous anastomoses and other major vascular defects can occur.

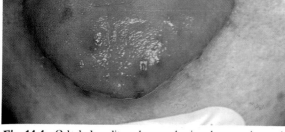

Fig. 14.4 Osler's hereditary haemorrhagic telangectasia; angiomata of tongue.

Angiokeratoma corporis diffusum (Anderson–Fabry disease)

This is a rare sex-linked disorder of sphingolipid metabolism seen mainly in males which leads to the deposition of glycolipid in small blood vessels in the skin and viscera. Multiple minute telangiectatic maculopapules appear in adolescence, particularly on the lower trunk and thighs. These are associated with episodes of excruciating pain in the extremities. Hypertension, coronary artery disease and renal failure may follow, causing early death from vascular accident or renal failure.

Ectodermal Dysplasias

These are disorders with a primary defect of ectodermal tissues, i.e. skin, hair, nails, sweat glands, etc. The best known is *hypohidrotic ectodermal dysplasia*, an X-linked recessive disorder characterized by absence of sweat glands, hypotrichosis and anodontia. The facies is distinctive.

Kyrle–Flegel disease

This is an uncommon but interesting genodermatosis which presents only in middle life, usually in women. A widespread, chronic papular eruption, partly follicular, consists of cone-shaped hyperkeratotic plugs, particularly involving the legs. The palms and soles are not involved.

Darier's disease (keratosis follicularis)

This fairly rare condition is inherited as an autosomal dominant trait with variable penetrance. Multiple yellow–brown crusted papules develop (Fig. 14.5), especially in flexures and 'seborrhoeic' areas. In severe cases, confluent, papillomatous malodorous masses of lesions form. Characteristic minute palmar pits are seen, as well as punctate keratoses. The fingernails are dystrophic and split, with longitudinal bands and jagged 'nicked' free ends. Onset is usually in the second decade. The course is chronic but the severity fluctuates. Mild cases require only emollients but in more severe disease etretinate 0.25–1.0 mg/kg daily is invaluable.

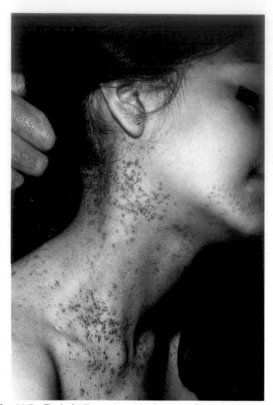

Fig. 14.5   Darier's disease in an adolescent Indian girl.

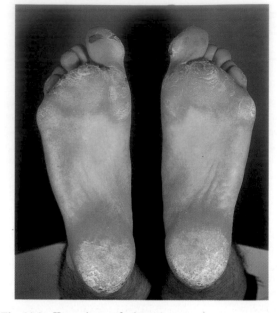

Fig. 14.6   Keratoderma of soles.

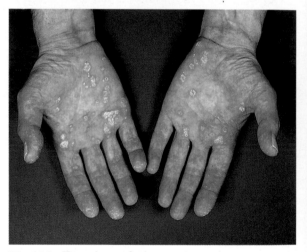

Fig. 14.7   Keratoderma of palms.

Keratoderma of palms or soles

Gross persistent hyperkeratosis of the palms and soles may be an inherited dominant or recessive trait. Persistent palmoplantar erythema in infancy may herald skin thickening. Sometimes the insteps and central palms are spared (Figs. 14.6 and 14.7). Punctate patterns may be seen.

— 15

Sunlight and the Skin

Apart from the eyes, the skin is the only organ exposed to the sun's radiation. The acute, subacute and chronic effects of light, alone or in combination with environmental chemicals, are described briefly.

Photobiology

The solar spectrum extends continuously from 250–3000 nm. It is divided into zones (Table 15.1). Ultraviolet C (UVC) is absorbed entirely by the earth's atmosphere, which is fortunate as it would be lethally damaging to our DNA. Much greater quantities of ultraviolet A (UVA) than ultraviolet B (UVB) are received by our skin, expecially in winter. Most of this UVA penetrates the epidermis to reach the dermis and beyond.

Ultraviolet B intensity increases with altitude. It is greatest in mid-summer and at mid-day. Ultraviolet B penetrates cirrhus cloud so that sunburn can occur on a cloudy day. Most UVB (80%) is absorbed by the stratum corneum but 20% reaches the viable epidermis and perhaps 10% reaches the dermis.

Light, including ultraviolet, can be reflected from the ground, intensifying its effects. Thus clean snow reflects 80%, sand perhaps 20% and water about 5%.

The cutaneous barrier

The keratinocytes of the stratum corneum, whilst mainly a physicochemical barrier (see Chapter 1), have a limited light-filtering effect. The main barrier to ultraviolet light is melanin, derived from melanocytes

Table 15.1 The solar spectrum.

Component	Wavelength range (nm)
Ultraviolet C (UVC)	< 290
Ultraviolet B (UVB)	290–320
Ultraviolet A (UVA)	320–400
Visible light	400–800
Infrared	> 800

(see Chapter 21). The keratinocytes of normal stratum corneum are packed with melanin granules.

The Biological Effects of Light on Skin

These can be divided into immediate, short-term and long-term effects (Table 15.2). Immediate pigmentation is due to photo-oxidation of melanin precursors. It fades in a few hours. Ultraviolet B also converts 7-dihydrocholesterol to vitamins D_2 and D_3 in the epidermis.

Sunburn

In sufficient dose UVB always causes erythema; the threshold dose is called the minimal erythema dose (MED) and is a useful parameter. Higher doses progressively cause oedema, blistering, severe itching and systemic symptoms. Itching and exfoliation accompany recovery. These effects begin 2–12 hours after exposure, according to dosage.

Prevention of sunburn requires graduated increasing exposures daily to allow protective tanning and stratum corneum thickening, the use of ultraviolet-

Table 15.2 Effects of light on skin.

Immediate	Thermal vasodilation
	Pigmentation
	Vitamin D synthesis
Short-term	Erythema (sunburn)
	Delayed pigmentation
	Epidermal hyperplasia
	Immunological suppression
Long-term	Ageing
	Melanocyte damage
	Carcinogenesis

blocking cosmetics and awareness of likely UVB exposure according to season, time of day and circumstances.

Delayed pigmentation

Melanogenesis is activated by UVA and UVB. It
begins after 2–3 days and peaks at 10 days. In Celtic
skin phaeomelanin is formed, which has little ultra-
violet-screening value and is quickly degraded. In
darker-skinned Caucasians eumelanin is formed which
absorbs UV and is thus protective.

Epidermal hyperplasia

This begins after 3–4 days causing thickening of
stratum corneum. It is less important than eumelanin
formation.

Immunological suppression

Epidermal Langerhans' cells are altered by UVB radiation and their immune functions suppressed, so that
allergic contact dermatitis is less likely to occur.

Ageing

Most (but not all) of the changes in the skin everyone
recognizes as 'ageing' actually occur on exposed skin
and are due to cumulative ultraviolet-induced damage
and not simply to the passage of the years. These
changes include dermal atrophy (loss of collagen), loss
of elasticity (solar elastosis), 'senile' purpura (increased
vulnerability of dermal venules to minor trauma
because of collagen loss) and epidermal atrophy.

Melanocyte damage

Eventually, irreversible damage to basal melanocytes
leads to patchy hyperpigmented marks (actinic lentigo)
and areas of diffuse hyper- or hypopigmentation on
exposed sites.

Carcinogenesis

The time course of photocarcinogenesis is measured in
years and decades. A fair, especially Celtic skin, outdoor work or lifestyle and residence in the tropics all
add to the hazards. Probably DNA repair mechanisms
are progressively damaged but reduced immune
responses may play a part. Ultraviolet B is the principal carcinogen but UVA may be a co-carcinogen.

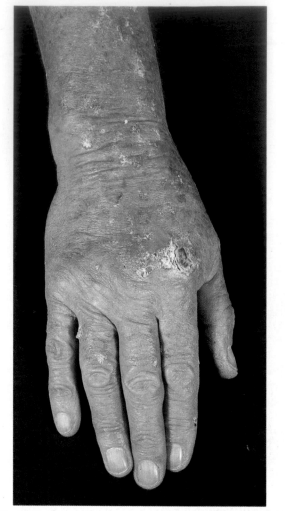

Fig. 15.1 Gross actinic keratosis in white skin after a lifetime in
the tropics.

Epidermal dysplasia is usually the first change,
causing actinic keratoses. White men who have led an
outdoor life in the tropics may have confluent masses
of keratoses on all exposed areas (Fig. 15.1). These
lesions are premalignant although the rate of conversion to squamous carcinoma is very low—perhaps one
per thousand per year. In addition, there is unequivocal evidence that cumulative ultraviolet exposure is of
central importance in the genesis of basal and squamous carcinoma, and of malignant melanoma.

The photodermatoses

These are skin diseases caused wholly or partly by

sunlight or artificial sources of similar radiation. Sun-beds and lamps and even ordinary white fluorescent tube lamps play an important role in inducing these diseases. Before describing the main syndromes, some important terms must be defined.

Photosensitization. This is the abnormal reaction to light (ultraviolet or visible) induced in the skin by a specific chemical 'photosensitizer' which absorbs particular wavelengths of light energy. The photo-sensitizer may be endogenous (e.g. porphyrins) or exogenous (by skin contact), for example industrial chemicals, cosmetics or in plants.

Phototoxicity. This is the damage induced in skin directly by the dissipation of energy absorbed by a photosensitizing molecule. No immunological mechanisms are involved. The morphological responses are diverse.

Photoallergy. This is the result of a cell-mediated immune response to a light-activated or light modified antigen.

Table 15.3 Drug-induced photosensitivity.

Phototoxic drugs	Tetracyclines
	Sulphonamides
	Chlorpromazine
	Amiodarone
	Psoralens
	Nalidixic acid
	Frusemide
Photoallergic drugs	Chlorpromazine
	Sulphonamide
	Halogenated salicylanilides
Drug-induced or -exacerbated disease	Porphyria
	Lupus erythematosus

Drug-Induced Photosensitivity

The main offenders are summarized in Table 15.3. A number of well-known drugs are phototoxic and each tends to induce its own pattern of disease. Thus tetracyclines tend to induce exaggerated sunburn reactions but may cause separation of the finger nails (photo-onycholysis). Sulphonamides can cause blistering reactions, as may nalidixic acid and (in high dosage) frusemide. Psoralens cause delayed-onset erythema and pigmentation (see PUVA therapy, p. 106). Amiodarone induces pigmentation as well as erythema. Benoxaprofen (now withdrawn) caused striking photo-onycholysis and bizarre immediate burning sensations in the skin.

The responsible wavelength (usually a UVA band) can be identified by monochromator studies. It is called the *action spectrum*. Interestingly, it may not correspond to the maximal *absorption spectrum* of the drug in vitro. One possible explanation is the intervention of a drug metabolite of different absorbance. Thus etretinate is not phototoxic but its metabolite, acetretin, is. Phenothiazine antihistamines (e.g. promethazine hydrochloride; Phenergan, U.K.), sulphonamides, halogenated salicylanilides (used as bacteriostats in soaps) and certain perfumes such as musk ambrette (in male toiletries) are potent photo-allergens.

The most important phototoxic chemicals are coal tar derivatives, certain dyes and plant-derived psoralens. Well-recognized clinical patterns of photo-contact sensitivity include phytophotodermatitis and Berlocque dermatitis.

Phytophotodermatitis

This is a striking linear, vesicular or bullous dermatitis of the limbs typically seen in children in summer after playing in weedy, grassy meadows. Psoralens occur naturally in many plants, especially the Umbelliferae, Rutaceae and Moraceae families. They are present in many plants sold as greengrocery and an outbreak of phytophotodermatitis has been described in celery handlers whose employer provided a recreational UVA-sunbed salon.

Berlocque dermatitis

This is a characteristic pattern of erythema followed by pigmentation, usually with an artefactual streaky pattern seen on the neck of women and due to photo-toxic perfumes containing psoralens (e.g. oil of bergamot) (Fig. 15.2).

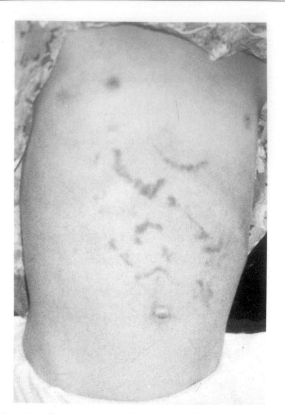

Fig. 15.2   Berlocque dermatitis; streaky artefactual pigmentation on belly of a child who spilled her mother's perfume, smeared her belly and then went in strong sunlight.

Glycine + Succinyl CoA

↓ ALA synthetase

Δ-Aminolaevulic acid (Δ-ALA)

↓ PBG synthetase

Porphobilinogen (PBG)
↓ UPG III synthetase
↓ UPG cosynthetase

8 COOH   Uroporphyrinogen III (UPG III)

↓ UPG decarboxylase

4 COOH   Coproporphyrinogen III

↓ CPG oxidase

2 COOH   Protoporphyrinogen IX (PPG IX)

↓ PPG oxidase

Protoporphyrin IX

Fe   ↓ Ferrochelatase

Haem

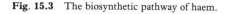

Fig. 15.3   The biosynthetic pathway of haem.

Light-Aggravated Metabolic Diseases

Porphyrias

The tetrapyrrolic porphyrin ring is capable of binding many metals. It binds ferrous iron as haem, which is central in all biological oxidation reactions. It binds magnesium as chlorophyll, on which solar energy utilization by plants depends.

The porphyrias are a group of disorders characterized by abnormalities in the biosynthetic pathway leading to production of haem (Fig. 15.3). As a result of various enzyme deficiencies, haem precursors (called porphyrins) accumulate in the bone marrow or liver and reach other organs via the bloodstream. They are particularly toxic in the central nervous system and are phototoxic in skin. Porphyrins have an absorption spectrum centred on 400 nm and this is precisely the action spectrum capable of inducing the abnormal responses in these patients. The abnormal quantities of porphyrins can be detected and measured in urine, faeces, plasma and red cells. Δ-ALA and porphobi-

linogen are not phototoxic so skin is unaffected in acute intermittent porphyria. Uro-, copro- and proto-porphyrins are phototoxic. The important porphyrias affecting skin are now briefly described.

Erythropoietic protoporphyria

Erythropoietic protoporphyria is inherited as a Mendelian autosomal dominant trait with very variable clinical expression. A deficiency of the enzyme ferrochelatase leads to an accumulation of protoporphyrin IX. Typically the disease begins in childhood. Light exposure causes immediate burning sensations in the exposed skin which becomes reddened and sometimes blistered. Eventually, characteristic thickening and scarring are seen on the nose, face and hands (Fig. 15.4). The diagnosis is confirmed by detection of excess protoporphyrin in red cells and plasma. Beta-carotene given orally is helpful in treatment.

Porphyria cutanea tarda

In this far from rare disease, a deficiency of uroporphyrinogen decarboxylase leads to an accumulation of uroporphyrinogen III. The abnormality can be acquired, particularly as a result of alcohol-induced liver disease or, rarely, may be inherited. The

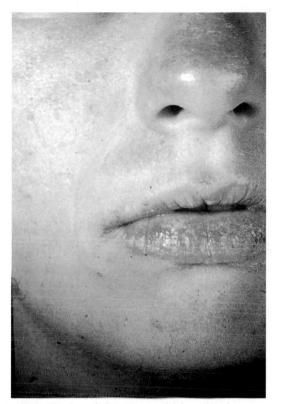

Fig. 15.4 Erythropoietic protoporphyria; chronic cutaneous changes.

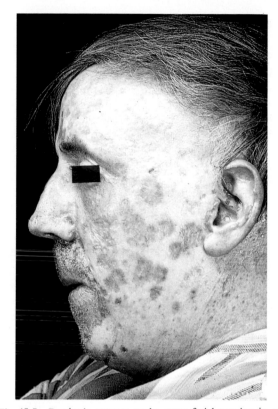

Fig. 15.5 Porphyria cutanea tarda; gross facial scarring in an outdoor worker.

cutaneous clinical picture is characteristic, with sun-induced blisters on the backs of the hands, healing with scarring (sometimes of bizarre pattern; Fig. 15.5), increased fragility of exposed skin, hypertrichosis, scarring alopecia and sometimes a scleroderma-like change in exposed skin. Porphyria cutanea tarda is seen in adult life and is occasionally precipitated in young women by oral contraceptives. Diagnosis requires the demonstration of increased plasma and urinary uroporphyrins and abnormal liver function. Iron metabolism is abnormal, with excess tissue stores.

Repeated venesections (500 ml every 14 days) lead to prolonged clinical and biochemical remission but repeated treatment may be necessary. Low dose oral chloroquine (200 mg twice weekly) is also safe and effective. Clearly, alcohol must be withdrawn.

Variegate porphyria

This autosomal dominant disease is very common in South Africans of Afrikaaner stock and all cases in South Africa have been reliably traced to a marriage in the Cape in the early 17th century. The disease is rare elsewhere in the world. It is due to a deficiency of the mitochondrial enzyme, protoporphyrin oxidase. The clinical picture combines the cutaneous features of porphyria cutanea tarda with the neuropsychiatric features of acute intermittent porphyria. The latter are particularly likely to be induced by certain drugs, for example barbiturates.

Pellagra

This common nutritional disease is due to dietary nicotinic acid deficiency but is occasionally induced by drugs, for example hydantoins or isoniazid. The triad of dermatitis, diarrhoea and dementia constitute classical severe pellagra. The rash is typically in light-exposed areas, especially about the neck, but may affect areas subjected to friction or pressure. Peripheral neuropathy may occur.

Hartnup disease

Pellagra-like photosensitivity and cerebellar ataxia are due to an autosomal recessive abnormality of tryptophan metabolism.

Idiopathic Photodermatoses

Polymorphic light eruption

This mysterious common disease of adults, commoner in women, is strictly confined to some or all exposed areas where itching erythematous papules and plaques develop within hours of solar exposure. In the severely affected it may be a problem throughout the summer. In others of higher threshold the disease constantly recurs on the first or second day of a holiday in the sun and clears within 2 or 3 days of the end of the holiday. Continuously exposed areas, such as the face and hands, may be 'hardened' and unaffected. The disorder tends to persist throughout life.

Investigation with an artificial light source (monochromator) reveals abnormal responses to UVB and sometimes to UVA.

Treatment

Sun protection and use of sunscreens are mandatory. Chloroquine or hydroxychloroquine (Plaquenil, U.K.), two tablets daily, have a photoprotective effect and may be given for up to 3 weeks to tide the patient over a holiday but are unsafe for use throughout the summer. Alternatively, the skin can be 'hardened' by a 3–6-week course of UVB or PUVA each spring.

Actinic prurigo

This rare disease of children and adolescents, known as Hutchinson's summer prurigo, is characterized by a chronic papular and nodular lichenification (prurigo) and intense itching. It is worse in summer and in exposed areas but may not disappear in winter, and sometimes lesions are seen on covered areas, for example the buttocks. It may disappear by adolescence.

Chronic actinic dermatitis

This uncommon disease (actinic reticuloid) typically affects men in the second half of life. Photosensitivity supervenes insidiously on a chronic dermatitis not particularly found in exposed areas. Papules and plaques form until the skin is grossly thickened. A universal erythroderma may supervene. Itching and discomfort are gross, and victims have been driven to suicide. The histology is of 'dermatitis' but with gross lymphohistiocytic ('reticuloid') dermal infiltrate. Monochromatic studies demonstrate photosensitivity throughout the ultraviolet and visible spectrum. Patch testing and photopatch testing may reveal contact or photocontact sensitivity to a plant oleoresin or a cosmetic ingredient such as musk ambrette in aftershave lotion. Whether such sensitivities are causative is controversial.

Treatment

Total avoidance of sunlight in a specially darkened room may be necessary, with extreme care out of doors. Topical steroids help and oral prednisolone may be needed. Azathioprine and PUVA 'hardening' are sometimes useful.

Solar urticaria

Rarely, urticaria can be induced by ultraviolet or visible wavelengths. It appears within minutes of exposure and settles in 1–2 hours in the shade. Urticaria may be a feature of erythropoietic protoporphyria and this must be excluded.

Diseases Aggravated by Sunlight

Lupus erythematosus is the most important. Sun exposure can aggravate both systemic and discoid lupus and can precipitate systemic disease. Light is one of the well-known triggers of herpes simplex on the face. Rosacea is often sun-aggravated. A minority of psoriatics are worsened by sun, suffering summer exacerbations in exposed areas.

External Photoprotection

Sunscreens reflect and disperse ultraviolet light by virtue of their inert powder content. Inevitably, the thicker the opaque powder layer the poorer is their cosmetic acceptability.

Sun filters absorb ultraviolet before it reaches the skin. Molecular manipulation may allow different wavelengths to be absorbed preferentially. Clearly, a satisfactory sun filter must be stable, non-irritating, non-allergenic and cosmetically pleasant.

Sun protection factors

These must be considered separately for UVB and UVA. For UVB, the protection factor can be determined simply by measuring the ratio of the minimal erythema dose (MED) with and without the agent under test. Complicated reference standards have been laid down by American (FDA) and German (DIN) regulatory authorities.

Assessing UVA protection is more complicated and has to involve quantitation of the immediate pigmentation phenomenon (see p. 123) or of a phototoxic response using oral psoralen.

Some of the main chemicals used as ultraviolet filters are shown in Table 15.4. Each has its own absorption spectrum. The best preparations combine UVB and UVA filters, if necessary with an opaque sunscreen added.

Table 15.4 Widely used ultraviolet filters.

Various esters of *para*-aminobenzoic acid (PABA)
Benzophenone
Cinnamate
Salicylate esters
Dibenzoyl methane

Vascular Disorders

These are numerous and defy rational classification. In this Chapter they are described in four main groups:
- The erythemas and other small-vessel disorders
- The vasculitides: small- and large-vessel arterial disease
- Venous disease in the leg
- Urticaria and angioedema

The Erythemas and Other Small-Vessel Disorders

Table 16.1 summarizes the erythemas and other small-vessel disorders.

Erythema

Erythema is redness due to vascular dilatation. Often it is macular but erythematous lesions will be palpable if there is accompanying dermal oedema (urtication) or cellular infiltration. It may be very transient, as in flushing, or last hours, days or much longer according to its cause. Many acute or subacute erythemas are due to microbial or drug antigens ('toxic erythema'). Such erythemas may resemble those of scarlet fever ('scarlatiniform'), measles ('morbilliform') or German measles ('rubelliform'). Occasionally, ringed patterns evolve centrifugally over weeks or months, for example the 'erythema chronicum migrans' of Lyme

Table 16.1 The erythemas and other small-vessel disorders.

Toxic erythema	Erythema ab igne
Flushing	Livedo reticularis
Telangiectasia	Raynaud's phenomenon
Venous stars	Perniosis (chilblains)
Spider naevi	Erythema nodosum
Purpura	Erythema multiforme
Capillaritis	Erythema induratum

borreliosis. In 'liver palms' the erythema may be fixed for years.

Flushing

Flushing is caused by *very* transient vasodilatation, usually of the face, ears, neck and upper trunk. It is a physiological response to overheating, exercise, embarrassment or other emotions, the latter especially in young women. Alcohol and other drugs, for example vasodilators such as amyl nitrate, may be responsible. Its occurrence in the menopause is well known. It may be a feature of various diseases including rosacea (p. 174), carcinoid syndrome and, rarely, phaeochromocytoma.

Telangiectasia

This is a fixed dilatation of dermal venules. It is a feature of rosacea, radiodermatitis, chronic actinic damage and excessive exposure to potent corticosteroids. Affecting larger venules, it is common on the legs in adult females, especially on the lower leg but sometimes on the thigh and lower back ('venous stars').

In spider naevi, an arteriole and its downstream capillaries are in fixed dilatation. Up to nine or ten may be seen in normal people, always on the face, neck or upper limbs. More may appear in pregnancy or in chronic liver disease.

Deft cauterization of the central vessel is possible without local anaesthesia. Telangiectasia is important in systemic sclerosis (p. 145) and in the inherited Osler's disease (p. 121), where the 3–4-mm red macules on the lips and tongue may provide the clue to the cause of epistaxes or a haematemesis.

Purpura

This blue–red macular discoloration of the skin is due to leakage of red cells out of small blood vessels. It may be due to faults in the blood itself or in the capillaries or perivascular collagen. 'Senile' and 'steroid' purpura are due to ultraviolet and steroid-induced dermal atrophy, respectively. The loss of 'lagging' around dermal venules allows easy tearing by any trauma. The exposed backs of hands, wrists, forearm and neck are the usual sites, since here the effects of ultraviolet light and oral or topical steroids will summate. This type of purpura may persist for many weeks because of poor inflammatory tissue response and weak phagocytosis in the elderly and steroid-treated. Chronic venous hypertension in the lower legs due to valvular incompetence or destruction often causes chronic purpura. The golden-brown colour of the lower leg skin is due to a mixture of fresh purpura and haemosiderosis derived from it (p. 136).

Capillaritis

Capillary leakage produces a characteristic punctate purpura. It may be due to infections, for example meningococcal septicaemia, or drugs. Dysproteinaemias may be responsible. Idiopathic capillaritis on the legs is occasionally seen.

Vascular Abnormalities Related to Heat or Cold

Erythema ab igne

This is a heat-induced reticular pattern of erythema and eventually pigmentation, typically seen on the anterolateral legs of women exposed to open fires or electric radiators. It occurs on the trunk if a hot water bottle is constantly held against the body to relieve pain, a sign which may indicate important internal disease.

Livedo reticularis

This is a characteristic pattern of cyanosis due to reduced arteriolar flow and consequent sluggish skin circulation. In its physiological form, due to cold, it is best observed on the thighs of senior British schoolgirls playing hockey in shorts on winter afternoons. A similar appearance can be caused by cutaneous arteriolitis (see p. 134).

Raynaud's phenomenon

Raynaud's phenomenon is virtually confined to the fingers where cold-induced arterial constriction induces pallor, cyanosis and, on warming, a reactive erythema. It may be physiological and life-long in some women but pathological causes include occupa-

tional trauma (pneumatic drills) or chemical exposure (vinyl chloride), drugs (e.g. beta blockers or ergotamines), arterial obstruction and systemic sclerosis. It predisposes to chronic paronychia. Nifedipine orally is of value.

Chilblains

In the United Kingdom, chilblains (perniosis) were extremely common up to 30 years ago. Since then, rising standards of living, improved social conditions and particularly the spread of central heating have made the condition very uncommon. In countries with much colder winters, such as the United States or Sweden, adequate heating had almost abolished perniosis much earlier. Chilblains are painful, itching, dark red swellings, typically seen on the fingers or toes. Less often, the lower calves can be affected (Fig. 16.1), especially in young women with plump legs. Miniskirts, when in fashion, may be responsible for

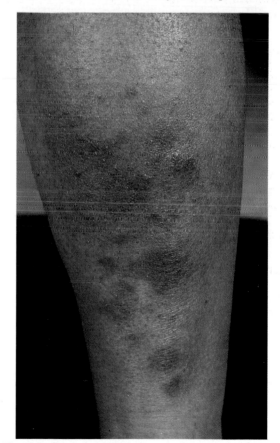

Fig. 16.1 Perniosis (chilblains) on the lower calves of a young woman. The lesions look inflamed but are cold to the touch.

chilblains on the upper outer thighs of fat girls, and stable-girls who exercise horses on cold winter mornings may have the same pattern, despite their riding trousers. Lesions may persist for weeks and occasionally ulcerate. Diagnosis is easy. To the touch, all inflammation is hot except chilblains which feel cold.

Erythema Nodosum

This is an uncommon, subacute, usually bilateral, tender painful erythematous nodular eruption, typically seen on the upper anterior and mid-shins in young adults, usually women (Fig. 16.2). Lesions may also occur lower on the leg laterally and, in florid examples, on the thighs and arms. When 'acute' the condition may be accompanied by fever and arthralgia. The nodules are diffuse, blue–red and fade over a few weeks, sometimes leaving bruising. They never ulcerate. The sedimentation rate is raised.

Drugs, especially sulphonamides, and sarcoidosis

(p. 33) are the commonest causes today but various infections, especially streptococcal and primary tuberculosis, can be responsible. A florid disseminated form may occur in leprosy (p. 200). It is probably an immunological reaction.

Differential diagnosis is from nodular vasculitis, superficial thrombophlebitis, perniosis, etc. A careful drug history, throat swab, blood count and chest radiograph are usually sufficient investigations to reveal the cause. Rest and analgesics are the essential treatment.

Erythema Multiforme

This is a dramatic hypersensitivity reaction, induced by infections or drugs. A bilateral, peripheral, symmetrical eruption affects hands and arms, legs and feet. Often lesions are clustered on the extensor aspects of the knees and elbows. The lesions are multiform, well-defined erythematous discs, often with marginal urtication, purpura and sometimes central necrosis leading to blistering. So called 'target' lesions are characteristic (Fig. 16.3).

In its severe forms, mucosae and mucocutaneous junctions are involved (Fig. 16.4), especially the mouth, lips, conjunctival margins and penile meatus. When fulminant the eruption becomes generalized, shades into toxic epidermal necrolysis and mucosal involvement may spread down the oesophagus and trachea. There may be renal involvement, secondary pneumonia and a fatal outcome. Usually, however, the process is self-limiting and heals spontaneously in 2–4 weeks. Recurrent erythema multiforme is not uncommon.

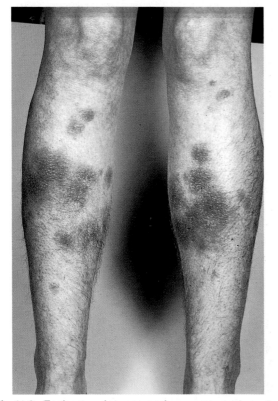

Fig. 16.2 Erythema nodosum; note the symmetry and anterior location. Perniosis never occurs at this site.

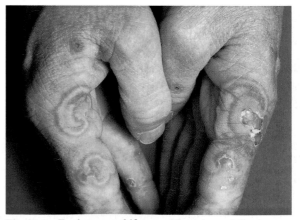

Fig. 16.3 Erythema multiforme; bilateral, peripheral, symmetrical.

Responsible infections include *Herpes simplex* and (in rural areas) orf. Streptococcal infection may be responsible, as may mycoplasma and other organisms. Many drugs have been implicated, amongst which penicillins, sulphonamides, barbiturates and piroxicam are the most important.

Treatment

Simple applications and mouth toilet may suffice for mild attacks. At the other end of the spectrum, fulminant attacks may necessitate the facilities of an intensive treatment unit. Given early, prednisolone, 60 mg daily initially, is valuable in severe attacks but is of little value if started later. The dose is reduced to zero over 3 weeks.

Erythema Induratum (Bazin's Disease)

This is now a rare disease in which painful, tender inflammatory nodules develop typically in the calves and may ulcerate. It is a hypersensitivity reaction to mycobacterial (tuberculosis) antigens. Histologically a nodular vasculitis is seen. A strongly positive tuberculin reaction at 1:10 000 and rapid and complete response to tuberculostatic drugs permit this diagnosis whether or not an active tuberculous focus is found.

Small-Vessel Arterial Disease

A summary is given in Table 16.2.

Table 16.2 The vasculitides: small- and large-vessel arterial disease.

Small vessel	Large vessel
Leucocytoclastic vasculitis	Atherosclerosis
Systemic lupus erythematosus	Buerger's disease
Polyarteritis nodosa	Kawasaki disease
Chronic cutaneous polyarteritis	
Livedo reticularis	
Nodular vasculitis	
Rheumatoid arteritis	
Temporal arteritis	
Wegener's granulomatosis	

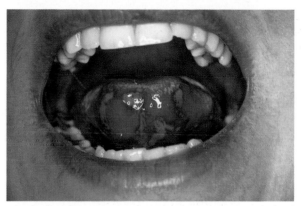

Fig. 16.4 Erythema multiforme; involvement of tongue.

Leucocytoclastic vasculitis

This is an acute chronic or recurring eruption typically seen in the legs and characterized by erythematous, purpuric and sometimes pustular, necrotic or papular lesions (Fig. 16.5). Malaise is slight and mucosae are

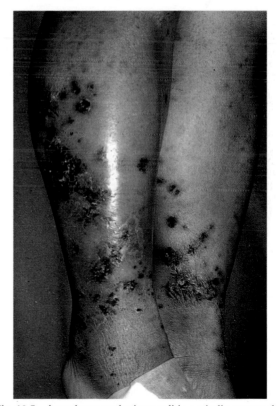

Fig. 16.5 Acute leucocytoclastic vasculitis, typically seen on the legs.

not affected. Drugs, infections or dysproteinaemias can be responsible but often no cause can be found. The histopathology is characteristic with necrotizing venulitis, perivascular infiltrate, fragmented polymorphs ('leucocytoclasia') and purpura. Immune complex deposition in small vessels may be responsible, and renal involvement with proteinuria and haematuria can occur. When this pattern of vasculitis occurs in children, associated with arthritis, enteritis and sometimes nephritis, it is sometimes called the Henoch–Schoenlein syndrome.

Mild attacks settle spontaneously. Severe episodes may require oral prednisolone 40 mg daily initially.

Systemic lupus erythematosus

Livedo reticularis, and ulceration, occasionally massive, may occur in systemic lupus erythematosus, fully described on p. 141.

Polyarteritis nodosa

Classical multisystem polyarteritis nodosa is rare but may be accompanied by cutaneous changes. These can include chronic urticaria, persistent erythematous urticated nodules and plaques (sometimes involving the mouth or lips), haemorrhagic papules or nodules, purpura and warty papules. Livedo reticularis is rare. Biopsy reveals a deep dermal arteritis with fibrinoid necrosis of vessel walls.

Chronic cutaneous polyarteritis

This uncommon syndrome has the histological features of polyarteritis nodosa but the disease remains confined to the skin, sometimes for many years. The main patterns seen are livedo reticularis and 'nodular vasculitis' in the legs. It is a disease of middle-aged women, and pain and swelling may be very troublesome. Long-term low dose prednisolone 5–10 mg daily may be required.

Livedo reticularis

Described earlier as a pattern of response to cold it may be due to cutaneous arteritis when fixed. Typically the feet and legs are involved and sometimes the upper limbs. Occasionally, ulceration or nodule formation accompanies the livedo. It may be part of the vasculitis of systemic lupus erythematosus, polyarteritis nodosa or chronic cutaneous polyarteritis. In Sneddon's syndrome, chronic livedo is associated with cerebrovascular disease and the presence of anticardiolipin antibodies.

Nodular vasculitis

Tender and sometimes painful hard inflammatory nodules can be palpated subcutaneously or deep in the skin, usually in the calves. Oedema is usual and the nodules may ulcerate. The disease is uncommon but chronic, and usually occurs in middle-aged women. Histologically the arteritis is in the deep dermis or in the fat. Management is difficult. Compression is important. Non-steroidal anti-inflammatory analgesics are often helpful, and occasionally dapsone or chloroquine seem to be useful. Severe pain, perhaps due to inflammation of vasa nervorum, may call for oral prednisolone. Often less than 10 mg daily will partly suppress the disease adequately. Sometimes azathioprine 50–100 mg daily has to be added and continued for years.

Rheumatoid arteritis

Very active nodular, seropositive rheumatoid arthritis may be accompanied by vasculitis, typically producing tiny haemorrhagic infarcts in the fingernail folds. Occasionally, nodular or ulcerated lesions affect the legs.

Temporal arteritis

This is an uncommon disease of elderly people. Cranial (mainly temporal) arteritis may produce local nodular inflammation and occasionally necrosis. Retinal arteritis may threaten blindness and 'polymyalgia rheumatica' may be associated. The sedimentation rate is raised. Prednisolone is the treatment of choice and a small permanent maintenance dose (2–5 mg daily) may be necessary.

Wegener's granulomatosis

Granulomatous and necrotizing arteritis, involving especially the upper respiratory tract, characterizes this rare and usually fatal disease. The kidneys, skin and other organs may be involved.

Large-Vessel Arterial Disease

The early diagnosis of peripheral arterial disease is of upmost importance, as stopping smoking tobacco,

Table 16.3 Risk factors implicated in peripheral arterial disease.

Cigarette smoking	Obesity
Hypertension	Family history
Diabetes mellitus	Physical inactivity
Hyperlipidaemia	Stress

control of hypertension or diabetes, weight reduction in the obese and reduction of hyperlipidemia may radically alter prognosis (Table 16.3).

Symptoms

Exertional leg pain, promptly relieved by rest (intermittent claudication), is often the first symptom. Occasionally rest pain, especially in bed, coldness of a foot, discoloration of a foot, discoloration of toes or nail dystrophy will be the presenting feature. Enquiry should be made for angina, diabetes, etc.

Physical signs

These are summarized in Table 16.4. Absence of peripheral pulses is central. Sometimes a weak dorsalis pedis or posterior tibial pulse will disappear if an ischaemic leg is exercised to claudication. Pallor may be obvious, especially on elevation of the leg to 45°. Delayed return of colour (≥ 10 seconds) after blanching of the pulp of the big toe by pressure is an unequivocal sign. If in doubt, this simple test can be repeated with the leg elevated. Cyanosis (rubor) on placing the leg in a dependent position is a late sign of gross disease. Auscultation for femoral or popliteal bruits should not be forgotten. In the male, loss of hair from the leg may be significant.

Table 16.4 Signs of peripheral arterial disease.

Absent or diminished peripheral pulses
Pallor of lower limb
Coldness of foot
Delayed filling after blanching a toe
Loss of hair
Bruits

Diagnosis

This depends on assessment of risk factors, symptoms and signs as described. Doppler ultrasound techniques confirm the diagnosis. Contrast arteriography is essential if vascular surgery is to be contemplated.

Differential diagnosis

The typical signs of venous disease are easily recognized (p. 136). Musculoskeletal pain may mimic claudication. Where ulceration is present, neuropathic and neoplastic causes must not be forgotten. The main causes of leg ulceration are listed in Table 16.5.

Atherosclerosis

Atheroma in the large vessels of a leg may eventually lead to thrombus formation and calcification, all contributing to narrowing of the vessel lumen. Conversely, media destruction may cause aneurysmal dilatation of the artery followed by thrombus formation and distal embolization.

Arterial emboli

Acute ischaemic pain with appearance of reticular livedo in the foot, followed by purpura and superficial ulceration, may be due to arterial embolization from an atheromatous plaque, for example in a popliteal aneurysm. The signs may mimic those of a local arteritis but other symptoms or signs of atheromatous disease, reduced or absent pulses, popliteal pulsation or an arterial bruit in the affected leg point to the diagnosis.

Table 16.5 Main causes of ulceration of a leg.

Chronic venous disease
Peripheral arterial disease—small and large vessel
Neoplastic—squamous or basal carcinoma, malignant melanoma
Neuropathic—diabetes, leprosy, etc
Haematological—e.g. sickle-cell disease
Acute coccal infection in diabetics and the immunosuppressed (ecthyma)
Chronic granulomatous infection—tuberculosis, gumma, deep mycoses

Buerger's disease

This is a rare disease of young men, invariably heavy smokers. As well as signs of arterial insufficiency, thrombophlebitis migrans may be a feature. Eventually, gangrene may require amputation of the limb.

Management of peripheral arterial disease

Attention to the risk factors is vital. Vasodilator and anticoagulant drugs are useless. Embolectomy may be needed in acute ischaemia. Reconstructive arterial surgery is possible in some patients and palliative sympathectomy, although usually disappointing, is worth trying in others. Smoking must be stopped.

Venous Disease in the Legs

Pathogenesis

The common mechanism is high venous pressure in the calf vein system. Previous deep vein thrombosis is the commonest cause, possibly decades earlier, provoked by prolonged bed rest, childbirth, surgical operations, trauma and occasionally the injection of sclerosants. Although thrombosed veins may eventually recanalize, the valves are permanently destroyed or damaged and become incompetent. Marginal valvular incompetence may be aggravated by obesity, arthritis or occupational stances which impair the efficiency of the calf muscle pump. Occasionally, valves may be congenitally incompetent.

The venous hypertension is transmitted backwards to the smallest venules and thus to the capillary bed. Increased capillary permeability follows, leading to oedema and accumulation of large molecules (particularly fibrinogen) in the tissues. If fibrinolysis is depressed, a pericapillary deposit of fibrin forms which impairs transfer of oxygen, nutrients, etc, out of capillaries, leading to cellular damage and necrosis. Chronic lymphoedema may follow.

Clinical picture

Most patients are over 40 years. In the elderly, the disease is commoner in women, probably because of postpartum deep vein thrombosis decades earlier. The presenting features may be any of the following (Table 16.6).
- Oedema, disappearing overnight initially, but eventually permanent. Progressive subcutaneous

Table 16.6 The six clinical features of chronic venous disease in a leg.

Oedema	Varicosities
Pigmentation	Ulceration
Dermatitis	White atrophy

fibrosis may harden the oedema and involve the fat (dermatoliposclerosis).
- Brown pigmentation of the lower calf skin due to deposits of haemosiderin, the result of chronic leakage of red cells from capillaries and a failure of the phagocytic system to clear the products of haemoglobin degradation. A mixture of fresh purpura and old haemosiderin may impart a golden-brown hue to the discoloration.
- Eczema (dermatitis) usually starts in the lower third of the calf and may gradually spread locally. Itching, scaling plaques may be exudative if acute or if provoked by irritant or allergenic applications. Secondary medicament-induced allergic contact dermatitis is common (see p. 87). With or without such sensitization, the eczema sometimes becoming disseminated, spreading to both legs and sometimes the arms or trunk.
- Varicose veins are variable. Sometimes gross varicosities of the saphenous system occur alone and may coexist with quite adequate venous return, in which case skin problems rarely arise. However, varicose veins may also indicate an incompetent deep venous or perforating vein system and a superficial collateral return pathway to the pelvic veins. Sometimes a 'blow-out' of multiple small veins is seen below the ankles and over the foot.
- White atrophy ('atrophie blanche'), representing small areas of scarring and devascularization, often with marginal telangiectatic vessels, may arise de novo around the malleoli in the absence of preceding ulceration.
- Ulceration ('venous ulcers') is common and the most serious consequence of venous incompetence. Neglected, such ulcers may become intractable and incurable and thus permanently incapacitating. Trauma, for example a kick or knock, or infection, may initiate an ulcer which fails to heal because of inadequate tissue perfusion. Venous ulcers occur in the lower third of the calf, usually laterally at first, often immediately above and behind the malleoli (Fig. 16.6). Eventually, neglected ulcers may be enormous and can circle

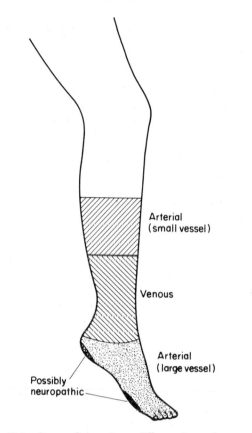

Fig. 16.6 Causes of ulceration at different sites on leg.

the calf. Bacterial colonization is usual and may cause frank infection, with the associated risk of cellulitis or thrombophlebitis.

Any number or combination of these six signs may be found. A 'full house' of all six is quite common.

Differential diagnosis

The causes of leg ulceration are listed in Table 16.5. The position of the ulcer is all-important. Cardiac, renal or hepatic oedema will be bilateral and possibly sacral. The dermatitis must be differentiated from psoriasis, lichen planus and endogenous nummular dermatitis.

Management

Reduction of leg venous hypertension and thus improvement in tissue perfusion is central. The principles of management involve:
- Effective compression to reduce, control and prevent chronic oedema
- Encouragement of exercise and use of the calf muscle pump
- Reduction of obesity where present
- Treatment of dermatitis, if present, and avoidance of sensitizing topical therapies
- Control of infection if ulceration or cellulitis are present
- Measures to promote ulcer healing
- Subsequent life-long supervision to prevent relapse

Mostly, these aims are best served by ambulant outpatient management. Rarely, hospital admission for bed rest, leg elevation, grafting, etc, will be unavoidable.

Treatment of venous dermatitis

Bland non-steroidal applications are of great value. Zinc and salicylic acid paste N.F. (Lassar's paste) is soothing and protective. It can be wiped off daily with arachis or olive oil. Other bland ointments are alternatives. Paste bandages may be useful (see p. 138). Lanolin-containing preparations and topical antibiotics carry a sensitization risk and should not be used. Sometimes, topical corticosteroid creams or ointments are necessary but should not be used if there is secondary infection or close to the edges of ulceration. Compressive bandaging must always accompany topical therapy.

Treatment of venous ulceration

Therapeutic aims are reduction in bacterial colonization, removal of necrotic debris and exudate, and induction of granulation followed by re-epithelialization. If there is much oedema and exudate daily cleansing is indicated. Normal saline, weak potassium permanganate solution, 1% aqueous phenoxytol and 10% aqueous povidone iodine (Betadine, U.K.) may all be useful for cleansing purposes. After gentle drying a sterile, non-adhesive absorbent dressing is applied and the leg compressed with an elasticated bandage from the toes to below the knee.

If progress is disappointing, debriding agent can be applied and left in situ after cleansing. Such agents include hydrophilic polysaccharide beads (Debrisan, U.K.), enzyme-containing preparations (e.g. Varidase, U.K.) or antiseptic starch gels such as Iodosorb (U.K.), brilliant green gel (Variclene, U.K.), silver sulphadiazine cream (Flamazine, U.K.) or an oxygen releaser (Hioxyl, U.K.).

Neomycin (or framycetin)-containing vaseline gauze (tulle gras) *should never* be used because of the risk of contact sensitization by the antibiotic, and indeed all topical antibiotics except chlortetracycline are best avoided. Neomycin-containing powders (e.g. Cicatrin, U.K.) are particulaly dangerous as they have caused deafness and renal damage after absorption from an ulcerated surface. Chlorhexidine tulle gras (Bactigras, U.K.) is permissible.

If exudate and oedema are minimal, occlusive medicated bandages left in place for 7–14 days are preferable. Such bandages may be impregnated with zinc paste (Viscopaste PB7, Zincaband, U.K.), coal tar (Coltapaste or Tarband, U.K.), ichthammol (Ichthaband, U.K.) or clioquinol paste (Quinaband, U.K.).

An occlusive, adhesive, compressive bandage (Poroplast or Lestroflex, U.K.) is then applied from the toes to the knee. In due course, plaster scissors with a flat lower surface should be used to cut through the dressing for removal.

Surgical measures

Grafting has a small but expanding place in intractable ulcers. Apart from conventional partial thickness or pinch grafts, cultured allografts offer great promise. Skin is obtained usually from breast or cosmetic surgery sources and maintained in culture until it loses its allergenicity, perhaps because of death of its Langerhans' cells. The graft probably does not survive but seems to promote revascularization and granulation.

Follow-up care

Once leg venous disease has been controlled, ulcers healed and eczema cleared, life-long vigilance is essential to prevent relapse. Elastic stockings may be needed indefinitely and ideally patients should be seen twice yearly.

Urticaria and Angioedema

Urticaria consists of transient pale dermal swellings (weals) on an erythematous background. It itches intensely. Individual lesions disappear leaving no residue within 15 minutes to 48 hours but the eruption may be widespread and recurring to run an acute, subacute or chronic course. Angioedema is the same process involving the subcutaneous tissues or mucous membranes.

Pathogenesis

The final common pathway involves sudden vascular dilatation and increased capillary permeability allowing escape of fluid from the circulation into the tissues. Release of histamine from the granules of mast cells is probably the usual cause of the acute inflammation but other vasoactive mediators may be involved, such as kinins and prostaglandins. Histamine release may be due to physical, chemical, pharmacological or immunological stimulation of mast cells.

Causes

Causes of urticaria are summarized in Table 16.7.

Trauma. Rubbing, firm stroking or scratching of the skin produces urticaria in 3–5% of otherwise normal people so that it is possible to 'write' on the skin. This is *dermographism*, which subsides within 30 minutes.

Pressure. Firm sustained pressure, for example to the hand from carrying a heavy case, or to the buttock from sitting on a hard bench, may lead to delayed urticaria after several hours which takes 24 hours or more to clear.

Cold. Exposure to cold, for example a biting wind, cold shower or swim, may induce urticaria. Acute, even fatal, anaphylactic shock due to histamine release could follow accidental immersion of the whole body in a cold-sensitive subject. Usually cold urticaria is idiopathic but, rarely, cold agglutinins or cryoglobulins are responsible secondary to myeloma, lupus erythematosus or an infection, such as syphilis.

Table 16.7 The causes of urticaria.

Trauma	Infection
Deep pressure	Collagen vascular disease
Cold	Lymphoma
Heat	Drugs
Light	Food additives
Water	Foods
Insect stings	Emotional stress

Heat. Warming the body either locally or generally by exercise may provoke urticaria, typically with very small weals and widespread erythematous flares. Release of acetylcholine from sympathetic nerve endings is responsible for this *cholinergic urticaria*.

Water. Contact with water at any temperature may induce transient itching and urticaria (*aquagenic urticaria*).

Light. Rarely, light exposure provokes urticaria. Either long ultraviolet or visible wavelengths can be responsible (p. 128).

Chemical. Contact urticaria is induced by direct inoculation of a chemical into the skin. Nettle rash, jellyfish stings and flea bites (papular urticaria) are examples.

Infections. Transient urticaria caused by minor viral infections is very common in children. Scabies can cause secondary dermographism. Rarely, intestinal parasites are culpable, when a blood eosinophilia is usual.

Systemic disease. Urticaria is a frequent component of the atopic syndrome (p. 89). It is an occasional feature of polyarteritis nodosa, systemic lupus erythematosus and other forms of vasculitis, as well as lymphoma. Sometimes the weals may be longer lasting (urticated erythema) and histologically more cells escape from dermal vessels or an urticarial vasculitis may be present.

Drugs. Codeine and other opiates, aspirin and other anti-inflammatory analgesics can be histamine liberators by pharmacological action on mast cells. Other drug-induced urticarias are mediated by immune reactions. Type I (IgE) reactions are commonest, as in penicillin urticaria. In Type III reactions, IgG and complement are involved, with immune complex formation.

Food and other additives. Azo dyes, for example tartrazine (E102), and preservatives, for example sodium benzoate, are occasionally responsible for chronic urticaria. Foods themselves may be culprits, such as nuts, shellfish or fruit. Type I hypersensitivity is the usual mechanism, often as part of a widespread atopic syndrome.

Emotional stress. This is certainly one trigger of cholinergic urticaria (see above). Rarely, psychological stress clearly underlies chronic urticaria.

Clinical picture

Urticaria may be localized or widespread, minor or florid. Close observation reveals a constantly shifting pattern of weals and erythema, recently resolved areas being refractory for a few days. Involvement of the lips, eyelids and penis may be alarming, and of the palms and soles very painful. It resolves without trace. The absence of scaling is important in differentiation from dermatitis (especially on the eyelids), and absence of purpura in excluding vasculitis.

Investigation

The cause of acute urticaria is often evident. A differential white cell count and ESR measurement help to identify systemic disease. The presence of eosinophilia points to parasitism and the appropriate tests. Diagnosis of the *physical urticarias* is usually clear from the history of cold, heat, light or pressure causation. Cold urticaria can be confirmed by application of an ice-cube firmly on the upper arm for one minute; localized heat urticaria is provoked similarly with a hot pad or rubber hot-water bottle. Immersion of both arms in a basin of water as hot as can be tolerated, or asking the subject to run up and down several flights of stairs, will demonstrate cholinergic urticaria over the rest of the body. Hanging a 5 kg weight from a broad band of cloth over the thigh for 30–60 minutes will confirm delayed pressure urticaria several hours later.

Superficial rubbing to reveal dermographism should always be done. Deliberate oral test dosing with food additives, aspirin or other drug suspects, is generally safe. It is most valuable when the disease is in remission. Rarely, keeping a food diary and selective inclusion or exclusion of food from the diet will reveal the cause of chronic urticaria. Skin tests for Type I allergy are virtually never of any value. In atopics, RAST tests for specific IgE antibody can be useful.

Treatment

Certain or suspected causative factors must clearly be removed. Topical therapy is ineffective except for the use of calamine lotion which reduces itching by skin cooling. H_1 antihistamines are more effective in reducing itching than wealing. Non-sedative drugs will be needed by day but a sedative antihistamine may be of advantage at night. Occasionally, addition of an H_2

blocker seems to be of value in chronic urticaria. Rarely, the severest cases may need oral prednisolone in short courses. Cold urticaria can be abolished by daily desensitization if the patient will tolerate progressively colder baths or showers under H_1 antihistamine cover.

Angioedema

This is a variant of urticaria where massive oedema involves subcutaneous tissues rather than the dermis. It may involve any part of the body surface especially about the lips, eyelids or penis, and more dangerously submucosal spaces in the tongue or larynx. It may be associated with urticaria from many causes but bee and wasp stings in sensitized subjects are particularly dangerous.

Management

Acute airway obstruction for example in urticaria or anaphylaxis, is best treated with immediate intramuscular adrenaline 1 mg, repeated after 5 minutes if necessary. Chlorpheniramine can be given intramuscularly at the same time. Rarely, tracheostomy may be unavoidable.

Patients who have had two or more episodes should be taught self injection with a preloaded adrenaline syringe (0.5 mg; Min-I-Jet-Adrenaline-IMS). Alternatively, use of a prescribed adrenaline aerosol (Medihaler epi-Riker) may suffice in less severe episodes. Desensitization to bee and wasp stings is possible.

Hereditary angioedema

This rare disease is caused by a quantitative or functional deficiency of C1 inhibitor, inherited as an autosomal dominant trait. The disease is characterized biochemically by persistent low serum levels of C2 and C4, normal C3 and increased serum esterase. Angioedema is due to a peptide derived by the action of plasmin on a complement fragment produced by cleavage of C2 and C4 by C1. Attacks are precipitated by trauma which activates Hageman factor, normally suppressed by C1 inhibitor.

Clinical picture

Attacks are infrequent in early childhood, common in adolescence and early adult life and later may subside. The typical story is of recurrent attacks of subcutaneous, laryngeal or intestinal oedema. Subcutaneous angioedema is not painful and does not itch. Intestinal oedema may cause severe abdominal pain, vomiting and diarrhoea. Laryngeal oedema may be obstructive and fatal. There is often a family history of sudden premature deaths.

Diagnosis

The finding of a low serum C4 with normal C3 is suggestive of the diagnosis, which is confirmed by demonstration of low serum C1 esterase inhibitor.

Management

In acute attacks, adrenaline is of little value. In life-threatening situations, fresh frozen plasma should be administered by intravenous infusion. Alternatively, a purified C1 esterase inhibitor concentrate can be given intravenously. When attacks have been frequent, preoperative prophylaxis is similar but long-term prophylaxis is with attenuated androgens, stanozolol (Stromba, U.K.) or danazol (Danol, U.K.) which inhibit pituitary gonadotrophin. These drugs stimulate hepatic synthesis of C1 inhibitor. The antifibrinolytic ϵ-aminocaproic acid and tranexamic acid are less satisfactory alternatives which prevent conversion of plasminogen to plasmin.

17

Autoimmune Diseases and Other Diseases of Collagen and Elastic Tissue

It is usual to group together several diseases which may overlap and in which autoantibody formation, collagen and vascular disorder occur. These are the 'collagen–vascular' diseases and they are described here, together with other minor disorders of dermal constituents.

Collagen

Collagen is a protein and is the major constituent of the dermis and many other tissues. It is made up of polypeptide chains which in turn are built from amino acids. The amino acid sequences vary in the different types of collagen found in various tissues. Collagen is synthesized by fibroblasts and various precursors evolve into mature collagen. The protein is organized in a fibrillar structure, strengthened by cross-linking covalent bonds. Side by side with synthesis, mature collagen is subject to degradation initiated by the enzyme collagenase. Several clinical situations where collagen is clearly abnormal are described later in this Chapter.

Lupus erythematosus

There are two major clinical patterns of this disease:
- Chronic discoid lupus erythematosus (DLE)
- Systemic lupus erythematosus (SLE)

They are not mutually exclusive. Discoid lesions are seen in some patients with SLE, and about 5% of patients presenting with DLE eventually develop SLE. Others with DLE have laboratory evidence, if not clinical evidence, of a systemic process.

Chronic discoid lupus erythematosus

This is a chronic benign disorder characterized by the development of well-defined erythematous, scaly plaques on exposed sites which progress to atrophy.

Aetiology

Discoid lupus erythematosus is twice as common in females. It usually begins between 30 and 60 years of age. Rarely it is familial. There are weak HLA associations with B7 or B8. Bright sunlight is an important initiating factor and an aggravating factor in the majority, once the disease is established.

Clinical picture

Typically, the disease affects the face, lesions being found on the cheeks, nose, chin, forehead or lips. Scalp involvement is common and leads to cicatricial alopecia. The ears, neck, upper trunk, hands and arms may also be involved.

The individual lesion is sharply defined and erythematous (Fig. 17.1). It may be macular at first, and oedematous if very acute. Later it develops scale which tends to be adherent and plugs the follicles ('carpet-tack' scale). Atrophy follows; eventually, scarring may be extensive and may destroy cartilage in the nose or ear (*lupus* = wolf). Pigmentary disturbance is usual and the hypopigmentation may be a major disfiguring factor in black and brown patients. In black people, gross hyperpigmentation is also sometimes seen. Comedones, set in scarred skin, provide a characteristic sign, especially in the ears. Infrequently, lesions are widely disseminated on the skin especially on the backs of the forearms, hands and fingers. Scarring and telangiectatic lesions may occur on the tips of the fingers and toes, and occasionally extensively on the palm and soles. Rarely the plaques are

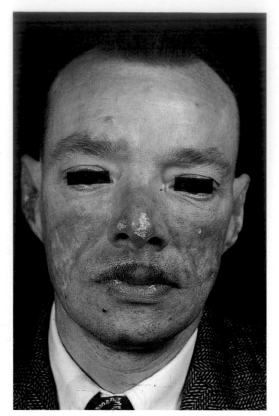

Fig. 17.1   Chronic discoid lupus erythematosus.

warty. Even in the absence of these peripheral skin lesions, it is not uncommon for patients with DLE to admit to cold extremities, chilblains or Raynaud's phenomenon.

Investigations

In a well-established lesion, skin biopsy typically reveals hyperkeratosis with follicular plugging, degeneration of the epidermal basal layer and a striking dermal infiltrate of lymphocytes and histiocytes, sometimes concentrated around the skin appendages. IgG and often C3 are demonstrable as bands at the epidermodermal junction of lesional skin. Raised ESR, hyperglobulinaemia or serum antinuclear factors (ANF) are found in 20–30% of patients.

Differential diagnosis

Dermatitis and psoriasis do not cause atrophy. Lichen planus may be confused histologically but is rare on the

face and scalp. Lupus vulgaris is now very rare in developed countries.

Treatment

Topical corticosteroids are central and the strongest may be needed. Steroid-medicated tape can be useful. Lesions should be screened from bright sunlight by appropriate clothing and sun-blocking applications. If these measures fail, mepacrine 200 mg daily is safer than hydroxychloroquine, although both drugs may be effective. The former causes yellow discoloration of the skin; the latter carries hazards for the retina. Both may occasionally cause lichenoid eruptions.

Prognosis

The disease is chronic over many years. Perhaps 50% eventually remit completely but where there is scalp and cold-sensitive hand disease, persistence is likely. Not more than 6% of patients will develop SLE but the disseminated form of DLE carries a 20% chance of eventual systemic disease.

Systemic lupus erythematosus

Systemic lupus erythematosus is a serious multisystem disease affecting vascular and connective tissues and characterized by autoantibody formation to DNA.

Aetiology

The female:male ratio is about 8:1. Black and Southeast Asian women are particularly at risk. Onset is classically in the second to the fourth decade and is rare before puberty. The genetic factor is more obvious than in DLE. Many drugs may precipitate a lupus erythematosus-like syndrome (Table 17.1), but the drug-induced syndrome may not be the same as 'natural' SLE. Bright sunlight is both a provocative and exacerbating agent.

Table 17.1   Main drugs which may precipitate a lupus erythematosus-like syndrome.

Hydralazine	Isoniazid
Anticonvulsants	Chlorpromazine
Procaineamide	Penicillamine

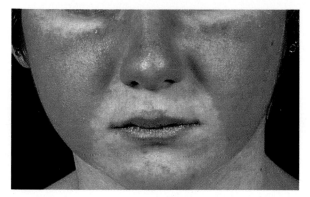

Fig. 17.2 Acute systemic lupus erythematosus in a 15-year-old girl; the disease was fatal within 4 years.

Table 17.2 Systemic disease in systemic lupus erythematosus.

Renal	Glomerulonephritis
	Arteritis
Cardiac	Myocarditis
	Pericarditis
	Libman–Sachs endocarditis
Cerebral	Infarction
	Thrombosis
	Psychosis
	Epilepsy
Musculoskeletal	Arthritis
	Tenosynovitis
Pulmonary	Atelectasis
	Pneumonitis

Clinical picture

The disease is often first manifest in the skin. A symmetrical fixed macular erythematous flush involves the cheeks and nose—the so-called 'butterfly eruption' (Fig. 17.2). Its margins are well defined. More extensive involvement may affect the forehead, chin and neck but there is usually circumocular and circumoral sparing. Redness of the palms is common and careful inspection of the fingertips may reveal dilated capillaries at the posterior nail fold, splinter haemorrhages and tiny infarcts. There may be diffuse hair loss. In later stages various clearly vascular lesions may appear in the skin, especially of the legs, such as purpura, livedo reticularis and ulceration.

Other symptoms and signs reflect the order of internal organ involvement (Table 17.2). Fever, lassitude, weight loss and joint pains are common. Effusion into joints, painful tenosynovitis, various cardiac or pulmonary changes all occur. Neuropsychiatric manifestations may include epilepsy and psychotic behaviour. Albuminuria is the usual initial manifestation of any renal involvement.

Investigations

In a skin biopsy some features of DLE may be present, but there are usually dermal oedema and collagen changes. Junctional immunoglobulins and complement are usually present in lesions and in uninvolved exposed skin, less often in non-exposed skin. Often IgG, IgM and IgA are all present and are sometimes found in blood vessel walls in various tissues. Leucopenia, thrombocytopenia and anaemia are common and a very high ESR is almost invariable. C-reactive protein is absent. Antinuclear antibodies are generally detectable and, in active disease, antibodies to double-stranded DNA are almost invariable. Detectable antibodies to various antigens [e.g. anti-SSA(Ro) and anti-SSB(La)] characterize various subsets of SLE (Table 17.3). False positive serological tests for syphilis may cause confusion; low serum complement levels imply increased consumption due to immune complex formation and disease activity.

Treatment

The important aspects of treatment can be summarized as follows:
- Avoidance of sunlight provocation
- Avoidance of drug provocation by penicillin and sulphonamides
- Oral prednisolone; sometimes very high dosage is needed to control disease exacerbations
- Oral hydroxychloroquine intermittently may be of great value
- Progressive and especially renal disease may require immunosuppressive use of azathioprine or cyclophosphamide in full dosage

The management of severe SLE taxes the resources of the most experienced and such cases are best managed in special units where possible. Plasmapheresis has proved disappointing.

Prognosis

The younger the patient, the more likely is severe progressive disease. In the middle-aged, the disease can be relatively benign. Overall, 5-year survival is probably over 90% and 15-year survival over 70%. Renal and central nervous system involvement imply a poor prognosis: renal failure, central nervous system vasculitis and infection are the commonest causes of death.

Uncommon variants of lupus erythematosus

Neonatal lupus erythematosus

This is rare but is now well recognized, presenting with erythematous and later atrophic skin lesions. Some of these babies prove to have heart block and other systemic abnormalities, for example thrombocytopenia.

The mother is usually clinically normal but anti-SSA(Ro) antibody is invariably present in her serum. Counselling on the risk to future pregnancies is crucial.

Chilblain lupus

A minority of women with DLE develop chilblain-like lesions on the extremities which may persist after the DLE has remitted. Their histology is of DLE. A few go on to develop SLE.

Rowell's syndrome

Occasionally, erythema multiforme-like lesions are seen in both DLE and SLE. The lesions last 2–4 weeks but may recur for years. This variant is associated with the presence of anti-SSB(La) antibodies.

Lupus erythematosus profundus

This is a form of panniculitis, occurring on the face, trunk or limbs. The deltoid region is a characteristic site. The overlying skin may be clinically normal but often shows histological evidence of DLE, and frank lesions of DLE may be found elsewhere. A deep biopsy is needed to demonstrate the panniculitis.

Subacute cutaneous lupus erythematosus

Widespread skin lesions may be associated with arthralgia, photosensitivity and other mild systemic features with a benign prognosis. Some patients are ANF-negative but anticytoplastic antibodies (SSA or SSB) are usually present.

SLE with severe Raynaud's phenomenon

Anti-RNP antibodies are found in this variant.

SLE with thrombotic episodes

A subset is now recognized characterized by a tendency to recurrent abortion, cerebrovascular episodes, livedo reticularis and even chorea. Such patients carry antiphospholipid (cardiolipin) antibodies and may give false positive serological tests for syphilis.

Scleroderma

Two forms of scleroderma are recognized and are more distinct than SLE and DLE:
- Morphoea (scleroderma circumscriptum)
- Systemic sclerosis

Morphoea

This is a purely superficial disorder in which circumscribed plaques or bands of sclerosis develop in the skin. The cause is unknown but the development of a similar picture in graft-versus-host reactions suggests an immunological cause. Typically, the disease presents with a round or oval plaque of induration and erythema which may have a heliotrope hue. Gradually the plaques become more indurated and shiny centrally as the epidermis becomes atrophic with an ivory-like appearance and loss of hair. After many years the lesion may resolve, leaving some pigmentation.

Morphoea tends to be centripetal, affecting the trunk (Fig. 17.3) or proximal portions of limbs. The female breast is a common site, inviting confusion with breast carcinoma. It is most often seen in young or middle-aged females (sex ratio 3:1) but a childhood form is far from rare and may be linear. Linear bands usually affect the limbs, are unilateral and may tether the subcutaneous tissues down to periosteum. A well-known but rare linear lesion affects the forehead or face 'en coup de sabre'. Very rarely, morphoea can be generalized but even this form may spare the hands (cf. systemic sclerosis) and feet.

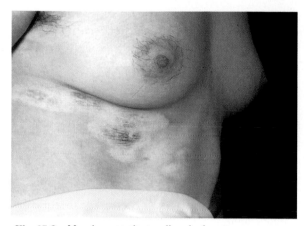

Fig. 17.3 Morphoea on chest wall under breast.

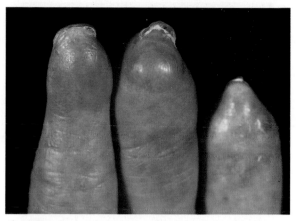

Fig. 17.4 Fingers in systemic sclerosis (acrosclerosis).

On biopsy, the epidermis is atrophic and the collagen of the dermis hypertrophic in the mature lesion. The collagen extends into the subcutis and appendages are progressively lost. There are no characteristic serum abnormalities. No treatment is of established value.

Systemic sclerosis

This disease is sometimes known as systemic scleroderma, acrosclerosis or CRST Syndrome. It is a systemic disorder in which Raynaud's phenomenon and acral sclerosis may be followed by gastrointestinal, cardiopulmonary or renal disease.

Aetiology

The disease is rare and affects mainly females (sex ratio 4:1). Onset is unusual before 30 years. Genetic and immunological factors probably play a part in pathogenesis.

Clinical picture

Almost always, Raynaud's phenomenon of increasing severity is the presenting symptom. Gradually permanent changes supervene in the fingers, particularly swelling and flexion deformity so that rheumatoid arthritis may be mimicked. Tapering of the finger pulps gives way to fingertip scarring and sometimes ulceration. Indolent paronychia is common, and osteolysis of the terminal phalanx may cause sagging of the nail bed and 'beaking' of fingernails (Fig. 17.4). Subcutaneous calcinosis may occur (Fig. 17.5) and rarely calcium deposits are extruded at the fingertips.

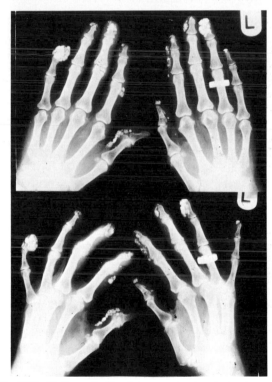

Fig. 17.5 Radiograph of hands in systemic sclerosis showing gross calcification of soft tissues.

Sooner or later the face is involved. Telangiectasiae develop on the skin of the face and neck. The facial skin loses its elasticity and becomes bound down. In advanced cases, the facies thus produced is characteristic with a wasting of the face, narrowing of the nose, 'crow's feet', furrowing at the corners of a small

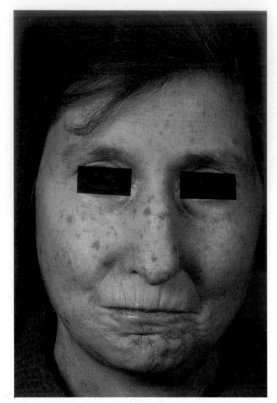

Fig. 17.6 Advanced systemic sclerosis; typical facies.

mouth and a smooth wrinkle-free forehead (Fig. 17.6). The lower eyelid may be difficult to evert.

Systemic manifestations appear in variable order and at widely differing tempos. Reflux is often the first symptom of oesophageal involvement. Advanced disease of the gullet may eventually cause dysphagia, stricture, hiatus hernia and aspiration hazards for the lungs. Small-bowel disease may present as a picture of malabsorption, subacute obstruction or a 'blind loop' syndrome. Exertional dyspnoea is the first symptom of lung disease. Progressive pulmonary fibrosis can lead to pneumothorax, bronchiectasis and cyst formation. Cardiac and renal involvement may be asymptomatic for years but eventually persistent proteinuria is followed by hypertension. Rapidly progressive renal failure is often the terminal event.

Pathology

In the skin, subtle alterations in the dermal collagen and ground substance may be associated with evidence of vasculitis and an inflammatory infiltrate. In the lungs there is progressive fibrosis in the alveolar-capillary spaces. Similar fibrosis occurs in the gut wall with endarteritis in some small vessels. Similar changes affect the heart. In the kidney, endarteritis of intralobar arterioles and fibrinoid necrosis in the glomerulus and the afferent arterioles are characteristic.

Investigations

Reduced capillary–alveolar transfer is the first indication of lung disease. Later, the chest radiograph becomes progressively abnormal. Oesophageal loss of motility and small-bowel disease may be evident radiologically. An abnormal ECG is common. Frequently present blood changes include a raised ESR and the presence of anti-Scl-70, and in the CRST variant, anti-centromere antibodies (Table 17.3).

Differential diagnosis

The cutaneous changes are centrifugal; in morphoea they are centripetal. In morphoea fingertips are always normal and Raynaud's phenomenon does not occur.

Treatment

No drug is of specific value. Smoking should be forbidden. Electrically heated gloves may be valuable. Low dose (under 10 mg daily) prednisolone is sometimes of limited value, especially if the hands are swollen and stiff. Intravenous infusions of prosta-cyclines and low molecular weight dextran may be of transient value, especially in promoting healing of ulcerated fingertips. Penicillamine and immuno-suppressive drugs are not of established value but may have to be tried.

Prognosis

The outlook is very variable. Occasionally, relentless progress can be fatal in a year or two. Conversely, disease apparently confined to the hands without systemic disease can persist for decades.

Variants of scleroderma

Occupational scleroderma

Occupational scleroderma can be caused by exposure to vinyl chloride. Apart from the acral changes, various systemic features are seen including bizarre emotional symptoms such as inappropriate laughter. Certain organic solvents and pesticides can cause similar milder scleroderma.

Drug-induced scleroderma

The antimitotic drug, bleomycin, can cause pseudo-scleroderma in the hands and even pulmonary fibrosis. These changes are slowly reversible.

Eosinophilic fasciitis

This condition presents as indurated, sometimes haemorrhagic and painful limb plaques, often associated with eosinophilia. Systemic involvement is not seen.

Lichen sclerosus et atrophicus

It is debatable whether this disease is related to morphoea. It may be seen in children as well as adults and has a predeliction for the anogenital region in females (Fig. 17.7) and the glans penis in adult males

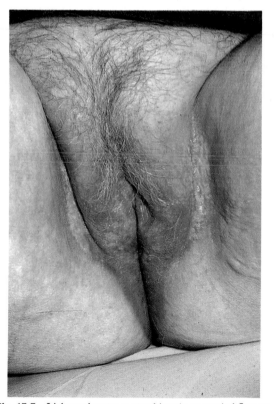

Fig. 17.7   Lichen sclerosus et atrophicus in anogenital flexures of a menopausal woman.

(balanitis xerotica obliterans). Rarely it may be on the trunk. White atrophic macules may become confluent in the female anogenital region, often at the menopause. Histologically, a hyalinized featureless upper dermis underlies an atrophic epidermis. Differential diagnosis from vulval intraepithelial dysplasia, psoriasis and lichen simplex is important. There is no treatment but 1% hydrocortisone cream affords relief from itching. Possible future sexual problems are important when prepubertal girls have genital disease. In men, meatal stenosis and sexual difficulties may be important.

Mixed connective tissue disease

This is an overlapping mixture of systemic sclerosis, dermatomyositis and lupus erythematosus, seen mainly in females. Antibodies to ribonucleoprotein antigen are detectable. Prognosis is better than in systemic sclerosis and oral prednisolone is of more value.

Scleredema of Buschke

This is a rare disorder in which massive induration, particularly of the upper trunk and neck, may appear over a few weeks. Its cause is unknown and it may persist for years, or resolve. It may be associated with IgA gammopathy.

Dermatomyositis

This is a rare disease in which a characteristic rash is associated with polymyositis. When it develops over the age of 40 years, about one-third of patients prove to have a carcinoma. It is commoner in females (2:1). It is the least rare of the collagen vascular diseases in childhood, where it is not associated with malignancy. Its cause is unknown but tumour-related disease probably has an immunological basis.

Clinical picture

The rash affects the face and often the extensor bony prominences of the shoulders and limbs, as well as the backs of the hands (Fig. 17.8). A fixed heliotrope erythema, without itching, is associated with variable oedema. Puffy red upper outer eyelids are characteristic (Fig. 17.9). The erythema is typically streaky over the knuckles and dorsal fingers, and gross dilatation of posterior nail fold capillaries ('pallisading') is usual and more ordered than in lupus erythema-

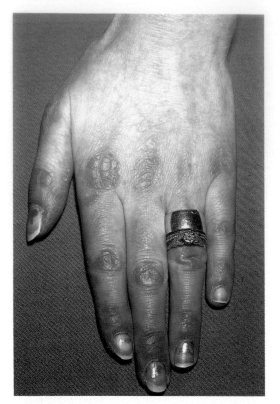

Fig. 17.8 Dermatomyositis on backs of hands; note the particular involvement of the skin over the joints.

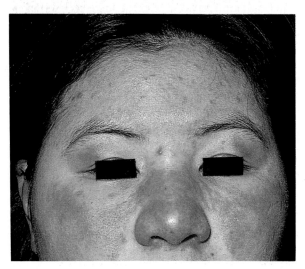

Fig. 17.9 Dermatomyositis in a 20-year-old Chinese woman; no underlying cause was evident.

tosus. Later the lesions may become atrophic and occasionally ulcerate.

Polymyositis may accompany or follow the rash. Occasionally it is mild and transient and may only be detected biochemically. Weakness of major proximal muscle groups is obvious in active myositis so that walking upstairs, lifting the arms above the head and getting out of bed are difficult. Proximal limb muscles may be swollen and tender. Rarely, involuntary muscles may be involved leading to potentially dangerous or even fatal difficulties in swallowing, breathing or cardiac action. Calcification in deep muscle planes is typical of chronic childhood dermatomyositis but is uncommon in adults. The lungs may be involved.

Diagnosis

The rash is instantly recognizable but muscle weakness may be subtle. Electromyography and muscle biopsy confirm the myopathy which is also revealed by raised blood levels of creatine phosphokinase, aldolase and transaminases. Search for a tumour is mandatory in the adult disease. The autoantibody anti-Jo1 is associated with pulmonary involvement.

Differential diagnosis

On the eyelids, contact dermatitis itches and may be weeping or scaly, features that are all absent in dermatomyositis. Occasionally oedema is gross so that angio-oedema may be simulated. Lupus erythematosus spares the eyelids and usually also the knuckles if the hand is involved.

Treatment

Active polymyositis with marked weakness calls for oral prednisolone, initially in doses of 40–120 mg daily according to severity. Rarely 'pulse' infusions of methyl prednisolone (1 g daily for 3 days) are necessary to initiate improvement. As the steroid dose is reduced, azathioprine should be added (2.5 mg/kg daily) and is likely to be needed long-term together with 5–10 mg daily of prednisolone. Methotrexate and cyclophosphamide are alternatives if azathioprine is ineffective in allowing steroid reduction.

Prognosis

Probably 50% of adults over 40 years die within 5 years, either from underlying malignancy or from the disease itself. In children the disease eventually burns out, usually leaving gross disability because of contracture and calcinosis.

Dermatological Features in Other 'Collagen' Diseases

Rheumatoid arthritis

Apart from the subcutaneous nodules of seropositive disease, vasculitis may occur causing small fingernail fold infarcts. Arteritis in the legs may lead to ulceration, particularly on the lateral mid-calves.

Still's Disease

A rare but highly characteristic shifting, chronic, patterned urticated erythema occurs in about 25% of patients.

Rheumatic fever

Erythema marginatum is an evanescent patterned shifting erythema which may come and go in a few hours.

Sjögren's syndrome

This is an autoimmune disease in which inflammatory cells infiltrate exocrine glands. Subsequent destruction of lacrimal and salivary glands leads to xerophthalmia and xerostomia. Anti-Ro and -La autoantibodies are detectable and malignant lymphoma may eventually supervene.

Other Disease of Collagen Alteration

Keloid

Excessive collagen production after skin injury or inflammation produces smooth hard nodules, seen most often around the shoulders, upper back or chest in adolescents or young adults (Fig. 17.10). Blacks have more keloidal tendency than whites and young black adults may suffer spontaneous multiple papular keloids at the nape, perhaps induced by ingrowing hairs (Acne keloid). Repeated intralesional triamcinolone injection may induce partial resolution. Excision only stands a chance of success if followed by radiotherapy or months of compression, which is most applicable to earlobes.

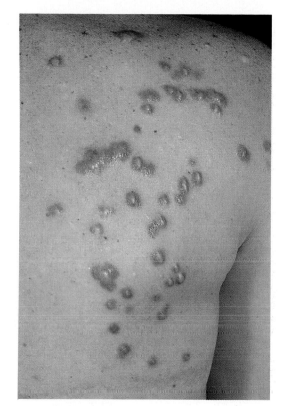

Fig. 17.10 Multiple keloid papules on upper back following acne.

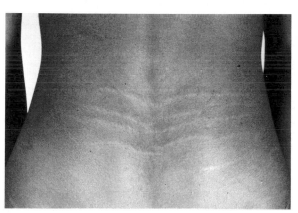

Fig. 17.11 Horizontal striae of back in adolescent boy.

Striae

Stretch marks due to dermal collagen stretching are physiological in adolescents as the shoulders expand in muscular boys and the breasts and hips in maturing girls. Horizontal linear striae across the lower back in young people are puzzling and may simulate the results of whiplashes (Fig. 17.11). Overexposure to oral or topical corticosteroids may induce striae, the latter typically on the inner thighs of atopic patients or at right-angles to the inguinal areas after flexural applications. Not surprisingly, they are seen in Cushing's syndrome.

Solar elastosis

The most obvious 'ageing' is seen in exposed skin due to progressive loss and degradation of collagen and elastic tissue. The inelastic, yellowish, wrinkled, thickened skin of gross 'elastosis' is readily recognized (farmer's neck, Berkshire neck, etc.).

Ehlers–Danlos syndrome

This syndrome is described with inherited disorders in Chapter 14.

Table 17.3 Auto-antibody aids to diagnosis in 'collagen-vascular' diseases.

Auto-antibody to:	Clinical associations:	Auto-antibody to:	Clinical associations:
ANA	Non-specific, infections	Sm *	SLE in black and yellow races
Double stranded DNA	SLE		
SSA (Ro) *	Sub-acute cutaneous LE Neonatal LE	Scl-70 (Topoisomerase I) *	Scleroderma (systemic sclerosis)
	Primary Sjogren's syndrome	Centromere (ANA) *	CRST syndrome (better prognosis)
SSB (La) *	Primary Sjogren's syndrome	Jo-1	Polymyositis (adult) Pulmonary fibrosis
Ribonucleoprotein (RNP) *	Mixed connective tissue disease	Phospholipid (cardiolipin)	Recurrent abortion Thrombosis Vascular accidents Livedo reticularis

* Soluble nuclear and cytoplasmic antigens (ENA); if ANA strongly positive, request 'DNA binding' (anti-dsDNA) and 'ENA' (extractable nuclear antigens).

18

Bullous Diseases

In Chapter 2 a vesicle was defined as a small blister (up to 5 mm in diameter) formed by the accumulation of fluid in the skin; a bulla is a larger blister over 5 mm in diameter. Vesicles or bullae can form at various depths in the skin according to the mechanisms involved.

The anatomy of blistering

Blisters can form at any of the levels indicated in Fig. 18.1 which can easily be identified on light microscopy. Electron microscopy, combined with immuno-fluorescence techniques, has allowed more precise localization of levels of cleavage in the area of the epidermodermal junction (see Fig. 1.6) which cannot be differentiated on conventional microscopy. All these changes appear subepidermal on ordinary microscopy. Table 18.1 lists a number of blistering conditions and indicates the level of cleavage in each.

The pathogenesis of blistering

In impetigo contagiosa and pustular psoriasis, internal epidermal inflammation and superficial leucocyte accumulation separate the stratum corneum, causing subcorneal blisters or pustules. Deeper in the epidermis the gross spongiosis of bullous dermatitis or acantholysis of pemphigus vulgaris (see later) cause intraepidermal blistering. Certain viruses such as *Varicella zoster* and *Herpes simplex* grossly damage epidermal keratinocytes which swell and vacuolate ('balloon degeneration') leading to blistering. A variety of immunopathological events at various levels (see Table 18.4) result in the blistering of the idiopathic bullous diseases which are the main subject of this Chapter. Various forms of genetically determined epidermolysis bullosa can now be precisely localized in terms of the level of trauma-induced cleavage (see Chapter 14).

Common Blistering Conditions

Common blistering conditions are summarized in Table 18.2.

Friction blisters

Everyone is familiar with the foot blisters induced by

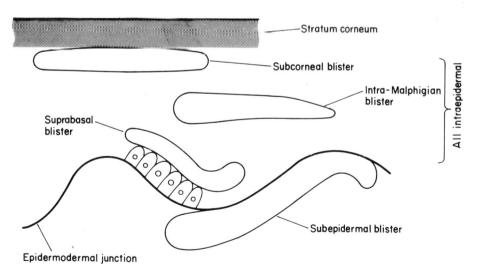

Fig. 18.1 Different levels of cleavage (blistering) in skin.

Table 18.1 Blistering diseases and their levels of cleavage.

Level of cleavage	Disease
Intraepidermal (subcorneal)	Impetigo contagiosa
	Pustular psoriasis
Intraepidermal (Malphigian cell layer)	Bullous dermatitis
	Friction blisters
	Herpes infection
	Pemphigus vulgaris
Intraepidermal (suprabasal)	Pemphigus vulgaris
Intraepidermal (basal cell damage)	Epidermolysis bullosa simplex
Junctional (lamina lucida split)	Junctional epidermolysis bullosa
	Bullous pemphigoid
Sub-basal lamina (dermal)	Dermatitis herpetiformis
	Dystrophic epidermolysis bullosa
	Acquired epidermolysis bullosa

Table 18.2 Common causes of blisters.

Friction	Dermatitis (contact)
Insect bites and stings	Impetigo
Burns	Drugs

prolonged walking in new boots or the hand blisters due to the first afternoon with the lawnmower in Spring.

Dermatitis

Pompholyx (p. 94) blistering on the palms or soles is well known but any fierce acute dermatitis may blister. Allergic contact dermatitis due to *Primula obconica* plants and phytophotodermatitis (p. 125) are particularly prone to gross blistering.

Impetigo

This coccal infection of the epidermis (p. 52) is particularly likely to be bullous in the neonate and in old age.

Insect bites

Gross blisters are sometimes seen, especially on the lower legs. The seasonal localization and history allow diagnosis easily.

Burns

Every housewife gets an oven burn blister on her wrist or arm at some time. Injudicious use of a hot-water bottle against the leg of a patient with sensory loss can result in a burn blister on the calf.

Drug reactions

Drug-induced bullae are described in Chapter 23.

The Uncommon Blistering Diseases

These are listed in Table 18.3. They include:
- Pemphigus in its various forms
- Pemphigoid and its variants
- Dermatitis herpetiformis and its variants

The four most important diseases are compared and contrasted in Table 18.4.

Pemphigus vulgaris

This is a potentially fatal mucocutaneous disease seen

Table 18.3 The uncommon blistering diseases.

Pemphigus vulgaris	Cicatricial pemphigoid
Pemphigus foliaceus	Dermatitis herpetiformis
Bullous pemphigoid	Linear IgA disease
Pemphigoid gestationis	

Table 18.4 A comparison of some blistering diseases.

Disease	Usual age (years)	Distribution	Cleavage	Acantholysis
Pemphigus vulgaris	20–50	Centripetal	Intra-epidermal	Yes
Pemphigus foliaceus	>60	Centripetal	Intra-epidermal	Yes
Bullous pemphigoid	>60	Centrifugal	Sub-epidermal	No
Dermatitis herpetiformis	20–50	Centrifugal	Sub-epidermal	No

equally in the sexes and usually in young or middle-aged adults. It is encountered worldwide but the incidence is increased in Jews. Its cause is unknown.

Clinical picture

The disease usually begins insidiously with the development of shallow flaccid blisters without much inflammation. The disease may start on the face or trunk but in about one-third of patients the onset is in the mouth (Fig. 18.2). As the blister roofs are rubbed off, raw 'weeping' erosions are left which fail to heal. In mild cases the lesions may remain small and discrete and even confined to the mouth for years. In severe untreated disease, spread is inexorable until large confluent erosions and generalized oropharyngeal blistering render life intolerable. Prior to the introduction of cortisone in 1950, 75% were dead within 4

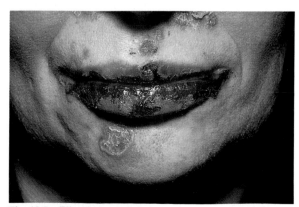

Fig. 18.2 Blistering acantholytic lesions on face and lips in pemphigus vulgaris.

years of onset. Death followed uncontrollable loss of fluid, proteins, etc, from the skin, gross interference with feeding, and secondary infection.

On examination the eruption is characteristically centripetal involving the trunk, neck, face and often the scalp but tending to spare the extremities. The blisters are thin-walled, flaccid, tend to rupture easily when touched and the surrounding skin is not inflamed. Blisters can often be enlarged by applying pressure with a finger—Nikolsky's sign. Pain and soreness rather than itching discomfort the patient.

Mucosal involvement is prominent. The lips, gingivae, sides and floor of the mouth as well as the palate may be eroded, red and raw, but bullae are inevitably transient. Discomfort is constant. Lesions may occur in the nasal vestibules, at the vulval introitus, at or near the anus or in the conjunctivae.

Internal organs are not affected and there is no systemic malaise until the secondary effects of severe disease take their toll.

Diagnosis

Expert cytology reveals the characteristic acantholytic cells (Tzanck test) to provide an instant diagnosis but skin biopsy should always be done for histology and immunofluorescence (see Fig. 3.5) to confirm the diagnosis. Serum samples allow the titre of circulating anti-intercellular substance antibody to be measured and subsequently monitored.

Pathology and immunopathology

The biopsy reveals intraepidermal, usually suprabasal blistering with acantholysis, i.e. the presence of rounded keratinocytes which have lost the ability to adhere to their fellows. Acantholytic cells are seen around the margins of the blister and floating free within it. Both direct and indirect immunofluorescence tests reveal intense intercellular IgG staining within the epidermis (Fig. 3.5).

Treatment

Topical therapy is ineffective. Severe cases require prednisolone 120–240 mg daily initially, the dose being reduced exponentially as control is achieved. A subgroup of milder cases can usually be controlled by much smaller doses (40–80 mg daily) but the clinician should not err by finessing the steroid dose, since failure to respond to initial dosage may necessitate a later large increase rendering the patient more liable to severe side-effects.

Addition of an immunosuppressive drug, normally azathioprine (1.5–2.5 mg/kg daily), is usual as the prednisolone dose is brought down below 50 mg daily. In time this has a steroid-sparing effect which should allow the prednisolone maintenance dose to be reduced to 10 mg daily and then very slowly by 1 mg decrements even lower. It is rarely possible to get below 7 mg daily and overambitious reduction may allow relapse, necessitating a large increase to re-establish control.

In the initial phase of very high steroid dosage, intensive care and monitoring is mandatory to prevent oral candidosis and to detect other opportunistic infections and side-effects as early as possible. Ranitidine or cimetidine is given to protect the gastroduodenal mucosa.

Maintenance treatment must be continued for many years with the lowest effective dosages of azathioprine and prednisolone. It is now known that some patients are eventually fully cured and do not relapse after treatment has been stopped. In one of the author's patients this was achieved after 23 years of treatment. Rarely, oral or parenteral gold or plasmapheresis combined with pulse cyclophosphamide therapy are used for resistant disease.

Prognosis

Modern therapy has transformed the outlook. Prednisolone alone has brought 70% 10-year survival albeit with much steroid-induced morbidity, especially from osteoporosis. The addition of azathioprine with its steroid-sparing consequences has now brought 90% 10-year survival and has enormously benefitted the patient's quality of life.

Variants of pemphigus

Pemphigus foliaceus

This is a rare, benign disease which generally does not affect mucous membranes. It is usually seen in an older age group than pemphigus vulgaris and is occasionally provoked by solar exposure. It presents as multiple small erythematous macular lesions on the upper trunk (Fig. 18.3) or head. The acantholysis is very superficial so that cleavage is high in the epidermis and often subcorneal. This results in a delicate blister roof which does not remain long intact, so that the inexperienced eye may not appreciate that this is a blistering disease.

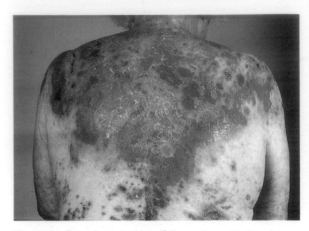

Fig. 18.3 Extensive pemphigus foliaceus in an elderly woman.

The glistening superficial erosions are characteristic, and histology and immunofluorescence are confirmatory.

Differential diagnosis is from dermatitis and psoriasis. In mild cases topical steroids alone suffice; if not, prednisolone 20–40 mg daily initially is usually adequate but sometimes azathioprine has to be added.

Brazilian pemphigus foliaceus

This is an endemic form of pemphigus foliaceus seen in lowland areas of Brazil and also known as fogo selvagem. It may be due to an infectious agent.

Pemphigus vegetans

This is a very rare chronic pustular and vegetating form of pemphigus vulgaris which affects the axillae and groins.

Pemphigus erythematosus

Pemphigus erythematosus, or Senear–Usher syndrome, is a rare form of pemphigus foliaceus affecting particularly the face, mimicking seborrhoeic dermatitis or lupus erythematosus. The immunopathology indicates a mixture of pemphigus foliaceus and lupus erythematosus features but SLE is not a hazard.

Pemphigoid

This is an uncommon chronic blistering disease of the elderly which largely spares mucous membranes. Its cause is unknown.

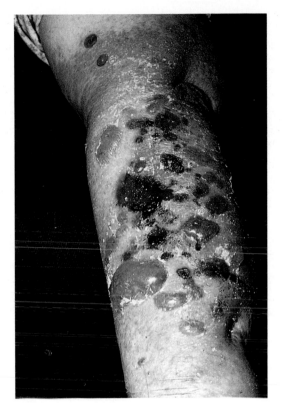

Fig. 18.4 Bullous pemphigoid; haemorrhagic subepidermal blisters.

Clinical picture

Occurring in an older age group than pemphigus vulgaris, the onset can be fairly rapid and even dramatic. Multiple tense, semispherical thick-walled durable blisters erupt on an erythematous and often urticated, patterned base (Fig. 18.4). The bullae are sometimes haemorrhagic. The distribution tends to be more centrifugal on the arms and legs, and may affect the hands and feet. Oral lesions are few or transient.

Diagnosis

The thick-walled tense blisters suggest subepidermal blistering in which the whole epidermis forms the roof. Haemorrhage confirms this localization.

Biopsy for histopathology and immunopathology provides confirmation and a serum sample allows detection of IgG anti-basement membrane zone antibody.

Pathology

The blister is subepidermal on light microscopy. Epidermal acantholysis is absent. IgG and C3 are demonstrable in a linear band at the epidermodermal junction. In sodium chloride-split skin preparations, the antibody binds to the roof of the split. The titre of anti-basement membrane zone antibody correlates with disease activity less clearly than in pemphigus vulgaris.

Treatment

Prednisolone 40–80 mg daily initially usually suffices and azathioprine 1.5–2.5 mg/kg daily is usually added. Dose reduction is pursued as with pemphigus, but the hazards of treatment in older, often immobilized, patients are considerable so that the disease has a mortality and carries a considerable risk of morbidity. Notwithstanding, expertly managed patients do well and treatment can often be stopped in 1–3 years.

Variants of pemphigoid

Benign mucous membrane pemphigoid

Cicatricial pemphigoid is a rare disease of middle life when blistering followed by scarring occurs particularly on the mucosae of the eyes, oropharynx, vulval introitus or anus. The cicatricial process can cause serious eye problems, oesophageal or laryngeal strictures and genital adhesions. The typical skin picture is one of localized recurrent blistering, typically on the scalp, with eventual scarring. The disease is not life-threatening but can be chronic, debilitating and mutilating when severe. The histopathology and immunopathology are that of pemphigoid.

Herpes gestationis

Herpes (or pemphigoid) gestationis is a fascinating but rare itching blistering disorder associated with pregnancy, hydatiform mole or choriocarcinoma. There is an association with HLA-DR3 and -DR4 as well as with autoimmune thyrotoxicosis. Epidemiological evidence suggests that an antigenic factor from the sexual partner may be relevant in a peculiarly immunoreactive woman. The morphology of the eruption, which begins in the second or third trimester, is of pemphigoid but the distribution is centripetal (often starting on the belly). The histopathology and immunopathology are of pemphigoid. The risk to the fetus is small but the disease tends to recur in subsequent pregnancies. Oral prednisolone is needed in severe cases.

Dermatitis herpetiformis

This is an uncommon chronic or recurring intensely itching disease of young adults in which a widespread herpetiform rash is associated with gluten enteropathy.

Clinical features

Onset is often in the third or fourth decade and there is a male preponderance (sex ratio 2:1). The patients are usually thin. The rash has a characteristic distribution, being found particularly on the extensor aspects of the limbs about the elbows and knees, on the buttocks and natal cleft, and over the shoulders, face and scalp. Lesions occasionally occur in the mouth and even in the larynx, causing hoarseness. Its morphology is herpes-like, i.e. grouped or clustered papules or vesicles are set on an erythematous and sometimes patterned urticarial base. Itching is intense and disabling. A large bullous variant can occur.

Pathology

Biopsy of the skin reveals a subepidermal blister. The earliest lesion is a microabscess in the tip of a dermal papilla. Immunofluorescence studies on perilesional skin show coarse granular IgA deposits at the dermoepidermal junction. C3 is also usually demonstrable.

Various serum antibodies may be detectable but are unimportant for diagnosis. More than 80% of patients are HLA-B8 positive.

In the gut, gluten enteropathy can be demonstrated by jejunal biopsy and varying degrees of malabsorption can be demonstrated biochemically.

Diagnosis

The pathology almost always confirms a confident clinical diagnosis. Tentative diagnoses of dermatitis herpetiformis are usually wrong. A therapeutic test with dapsone dramatically reduces itching in 72 hours, often providing confirmation before the biopsy result is available.

Treatment

Dapsone 100–300 mg daily or sulphapyridine 1000 mg daily are the treatments of choice, the minimum effective dose being continued long-term. Problems with these drugs are few but dapsone always shortens red cell life and rarely causes acute haemolytic anaemia. Neither drug can be given to a patient with glucose-6-phosphate dehydrogenase deficiency. Dapsone particularly may not be well tolerated by the elderly with cardiac or respiratory disease.

Where feasible, a gluten-free diet should be instituted. Strict adherence to the diet may slowly reduce drug requirements.

Prognosis

Treatment has to be continued life-long. Relapse is usually rapid if the drug is stopped.

Variants of dermatitis herpetiformis

Linear IgA disease

This disease of adults may resemble dermatitis herpetiformis or pemphigoid but a characteristic pattern of peripheral vesiculobullous lesions about a red central area may allow clinical recognition. The blister is subepidermal and immunofluorescence demonstrates a linear IgA band at the dermoepidermal junction, in contrast to the granular papillary IgA deposits of dermatitis herpetiformis. Gluten enteropathy is absent and there is no association with HLA-B8; the condition may not respond to dapsone so that prednisolone may be needed. Probably it is a separate entity unrelated to dermatitis herpetiformis.

Benign chronic bullous dermatosis of childhood

This is a rare acquired disease of childhood in which a dermatitis herpetiformis-like or pemphigoid-like eruption is concentrated about the pelvic regions, belly, scalp and face. It is relatively commoner in Asia and Africa. The blister is subepidermal and a linear IgA band at the dermoepidermal junction is demonstrable. Low titre circulating IgA anti-basement membrane zone antibodies may be demonstrable. HLA-B8 is associated although not as strongly as with dermatitis herpetiformis. Gluten enteropathy is absent. Possibly it is the childhood form of linear IgA disease.

Tumours of the Skin

This Chapter is devoted only to common and important tumours, although a few rare ones of special interest are mentioned briefly. Many rare tumours for example of epidermal appendages, nerve sheaths, etc, are not mentioned.

Carcinogenesis

Table 19.1 lists known carcinogens in skin. The role of ultra-violet light is discussed on p. 124. Chemical carcinogens are less important but industrial hydrocarbons have been recognized as carcinogens since scrotal cancer was described in chimney-sweeps by Percival Pott in 1775 and by Von Volkman in tar workers a century later. In the United Kingdom financial compensation for occupational tar-induced cancer was introduced in 1907.

Chemicals taken internally may be important. Inorganic arsenic (sodium arsenate) is the best known, used widely until 30 years ago in the treatment of psoriasis and as a 'tonic' in childhood. Lastly, infrared radiation (e.g. in blast furnace workers) and X-irradiation in medical and nursing personnel, miners of radioactive ores, etc, may both cause skin cancer.

Lastly, genetically determined disorders of DNA repair, for example in xeroderma pigmentosum, may predispose to premature carcinogenesis from ultraviolet damage.

Tumours of the Epidermis

In addition to the clearly benign or malignant lesions (Table 19.2), several intermediate conditions which have malignant potential are included (see Table 19.7).

Table 19.1 Known carcinogens in skin.

Ultraviolet light
X-irradiation
Heat
Arsenic ingestion
Industrial hydrocarbons

Table 19.2 Tumours of the epidermis.

Benign	Malignant
Basal cell papilloma	Basal cell carcinoma
Squamous papilloma	Squamous cell carinoma
Clear cell acanthoma	Malignant melanoma

Benign Epidermal Tumours

Basal cell papilloma

These lesions, also called seborrhoeic warts, seborrhoeic keratoses or senile warts, are almost universal in the second half of life. They develop in both sexes particularly on the upper trunk, brow, temples and face. The lesions are grey–brown, brown or almost black and often have a greasy appearance. They are round or ovoid and may reach diameters up to 3 or even 4 cm. They may be almost flat or raised or sessile nodules, or may even be pedunculated. The surface is irregular and papillomatous. Differential diagnosis is from moles, pigmented basal cell carcinoma, lentigo maligna and malignant melanoma.

Cryotherapy with liquid nitrogen is effective. Very large and numerous lesions are best curetted off flush with the skin surface. Local anaesthesia is often unnecessary. Very light galvanocautery suffices for haemostasis. Healing is rapid and should leave little scarring.

Squamous papilloma

Solitary wart-like papillomata are sometimes seen in the elderly, usually on the face. They rarely grow larger than 5–7 mm. They can be destroyed by liquid nitrogen or curetted out and cauterized under local anaesthesia. Some are probably viral warts.

Clear cell acanthoma

This is a very rare, usually solitary nodule (Degos' acanthoma) which develops slowly over many years or even decades, usually on the anterior or lateral aspect of the lower leg. Its surfaces may be scaly or may appear eroded or translucent. Histologically, the acanthotic epidermis shows characteristic areas of 'clear' cells which contain glycogen. Excision biopsy is the treatment.

Cysts of the epidermis

Epidermoid cysts

These are commonly misnamed 'sebaceous cysts'. They can occur on any part of the body, presenting as cystic swellings with a smooth overlying epidermis usually showing a central punctum. The cyst contains keratin, not sebum, produced by the endothelial lining which shows normal maturation, including granular layer formation. Surgical excision is the treatment of choice. Epidermoid cysts are associated with intestinal polyposis in Gardner's syndrome which is inherited in an autosomal dominant fasion. Malignant transformation of the polyps is not uncommon.

Pilar (trichilemmal) cysts

Better known as 'wens', these are usually multiple and occur on the scalp. They may be familial. The cyst is tense, smooth and does not show a punctum. Its epithelial lining resembles the outer root sheath of hair follicles. The contents are keratinous but a granular layer does not form. Treatment is by excision.

Milia

These are pin-head epidermoid cysts commonly seen on the upper cheeks and around the eyes in young adults. Each milium is seen as a glistening white 1–2 mm papule which can be lifted out with the point of a sterile hypodermic needle. The development of milia may be secondary to trauma and inflammation, particularly following subepidermal blistering. Such milia are seen in the scars of epidermolysis bullosa dystrophica, bullous pemphigoid and porphyria cutanea tarda.

Malignant Epidermal Tumours

Three potentially invasive tumours may arise from epidermis. Basal cell carcinoma is much the commonest, and malignant melanoma the least common. Malignant melanoma and squamous carcinoma may metastasize.

Basal cell carcinoma

A basal cell carcinoma is a slow-growing, locally invasive tumour usually arising during middle or old age, and usually found on the face. The cheek (especially near the inner canthus), forehead, temple, nose and neck are all common sites. Less commonly they occur on the trunk or limbs but never on palm, sole or glans penis. The ear is also an unusual site. Rarely, multiple tumours occur in the hairy scalp in old people who underwent X-ray epilation for tinea capitis half a century earlier, or along the mid-line of the back after X-irradiation of the spine for ankylosing spondylitis long ago. Multiple lesions of non-exposed areas are also the predominant tumours induced by previous inorganic arsenic administration. Men are more frequently affected, usually because of occupational solar exposure.

There are three main clinical patterns:
- A slow-growing papule or nodule
- Early ulcerated lesions
- Self-healing flat lesions ('morphoeic')

Usually the lesion commences as a small, hard, painless, superficial nodule which, during a course of one to several years, slowly enlarges until it becomes about a centimetre or more in diameter. Eventually central necrosis leads to ulceration. At this stage it has a hard, raised, pearly, telangiectatic edge which forms the rim of the crateriform ulcer (Fig. 19.1), the centre of which is covered by a brownish crust. When the crust is removed a reddish area of pseudo-granulation tissue is exposed. The lesion is usually circular or oval.

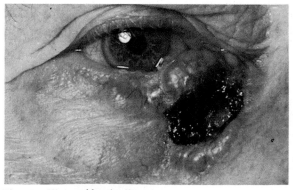

Fig. 19.1 Ulcerated basal cell carcinoma at atypical site.

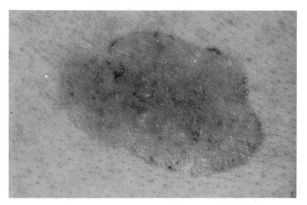

Fig. 19.2 'Morphoeic' basal cell carcinoma with slightly raised pigmented rim.

If left untreated the growth erodes the deeper tissues, may destroy cartilage and invades bone. In the later stages of neglected tumours, relentless spread in bone and under periosteum may render the disease incurable. Sometimes, localized superficial ulceration which refuses to heal is the first change the patient notices, especially on the nose. Careful inspection may reveal the tumour to be much larger than initially suspected. The 'morphoeic' type is the most insidious of all and may have been present for years before being brought to medical attention or noticed incidentally during medical examination (Fig. 19.2). Trunk lesions are often morphoeic and present as a red scarred plaque, not raised and often slightly depressed. There may be a thread-like raised translucent rim and a self-healing central zone, although the latter can easily be eroded by rough handling. A superficial resemblance to morphoea accounts for its name. This form of carcinoma produces a considerable fibrous reaction which may cause atrophy of the cancerous tissue and partial healing. Sometimes nodular lesions are unusually translucent and white, simulating cysts (Fig. 19.3). Small venules can be seen on the surface of the nodule. Haemorrhagic (pigmented) lesions may be confused with malignant melanoma.

The diagnosis should always be confirmed by biopsy unless a skilled cytologist is available. In expert hands, exfoliative cytology of scrapings from the tumour is 99% accurate and furnishes a definitive diagnosis in 30 minutes (Fig. 3.3).

Treatment

Surgical excision, radiotherapy, curettage and

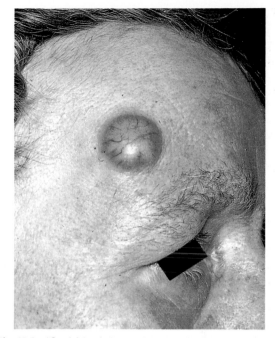

Fig. 19.3 'Cystic' (non-ulcerated) basal cell carcinoma.

electrodesiccation and cryotherapy all have a place according to the patient's age and state of health, and the site, type, size, etc, of the tumour. All have a 5–10% recurrence rate. The best results are obtained where difficult therapeutic decisions can be taken by a plastic surgeon, radiotherapist and dermatologist working together in a combined clinic. Mohs surgery, guided by frozen sections, is tissue-sparing but time consuming.

Basal cell naevus syndrome (Gorlin's syndrome)

Multiple tumours may be part of a genetic disorder which includes palmoplantar pitting, jaw cysts and defects of ribs and vertebrae. Multiple basal cell tumours develop in adolescence or early adult life, particularly on the face and brow but sometimes the trunk. Most do not behave aggressively. Bony defects in the skull confer a characteristic facies and radiographs are likely to reveal dental cysts, calcification of the falx cerebri and broad or bifid ribs. A variety of other skeletal and neurological defects may occur.

Squamous cell carcinoma

This malignant growth is capable of metastasizing, usually via the lymphatic channels. Most tumours

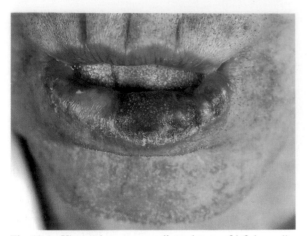

Fig. 19.4 Ulcerated squamous cell carcinoma of left lower lip. The whole of the lip was grossly dysplastic.

occur in men. The face and lower lips (Fig. 19.4) are the sites of election, i.e. sun-exposed areas, but these tumours may be found elsewhere, for example on the ear, back of the hand, forearms or shins. They may arise from actinic thermal, arsenical, X-ray or hydrocarbon keratoses or from the dysplastic epithelium of leukoplakia as well as from areas of Bowen's disease. Rarely, they arise in the margin of a chronic leg ulcer. Pipe smokers, especially those who use clay pipes, may develop the tumour on the lip or tongue.

Squamous carcinomata are seldom seen in persons under 45 years of age. At presentation, the duration is measured in weeks or a few months, unlike the many months or years of a typical basal cell carcinoma.

Histopathologically, the epidermis is grossly thickened with downward invasion of the dermis by abnormal epidermal cells. The clear-cut epidermodermal junction is lost and clumps of neoplastic epidermal cells are present in the dermis. Mitotic figures, many abnormal, are frequent and 'cell nests' of deeply keratinized cells are often scattered in the undifferentiated neoplastic epidermis. The surface layers are 'warty' with hyperkeratosis.

Macroscopically the tumour commences as a nodule which grows fairly rapidly and forms an oval or circular tumour, raised a few millimetres above the level of the surrounding skin. Ulceration may occur and the edges of the fully formed lesion are everted. If left untreated, a fungating tumour develops and erodes all the adjacent tissues; metastases form in the draining lymphatic glands, and may spread to distant organs.

Differential diagnosis

On the face, keratoacanthoma has to be distinguished. Basal cell carcinoma does not keratinize. Rarely, warty granulomata can be confusing, and even non-pigmented malignant melanoma. A syphilitic chancre may have to be considered and atypical basal cell papillomata can also cause confusion at times.

Diagnosis

Excision biopsy of small lesions or incisional biopsy of larger ones is essential for accurate diagnosis. Cytology is not reliable. Thorough clinical (and if necessary histological) examination of regional lymph glands is essential.

Treatment

Radical surgery and radiotherapy are both effective and the choice depends on age, site, fitness for anaesthesia, etc. Curettage is dangerously inadequate. Mohs surgery has a place in special centres. It should be remembered that the underlying carcinogenic factors may lead to further primary tumours in the future, so patients with basal or squamous carcinomata should be checked regularly for at least 5 years and the whole of the skin examined on each occasion.

Malignant melanoma

This is a malignant tumour arising from melanocytes. It can arise from previously normal epidermis, presumably from malignant transformation of one epidermal melanocyte or from a pre-existing melanocytic naevus (mole) where the cells are on the dermal side of the epidermodermal junction.

Risk factors

Three important precursor lesions are now recognized. These and other risk factors are listed in Table 19.3.

Giant congenital melanocyte naevi. These are described on p. 182.

Lentigo maligna. This is an uncommon macular pigmented lesion arising in elderly people on sun-

Table 19.3 Precursor lesions and risk factors for malignant melanoma.

Precursor lesions	Lentigo maligna
	Congenital giant melanocyte naevus
	Dysplastic naevus syndrome
Other risk factors	Gross regular or intermittent solar exposure
	Very large numbers of moles
	Family history of melanoma
	Trauma, e.g. to the feet in Africans

damaged skin, usually on the face. The contour (border) and pigmentation are characteristically irregular (Fig. 19.5). Partial regression may occur. Eventually (after 5–30 years), invasive lentigo maligna melanoma develops (Fig. 19.6) (see below).

The diagnosis is confirmed by incisional biopsy through the darkest part of the lesion, which reveals

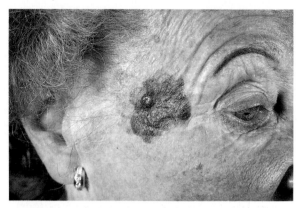

Fig. 19.6 Nodular malignant melanoma arising from longstanding lentigo maligna.

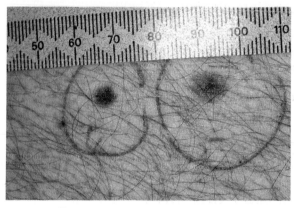

Fig. 19.7 Dysplastic naevi in a 35-year-old man with a malignant melanoma elsewhere on skin.

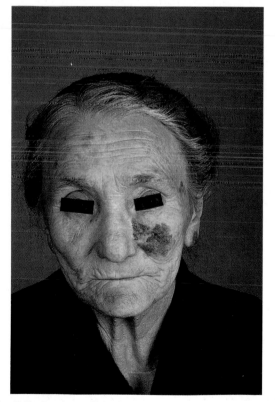

Fig. 19.5 Lentigo maligna (malignant melanoma pre-invasive or in situ).

atypical melanocytes spreading along the basal epidermis and often down hair follicles and appendages. A mononuclear dermal infiltrate is usually present. There is thus malignant melanoma in situ but without invasion.

Differential diagnosis is from simple and actinic lentigo. Basal cell papilloma superimposed on a lentigo should not be mistaken for nodular melanoma.

Treatment. In the very aged in poor health, no treatment is needed. Otherwise complete surgical excision (with grafting, if necessary) is curative. Cryotherapy and dermabrasion are not yet of proven value.

Dysplastic naevus syndrome. The dysplastic naevus is only a recently recognized entity. It is a clinically and histologically atypical pigmented naevus with irregular or indistinct borders, varied colour shades and a barely raised surface (Fig. 19.7). Such naevi may

appear in adolescence and continue to appear thereafter. Less than 2% of white adults have such naevi but
of those with sporadic malignant melanoma, 30% have
one or more dysplastic naevi. Of melanoma patients
with a family history of melanomas, over 70% have
dysplastic naevi, as do over 30% of their close relatives.

Dysplastic naevi may be sporadic or familial, the
latter showing autosomal dominant inheritance. Their
malignant potential has been established beyond doubt
by observed development of melanoma in previously
photographed lesions.

Management. A suspected dysplastic naevus should
be excised for histopathology. The whole body should
be examined. Other highly suspected lesions should
also be excised. Less suspicious ones ideally should
be photographed and the patient followed up by
6-monthly examinations. If possible, first-degree relatives should be examined; if not, family history for
melanoma is mandatory.

Other risk factors. Epidemiological studies, especially
in Australia, have established the importance of solar
exposure as a risk factor. Such exposure, as a result of
the cult of sunbathing, made possible by rising
affluence and modern air transport, is probably the
main reason for the quadrupled incidence of malignant
melanoma in the last 30 years in white people. A family
history of malignant melanoma is an important risk
factor, as is a large number of moles (> 100) or trauma
(Table 19.3).

Age and sex distribution

Most melanomas arise in the second half of life but
onset in the third and fourth decades or even earlier is
by no means rare. In the United Kingdom, there is
slight female preponderance. There are also several
differences in distribution. In women, the leg is much
the commonest site whereas in men, tumours on the
trunk are more common. In black Africans who walk
barefoot, the sole is much the commonest site.

Classification

Four main clinicopathological variants are now recognized.

Superficial spreading malignant melanoma (Fig. 19.8).
This is the commonest type and tends to spread
laterally, sometimes with central regression. Eventually it may become nodular as vertical invasion
develops.

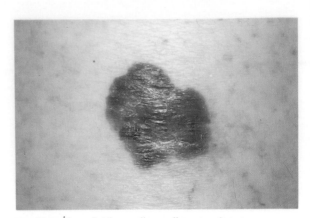

Fig. 19.8 Superficial spreading malignant melanoma.

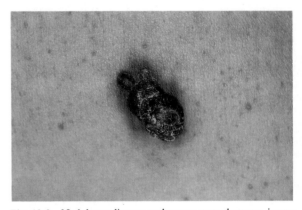

Fig. 19.9 Nodular malignant melanoma; note the gross irregularity of profile and colour.

Nodular malignant melanoma (Fig. 19.9). This is the
most dangerous and rapidly spreading type. It is
nodular, variably pigmented and may ulcerate quickly.
Some lesions are very uniformly pigmented and almost
black. Vertical invasion is an early feature.

Acral lentiginous malignant melanoma. These tumours
arise on the palm or sole and occasionally around or
under a nail. Any central nodular lesions may have a
surrounding area of macular pigmentation representing very superficial lateral spread.

Lentigo maligna melanoma (Fig. 19.6). This is invasive
melanoma arising in an area of lentigo maligna (see
above). The appearance of a papule, nodule or plaque
signals the conversion to invasive tumour.

Physical signs

Any pigmented lesion which has grown rapidly, or changed its shape or colour, should be examined carefully for the following.

- Irregularity of contour (Fig. 19.8). As with Bowen's disease, this points to uncontrolled, i.e. neoplastic growth, in the horizontal plane. Sometimes one or more notches are seen in the contour. This sign is seen best in superficial spreading tumours.
- Irregularity of profile (Fig. 19.9). This betrays uncontrolled growth in the vertical plane. It is seen best in nodular lesions.
- Irregularity of pigmentation (Fig. 19.9). Close examination will reveal variable shades and depth of colour in most tumours. Areas of dense, almost black pigmentation may adjoin paler blue, grey, light-brown or even red areas. However, nodular malignant melanoma may be uniformly black or dark blue.
- Erosion and ulceration are *late* signs (whose absence means nothing) indicating complete invasion of the epidermis, by which time spread in the dermis is likely to be substantial. However, slight 'weeping' of a pigmented lesion should never be ignored.
- Satellite pigmented papules and enlarged regional glands are late disaster signs, betraying lymphatic invasion by tumour cells.

Subungual melanoma

Although rare, these tumours are easily missed. Macular pigmentation spreading proximally or laterally from the nail fold in a Caucasian should always arouse suspicion. The nail may become distorted or otherwise dystrophic. Longitudinal bands of pigmentation in the nail may cause particular difficulty. Subungual haemorrhage due to trauma must be differentiated (e.g. black heel, tennis toe). Pigmentation arising distally in the nail bed is unlikely to be due to melanoma.

Pathology

In lentigo maligna, malignant melanocytes spread laterally along the basal epidermis. In superficial spreading melanoma, there is invasion of the epidermis and the dermal papillae. Nodular lesions spread deeply in the dermis.

Table 19.4 Levels of invasion of malignant melanoma (Clark's levels).

Level I	Intraepidermal (not invasive)
Level II	Reaching but not filling the papillary dermis
Level III	Filling the papillary dermis
Level IV	Reaching reticular dermis
Level V	Penetrating subcutaneous fat

Because convincing evidence has accumulated that prognosis is directly related to depth of invasion, i.e. to the thickness of the tumour, histopathologists now express this precisely, either by stating a Clark's level (Table 19.4) or a Breslow thickness, which is the distance in millimetres from the stratum granulosum of the epidermis to the level of the deepest tumour cells seen.

Diagnostic procedures

The procedure of choice is excision biopsy. If the lesion is large and there is diagnostic doubt, incisional biopsy is permissible. Cytology is not reliable. Acquired longitudinal pigmented nail bands in a white adult call for the removal of the nail, reflection of the posterior nail fold and adequate biopsy of the nail matrix.

Differential diagnosis

Basal cell papilloma rarely causes difficulty. Pigmented basal cell carcinoma may be more testing. Eroded nodular amelanotic melanoma can easily be confused with granuloma telangiectaticum or other angiomata.

Prognosis

This depends upon clinical and histological staging (Table 19.5). For Stage III patients (with distant metastases) the outlook is grim, median survival barely exceeding one year. Perhaps 30% of Stage II patients survive 5 years, and hardly any 10 years. Survival for Stage I patients correlates best with Breslow thickness of the tumour (Table 19.6).

Treatment

Wide surgical extirpation is mandatory. Often this will

Table 19.5 Clinical staging of melanoma.

Stage I	Primary tumour only, no abnormal palpable lymph glands
Stage II	Clinical involvement of regional lymph glands
Stage III	Distant metastases

Table 19.6 Tumour prognosis related to Breslow thickness (Stage I disease).

Tumour thickness (mm)	Five-year survival rate
<0.85	99%
0.85–1.69	90–95%
1.70–3.64	60–80% (depending on size)
>3.65	about 30%

Table 19.7 Intermediate epidermal lesions.

Keratoses	Actinic including PUVA keratoses
	X-irradiation
	Thermal
	Arsenical
	Hydrocarbon (pitch, tar, etc)
Leukoplakia	
Intraepidermal carcinoma	Bowen's disease
	Erythroplasia of Queyrat
	Paget's disease of the breast
	Extramammary Paget's disease
Keratoacanthoma	

necessitate grafting. Radiotherapy is of no value. Adjuvant chemotherapy with vindesine and imidazole carboxamide is added for tumours with poor prognosis or where there is known metastatic disease.

The value of routine regional lymph node removal in deeper tumours is controversial. Malignant melanoma patients are at significant risk of developing a second primary tumour and long-term surveillance is advised.

Intermediate Epidermal Lesions

These lesions are grouped together (Table 19.7) because they are neither utterly benign nor unequivocally malignant. The various keratoses, Bowen's disease and leukoplakia have variable malignant potential. Keratoacanthoma occasionally overlaps with squamous carcinoma. Paget's disease of the nipple is really epidermal invasion by an underlying ductal carcinoma.

Actinic keratosis

The lesions of actinic (or solar) keratosis are usually multiple and occur on exposed skin. Their development and number are directly proportional to the fairness of the patient's skin, the age, and the amount and intensity of sunlight to which the skin has been exposed. They may be profuse and gross in white skin

after a lifetime in the tropics. The lesions are palpable, scaly and rough to touch, and often brownish in colour. The scale is adherent. The lesion is usually discrete but after decades of gross sun exposure virtually the whole of the exposed skin may be dyskeratotic (Fig. 15.1); some lesions are very warty or may form cutaneous horns.

Histologically, grossly disordered epidermal maturation accompanies other actinic changes. Squamous cell carcinoma may slowly develop in a very small proportion (perhaps one per thousand per year) but is not usually aggressive, i.e. metastasis is slow.

Treatment

5-Fluorouracil 5% cream is the treatment of choice, applied twice daily for up to 14 days to small areas at a time. Marked inflammation may be induced, about which the patient must be warned. Used properly, it can literally rejuvenate the epidermis of the head and face but is ineffective on the hands. Cryotherapy, curettage and even dermabrasion of localized lesions have their place. Freezing is particularly appropriate for solitary or few lesions.

X-irradiation keratoses

Multiple keratoses may develop on the hands, arms and face of elderly dental surgeons, radiologists, radiographers and others exposed to X-rays in their younger days when radiation control was less strict. Bowen's disease or invasive carcinomata may supervene.

Thermal keratosis

Blast-furnace workers in the steel industry may be affected. Squamous carcinoma has supervened on chronic erythema ab igne with keratoses.

Arsenical keratosis

Multiple punctate keratoses of the palm and soles may develop 10–30 years after exposure to inorganic arsenic. Larger papular and nodular keratoses slowly evolve and clinical differentiation from squamous carcinoma can be difficult. Bowen's disease and basal or squamous carcinomata are liable to develop elsewhere.

Hydrocarbon keratosis

These lesions ('pitch wart') are common in workers habitually exposed to various coal tar products, usually after a latency period of 5–15 years. The keratoses are usually tiny and flat and occur on the face, backs of the hands and forearms, ankle and foot and scrotum. Occasionally larger keratoacanthoma-like lesions are seen.

If exposure is gross, associated inflammatory effects of tar may be evident such as photosensitive erythema, folliculitis, comedones and conjunctivitis. Hyperpigmentation and poikiloderma may develop. Periocular benign fibromas are common.

Keratoses and 'warts' may continue to appear years after the man has left the industry. Fortunately, evolution to squamous carcinoma is uncommon and metastasis is unusual except for scrotal cancers which are invariably invasive.

Leukoplakia

This is a particular pattern of hyperplasia of the skin or mucous membranes characterized clinically by the formation of thickened, whitish-grey, well-defined plaques and histologically by hyperkeratosis and acanthosis with dysplasia of the epidermal cells. It may proceed to squamous cell carcinoma. It is seen in the second half of life and external irritants play a role in its development. It is seen in the mouth or the lip, buccal mucosa or tongue. It is also seen in the anogenital region in women, at which site it has been renamed vulval intraepithelial neoplasia (VIN) and graded histologically. HPV-16 and other wart viruses may play a part in its genesis. In oral leukoplakia, smoking, ill-fitting dentures or abnormal teeth may be responsible. Discharges, maceration and friction may be relevant in genital lesions.

In the mouth, differential diagnosis is from simple mucosal hyperplasia due to gum biting and chewing, from lichen planus and from white sponge naevus. Anogenital leukoplakia (VIN) must be differentiated from lichen sclerosus et atrophicus, lichen planus, lichenified eczema or psoriasis.

Histologically unequivocal lesions should be excised surgically. Irritant factors must be removed.

Bowen's disease

Bowen's disease (intraepidermal carcinoma) is an uncommon, usually solitary, condition seen in the second half of life. It can occur anywhere on the body. Usually it develops de novo but may be caused by solar damage, X-irradiation and previous oral therapy with inorganic arsenic.

The lesion presents as a fixed psoriasis-like or eczema-like plaque, spreading very slowly over many years and with a characteristically irregular contour (Fig. 19.10). It may reach several centimetres in diameter. It is scaly and quite unresponsive to topical steroids. Itching is usually minimal. Histologically, acanthosis, disordered epidermal maturation with individual cell keratinization, and the presence of large keratinocytes with big 'nuclei' (often with abnormal mitotic figures) allow easy recognition. Evolution into invasive squamous cell carcinoma is very unusual but may eventually occur.

The diagnosis is confirmed by biopsy. Surgical excision is the treatment of choice but cryotherapy, radiotherapy or curettage may be more appropriate in some cases.

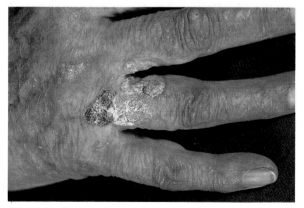

Fig. 19.10 Bowen's disease (intraepidermal carcinoma) of finger.

Erythroplasia of Queyrat

The term should be discarded: this is Bowen's disease occurring on the penis. It is commoner in the uncircumcized and usually straddles the glans and adjacent distal shaft. The affected zone is bright red and glazed and often sore. After biopsy confirmation, radiotherapy is the treatment of choice. Differential diagnosis is from psoriasis, lichen planus and plasma cell balanitis of Zoon.

Paget's disease of the breast

In this rare disease a unilateral eczema-like eruption develops in the skin of the nipple and slowly spreads centrifugally on the breast. The surface of the plaque is moist and crusted, and the disease is unresponsive to topical corticosteroids. Differential diagnosis is from dermatitis and is confirmed by biopsy which reveals Paget's cells in the epidermis. These are malignant cells arising from an underlying intraductal carcinoma of the breast. The treatment is simple mastectomy.

Extramammary Paget's disease

This rare condition arises from the adnexal apocrine structures and occurs in the anogenital region or axilla. Underlying carcinoma must be excluded.

Keratoacanthoma

Keratoacanthoma, or molluscum sebaceum, is a rapidly growing but self-healing tumour thought to arise from a hair follicle. It is generally solitary and on the face or arm. A rapidly growing papule matures in a few weeks into a domed, firm nodule up to 2 cm in diameter. As the lesion develops its sides show a bulging convexity and its crown may have a whitish appearance with a central horny plug (Fig. 19.11). Later, the horny plug may fall out, leaving a crateriform nodule. It reaches its maximum size by 8 weeks, then remains stationary for weeks or months before involuting (if left untouched), often leaving a depressed scar.

For small lesions (up to 1 cm), excision biopsy provides the best histological material. Where primary closure would be difficult, for example on the nose, or with larger lesions, very deep curettage in one piece is simple to perform and rarely causes histological difficulty. Under low power magnification the architecture is characteristic but the histology of a rapidly growing lesion in a small biopsy may be impossible to distin-

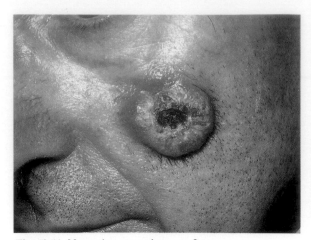

Fig. 19.11 Mature keratoacanthoma on face.

guish from that of squamous cell carcinoma. Occasionally lesions recur after curettage and may cause anxiety. Rarely, tumours clinically and histologically indistinguishable from keratoacanthoma, subsequently behave as metastasizing squamous cell carcinoma.

Benign Tumours of the Dermis

Derived from fibroblasts

Histiocytoma (dermatofibroma)

These are common lesions, more often seen in females particularly in middle life and usually on the legs. They may be solitary or multiple and are generally symptomless. The clinical features are quite characteristic, revealing a small 5–10-mm hard papule or nodule, often rather flat and with a 'button-like' shape on palpation. The lesion is firmly attached to skin and its surface is bound down. The colour is usually pale or deeper yellow–brown. It grows very slowly and then remains stationary for years. Some of these lesions may arise from insect bites.

Histologically, a well-circumscribed mass of fibroblastic cells is seen in the dermis. Often the over-lying epidermis shows modest basaloid hyperplasia. Treatment when requested is excision.

Derived from vascular tissue

Granuloma telangiectaticum

This common lesion, also called pyogenic granuloma, usually occurs at sites of trauma and is seen on the hand, finger, face or occasionally the lip. It presents as a rapidly growing friable papule which bleeds easily. Large lesions may reach a diameter of 10–15 mm and become pedunculated. More often, the lesion sits in a ring of sodden epithelium, like an acorn in its cup. Long-lasting lesions grow a surface epithelium and become less friable. Histologically, a mass of proliferative small blood vessels is set in a stroma infiltrated with inflammatory cells.

Bleeding is brisk after curettage but can be controlled by cauterization and pressure. However, sometimes the lesion will partly respond to an antibiotic ointment. Cryotherapy may also be effective. Curettings should always be examined histologically.

Cherry angioma (Campbell de Morgan spot)

These lesions are very common in the second half of life and increase in size and number with advancing age. They are found mainly on the trunk as 2–5-mm firm, regular red vascular papules with a smooth overlying epidermis. Some people have 20 or more. Only reassurance is required but they can be destroyed by cauterization if the patient insists.

Haemangioma simplex

Simple haemangiomata may develop in later life. The lower lip is probably the commonest site. Small lesions can be destroyed by electrocautery but larger ones should be excised.

Glomangioma

This tumour arises from the glomus body of the dermis, which is a specialized arteriovenous shunt bypassing the papillary capillaries (see Fig. 1.8). The central vessels are lined by glomus cells derived from smooth muscle.

The glomus tumour is usually a solitary blue–red soft papule which is tender on compression and which may be spontaneously painful. It is generally found peripherally on a limb and may occur on the nail bed. The treatment is surgical excision.

Derived from lymphatic tissue

These are probably hamartomatous malformations rather than true neoplasms.

Lymphangioma circumscriptum

These lesions usually appear in childhood, most often on the head, neck or around the shoulders. They are made up of masses of small vesicles deeply set in the skin, resembling frogspawn. There may be deeper subcutaneous lymphatic cisterns. These hamartomas are best left alone; attempts at surgical extirpation usually fail.

Diffuse lymphangioma

This is fortunately a rare condition in which extensive lymphangioma is associated with serious impairment of lymphatic drainage. A whole limb may be involved, sometimes a leg with genital lymphoedema. Major amputation or plastic surgery may become inevitable. Recurrent streptococcal lymphangitis tends to complicate the situation, necessitating life-long penicillin V prophylaxis.

Malignant Tumours of the Dermis

Secondary deposits

The skin may be the seat of metastatic deposits from an internal carcinoma. The breast is the usual primary site but tumours of the gastrointestinal tract and bronchus are occasionally responsible. The lesions are usually multiple, painless hard nodules in the dermis and subcutis. The diagnosis is confirmed by biopsy.

Kaposi's sarcoma

In its classical form this is a rare tumour of elderly men, also called idiopathic haemorrhagic sarcoma. It is particularly seen in Ashkenazi Jews but is now known to occur throughout the world and to be particularly common in parts of Africa. Multiple blue–red, firm, rather warty plaques and nodules usually begin on the skin of the foot and slowly spread up the leg (Fig. 19.12). Eventually, scattered nodules affect the thighs, arms, head or trunk. The disease causes increasing oedema of the lower limbs due to lymphatic obstruction and may spread to the lymph glands and systemic organs. It is a tumour of multicentric origin with vascular endothelial and fibroblastic elements. After a course of up to 10 years, it is eventually fatal but can often be contained by judicious local radiotherapy.

The dramatic arrival of AIDS on the world scene has brought with it a quite different pattern of Kaposi's sarcoma, typically seen in young HIV-positive homo-

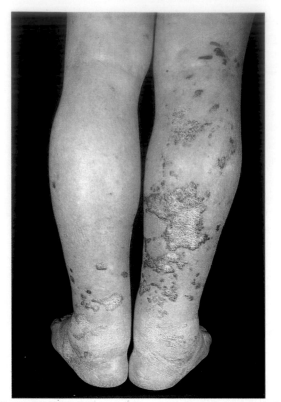

Fig. 19.12 Classical Kaposi's sarcoma of legs and feet in an elderly patient.

sexual men. Multiple round blue–red nodules develop widely on the trunk, limbs and face. Lesions of the tip of the nose, neck and buccal mucosa are common (see p. 50).

Angiosarcoma and lymphangiosarcoma

Malignant angioendothelioma is a rare tumour, usually seen on the head in the elderly and arising in cutanous blood vessels. A lymphangiosarcoma may arise in a chronically lymphoedematous limb, for example in the arm after a radical mastectomy (Stewart–Treves syndrome).

Lymphoma and Leukaemia

Aetiology

Some known factors may contribute to these neoplastic disorders (Table 19.8).

Heredity. If an identical twin develops leukaemia, the

Table 19.8 Aetiological factors in lymphoma and leukaemia.

Heredity
Chromosomal abnormalities
Virus infections
X-irradiation
Autoimmune disease

co-twin has a 20% chance of doing so, often quite quickly.

Chromosomal abnormalities. The link between chronic myeloid leukaemia and the Philadelphia chromosome is well known. Children with Down's syndrome are at special risk of leukaemia, as are those rare children with Bloom's syndrome (p. 120).

Virus infections. The Epstein–Barr virus is almost certainly implicated in Burkitt's lymphoma. HTLV-I virus is now recognized as the cause of certain fatal leukaemias.

Autoimmune disease. Increased risk of lymphoma is a recognized hazard in these diseases and in immuno-suppressed patients, for example those given renal allografts or on long-term immunosuppressive drugs for various diseases.

Cutaneous involvement

This may be specific, i.e. with histologically demonstrable neoplastic cells, or non-specific. The latter 'markers' of lymphoid malignancy are described in Chapter 14.

Cutaneous T-cell lymphoma

This disease, formerly known as mycosis fungoides, is a very slowly evolving infiltration of the skin by T-helper lymphocytes, only terminally becoming systemic. Its various forms were classically described by successive French physicians throughout the 19th century.

Pathology

Typically a dense upper dermal lymphocytic infiltrate is associated with epidermal invasion by lymphocytes to form 'Pautrier abscesses'. Many of the lymphocytes have densely stained convoluted nuclei—the Lutzner cells. Surface marker studies indicate that the T-helper cell is in the majority and that T-suppressor cells are sparse. All these changes may be less obvious in early disease and repeated biopsies at intervals of several months may be needed to establish the diagnosis.

Clinical staging

The author does not find the various classifications of the pundits useful, especially for undergraduate teaching purposes, and prefers the following simple divisions (Table 19.9).

Stage 1. Eczema-like or psoriasis-like lesions are seen, often with troublesome pruritus. The lesions may be fixed or a shifting pattern is seen. Often lesions have unusual (e.g. polycyclic) shapes (which arouse suspicion), and are likely to be on the trunk or proximal parts of the arms or legs. Relative lack of responsiveness to topical corticosteroids may also be a feature. Poikiloderma may be seen on the trunk. Biopsy may not provide absolute confirmation although surface marker studies are allowing earlier diagnosis. This stage may persist for many years.

Stage 2. The Stage 1 disease has evolved into fixed infiltrated plaques often with bizarre shapes, the partial horse-shoe shape being characteristic (Fig. 19.13). The disease may or may not be more widespread. The palms or soles may be involved. Biopsy confirms the diagnosis. Treatment may contain the disease at this stage for many years.

Stage 3. This is late disease. Nodules, tumours or ulcers have developed but the disease remains confined clinically to the skin. The prognosis is grim.

Stage 4. Lymph node or systemic organ involvement is

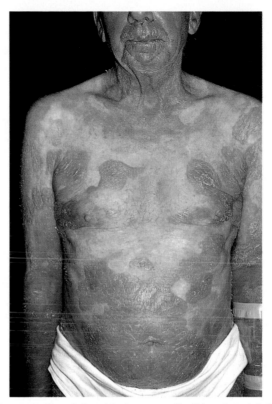

Fig. 19.13 Mycosis fungoides (cutaneous T-cell lymphoma). Infiltrated erythematous plaques in bizarre patterns.

evident and the disease is terminal. One variant of Stage 4 is erythroderma with atypical 'Sezary' cells demonstrable in the blood.

Clinical variants

Erythroderma occasionally develops early. A widespread atrophic poikiloderma, especially of the buttocks, belly and breasts, is another unusual presentation. Almost macular hypopigmented lesions are rare. Follicular mucinosis, in which erythematous plaques form with loss of hair follicles (which histologically show mucinous degeneration), may precede the lymphoma by months or years. Rarely multiple boil-like lesions mimic staphyloderma.

Diagnosis

Apart from skin biopsy, peripheral blood smears must be examined carefully for circulating Sezary cells. The bone marrow biopsy should be normal. A chest radiograph is necessary. Abnormal lymph glands

Table 19.9 Stages of cutaneous T-cell lymphoma.

Stage 1	Eczematoid or psoriasiform erythematous lesions
Stage 2	Infiltrated plaques
Stage 3	Nodules, tumours, ulceration
Stage 4	Lymph node involvement with or without systemic dissemination

demand biopsy but routine lymph gland removal for staging is pointless, as is lymphangiography for the same purpose. Ultrasound scanning of liver and spleen is non-invasive and probably worthwhile.

Treatment

In Stage 1 disease topical steroids may suffice for years, perhaps supplemented by intermittent UVB therapy. Small doses of oral prednisolone (5–10 mg daily) may be useful in suppressing pruritus and inflammation.

Once the diagnosis is beyond doubt (Stage 2) it is usual to offer PUVA therapy (see p. 106). PUVA is extremely effective in suppressing the disease although histological persistence is common and plaques may persist in inaccessible sites. Topical application of nitrogen mustard is an alternative for Stage 2 disease but is more difficult to handle than PUVA therapy.

Eventually the disease escapes from the control of these therapies. Localized nodules or tumours respond very well to conventional radiotherapy. In more widespread Stage 3 disease, electron beam therapy may induce temporary remission. Combination chemotherapy is disappointing.

Prognosis

Patients with Stage 1 or Stage 2 disease may survive in reasonable health for many years. The elderly may eventually die of other causes. If they survive long enough advanced disease eventually develops, whatever the treatment, and death within a year or two is likely.

There is no evidence as yet that very aggressive regimes which attempt to eradicate the abnormal cells entirely offer a better alternative, and indeed may simply execute the patient before his time!

Skin lesions in leukaemia

Various specific and non-specific changes may occur, especially in monocytic leukaemia. Purpura is common in acute leukaemia.

Other lymphomas

The Sezary syndrome

This is a rare disease of elderly males who develop erythroderma or rapidly progress to it from cutaneous T-cell lymphoma. There is a tendency to lymphadenopathy and abnormal T-helper cells (Sezary cells) are found in the blood, often comprising 10% or more of the circulating lymphocytes. Skin biopsy reveals similar cells in the dermis. A frank T-cell leukaemia with skin tumour formation may be a terminal event. PUVA, chemotherapy or leucapheresis may be of temporary value but few survive more than a year.

Lymphomatoid papulosis

This is a rare condition in which erythematous papular lesions evolve, scale and disappear over a few weeks. The disease resembles pityriasis lichenoides chronica but the histopathology is lymphoma-like.

Usually the course is benign but perhaps 10% of patients eventually develop true lymphoma (cutaneous T-cell lymphoma).

Crosti's indolent lymphoma

This is a rare disease of elderly men in which a solitary nodule of T-cell lymphoma develops, usually on the back. Radiotherapy is curative. Differential diagnosis is from a B-cell lymphoma with an entirely different and sinister prognosis.

Pagetoid lymphoma (Woringer–Kolopp disease)

A solitary, scaly indurated plaque slowly extends on a palm or sole in a young adult. Histologically abnormal cells of uncertain lineage invade the thickened epidermis.

B-cell lymphoma

Skin lesions are not uncommon. Smooth-surfaced dermal nodules and plaques, often with unusual shapes, may be a presenting feature. The writer has seen them on the trunk, upper arms and scalp.

Full assessment and staging by a haematologist –oncologist is essential. Initially at least, the skin lesions tend to be very radiosensitive.

Burkitts lymphoma

The skin is not involved in this form of lymphoma seen in African children and thought to be caused by the Epstein–Barr virus.

Acne Vulgaris, Rosacea, Perioral Dermatitis

Acne Vulgaris

Acne is one of the commonest of the diseases of skin. Because it is mainly a disease of adolescence it has attracted less interest than it deserves until recently and, because it does not threaten life or limb, its efficient treatment is often neglected. In fact, the sum of unhappiness directly caused in young people by acne is enormous and its successful treatment gratifies both patient and physician.

Pathogenesis

Acne vulgaris is a chronic disorder of the pilosebaceous apparatus, particularly in the skin of the brow, face, shoulders and upper trunk. It is characterized by the formation of microcomedones, excessive amounts of sebum, by obstruction of its outflow and by the release of mediators which cause inflammation in and around the dilated obstructed sebaceous glands. Rupture of the swollen pilosebaceous unit then leads to escape of fatty materials into the surrounding dermis or subcutis, provoking an inflammatory tissue response. Immune mechanisms probably play a part in this inflammation.

True seborrhoea, or excessive production of sebum, has been demonstrated to be a feature of acne subjects when their sebum output is compared with suitably matched controls. The cause of the seborrhoea is debatable. Sebaceous glands are under the control of the sex hormones, the androgenic ones stimulating increased gland size and sebum production, and the oestrogenic ones having an antagonistic effect. Although acne is a feature of syndromes characterized by excessive circulating androgens, for example Cushing's and Stein–Leventhal syndromes, the bulk of female acne subjects do not have raised circulating androgen levels, although a minority do have minor abnormalities of plasma testosterone or its carrier protein, sex-hormone binding globulin. In addition, androgen metabolism can occur in the skin. Thus testosterone can be metabolized in the skin to the more active dihydrotestosterone, a reduction catalysed by the enzyme $5\text{-}\alpha\text{-reductase}$. This supports the hypothesis that excessive androgenic activity may develop locally around the sebaceous glands and possibly about the hair follicles in 'idiopathic' female hirsutism.

The reasons for the obstruction to outflow are also complex. The amount of sebum, its viscosity, the degree of stratum corneum hydration, and poral hyperkeratosis induced by androgens may all be important. Certainly the comedone, or blackhead, is not simply a 'bath plug' causing obstruction; indeed, its formation may be a consequence rather than a cause of the sluggish sebum flow.

The chemical changes within the retained sebum are better understood because such sebum can be obtained and analysed. Normal sebum consists mainly of triglycerides with smaller amounts of fatty acids, cholesterol, lecithin and phospholipids. Retained acne sebum contains a higher than normal proportion of free fatty acids. Almost certainly these fatty acids are derived from the breakdown of neutral triglycerides by lipases released by the commensal bacterial residents of the pilosebaceous unit, namely *Proprionobacterium acnes* and *Staphylococcus albus*. However, it has not been convincingly shown that the commensal flora of the acne patient differ quantitatively or qualitatively from the normal.

Trauma by squeezing, overhydration of the stratum corneum in hot, humid conditions or overuse of cosmetics probably all contribute to gland rupture at different times and the consequent fierce, chemically induced inflammation.

Pathology

The lesions of acne are pleomorphic, falling into three groups. Blackheads, or comedones, consist of masses of cornified cells arranged somewhat like the layers of an onion and enclosing inspissated sebum and perhaps a vellus hair. The external part is black, due to the presence of melanin. Whiteheads are distended sebaceous glands without a pore. Acne cysts are larger, deeper masses of retained sebum.

All the above are essentially non-inflammatory. The second category of lesions is the consequence of inflammation and includes papules, pustules and abscesses. Postinflammatory scars of various types constitute the third type of lesion.

Clinical picture

Acne begins at puberty when hormonal activity wakens the latent sebaceous glands of childhood. Sometimes the first comedones appear at 8 or 9 years and parents are reluctant to accept that this heralds the onset of puberty. The peak incidence is in the years of adolescence but the disease is by no means uncommon in the twenties, nor rare in the thirties. In adolescence the sexes are equally affected but later chronic papular acne on the face, and especially the chin, may persist in women. In a few men severe nodulocystic acne of the face, neck and back may endure into the forties. The face, including the brow, shoulders, nape of neck and the upper trunk in a V-shape are the sites involved, although the disease may be localized in any of these areas.

In early adolescence blackheads and whiteheads often predominate without obvious inflammation and with only very superficial pinhead papules and pustules. Such acne can nevertheless leave distressing scarring. In more inflammatory disease the above are combined with larger papules, pustules, abscesses (Fig. 20.1) and cysts. Sebo-pus may track to produce elongated fluctuant abscesses. Occasionally the disease is grossly inflammatory, reducing the face and upper trunk of the hapless patient to a florid mass of pleomorphic lesions (Fig. 20.2).

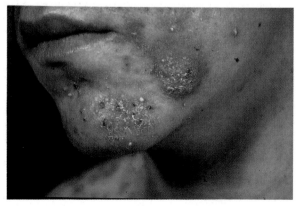

Fig. 20.1   Acne abscess on chin.

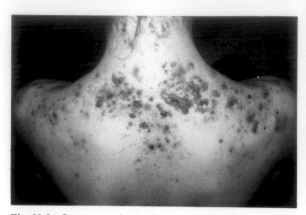

Fig. 20.2   Severe necrotic acne in a 12-year-old boy.

A very rare variant is called *acne fulminans*, seen almost exclusively in boys in early adolescence. The lesions become necrotic and form haemorrhagic crusts. Malaise, fever, arthralgia and even frank arthritis or an immunocomplex vasculitis can complicate acne fulminans and the ESR is very high. Such acne, if allowed to progress, may leave grossly disfiguring and irreversible scarring.

Fortunately, some scarring is reversible and the younger the patient, the better the prognosis in this regard. If the disease persists after adolescence, blackheads tend to be less evident and the disease tends to become more monomorphic. A recognizable subset of acne is seen in very tall white males who develop persistent severe nodulocystic acne (sometimes called acne conglobata), often with frequent multiple abscess formation. The disease shows no sign of spontaneous regression with the passing years.

The clinical evidence of the seborrhoea is very variable. Patients may complain that the affected skin in whole or in part is very greasy, and direct questioning usually, but not always, elicits the fact that the hair has to be washed daily because of its oiliness.

Acneiform eruptions

Acne due to oral corticosteroids (or Cushing's syndrome) has a different clinical pattern. Comedones, whiteheads and cysts are absent and typically a monomorphic mildly inflammatory papular acne appears on the shoulders and upper trunk with relative sparing of the face.

Isoniazid-induced acne does affect the face and is more like the natural disease but can be florid and pustular. Iodides and bromides can induce a similar picture.

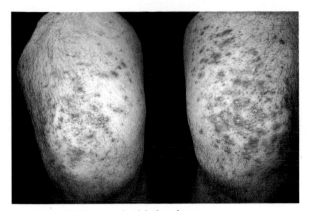

Fig. 20.3 Oil (hydrocarbon)-induced acne.

Table 20.1 Management of acne vulgaris.

	Mild	Moderate	Severe
Topical	Sulphur	Sulphur	Sulphur
	Benzoyl peroxide	Benzoyl peroxide	Benzoyl peroxide
		Retinoic acid	Retinoic acid
		Erythromycin	Erythromycin
			Clindamycin
Systemic		Tetracylines	Minocycline
		Erythromycin	Doxycycline
			Dianette
			Isotretinoin
			Steroid injection of abscesses

Pin-head acne is sometimes seen in infants on the cheeks but tends to disappear after the first year. Rarely, infantile acne is cystic.

Oil acne is a recognized industrial disease due to oils and other hydrocarbons. It is typically seen on the thighs and knees of apprentice engineers due to prolonged contact with oil-soaked trousers and aided by lack of attention to hygiene (Fig. 20.3). Chloracne is a severe form of chemical acne due to chlorinated hydrocarbons.

Treatment

The prognosis is a function of the natural severity and longevity of the disease process and the efficacy of treatment. Management (Table 20.1) depends entirely on the severity of the disease but a long-term view must always be taken. Diet is probably irrelevant but many acne patients insist otherwise, and selective withdrawal of sweets, chocolates and cream from the diet is beneficial for other reasons and need not be discouraged by the physician. The affected parts should be washed with ordinary soap not more than twice daily, and squeezing of lesions should be strongly discouraged. Saunas, Turkish baths and other forms of 'steaming' are contraindicated and may lead to acute poral occlusion and gland rupture. Ultraviolet B is usually helpful whether natural, when the climate allows, or artificial.

Topical therapy should be the first approach. Preparations containing sulphur or benzoyl peroxide should be used and many proprietary lotions, gels and creams contain variations and combinations of these substances. Retinoic acid (Retin A, U.K.) is also useful, although very slow to act. All these preparations are potentially irritant and drying, so patients must be warned and instructed to build up the frequency and duration of exposure gradually. One- or two-hour applications are safest initially. This is particularly important in brown- or black-skinned girls where overuse can lead to an irritant dermatitis leaving gross hyperpigmentation in its wake which may take months to subside. Although topical erythromycin or clindamycin can be effective, their use should be discouraged because of the possible epidemiological consequences of transferred bacterial resistance.

If topical therapy has failed, systemic therapy on a long-term basis is needed where more than mild inflammation is present or scarring is threatened or is occurring. Erythromycin or tetracycline can be used in a dose of 1 g daily (in divided doses) for more severe cases, 750 mg for moderate cases and 500 mg daily for mild ones. Whichever drug is chosen the trial should last not less than 3 months and sometimes 6 months is needed for optimum benefit. If one has failed, the other can be tried.

Milk and milk products interfere with the absorption of tetracycline (as does oral iron) so the drug should be taken with water 30–45 minutes before meals. Pregnancy is an absolute contraindication to tetracycline therapy and girls must be warned accordingly.

If both drugs have failed, minocycline (Minocin, U.K.) 50 mg twice daily, doxycycline (Vibramycin,

U.K.) 50 mg daily or co-trimoxazole (Septrin, Bactrim, U.K.) two tablets daily, can be tried in turn in the same way. If successful, any of these drugs can safely be continued on a long-term basis. Probably all of these antibiotics act by inhibiting the lipase-producing commensal bacteria of the pilosebaceous follicles. They are suppressive and not curative and, if disease activity remains, relapse will follow withdrawal of the drug. A pustular folliculitis of the face due to Gram-negative superinfection is a rare complication of long-term antibiotic therapy.

One of these drugs will control acne in 90% of patients if supported by suitable topical therapy. Occasionally, severe and persistent acne in young females, resistant to all other treatment, requires the administration of an oestrogen-containing drug. A combination of ethinyloestradiol 35 μg and cyproterone acetate 2 mg (Dianette, U.K.) taken for 21 days each month starting on the fifth day of each cycle is sometimes helpful but a 6-month trial is needed. The physician should be certain that there is no gynaecological or other contraindication to this treatment. Locally applied oestrogen cream is useless. Oral spironolactone has an antiandrogenic action. Trial of 100–200 mg daily may be justifiable but in females only.

Acute acne abscesses and cysts are best treated by intralesional injection of 0.05–0.1 ml triamcinolone suspension (Lederspan or Adcortyl, U.K.) (5–10 mg/ml) which brings about resolution within 3 days. Surgical incision should be avoided and can result in horrific scars. In acne fulminans oral prednisolone, 20–40 mg daily, may be needed initially until concomitant isotretinoin has started to act.

The arrival of the retinoid, isotretinoin (Roaccutane, U.K.; Accutane, U.S.A.) has revolutionized the treatment of very severe acne. It is indicated in acne fulminans, gross persistent nodulocystic acne in either sex and, indeed, any very severe inflammatory acne which has resisted thorough oral antibiotic treatment. It is best given in a dose of 1.0 mg/kg daily for 16–24 weeks. Lower doses may be effective but the relapse rate is much higher. The patient must be warned about the inevitable marked dryness of the skin and mucous membranes, especially the lips, the likelihood of minor nosebleeds and increased liabilities to chapping or sunburn. Paronychia, meatitis in the male and contact lens problems due to eye dryness are other occasional problems. Staphyloderma is common, as is coccal colonization of the nostrils. Those who take vigorous physical exercise should be warned about the possibility of aching discomfort in muscles and joints. Most important of all, the drug is teratogenic and pregnancy must be excluded before treatment and reliably prevented during and for one month after treatment. Abnormalities of serum lipids and liver function tests should be excluded before treatment and sought after 4 and perhaps 8 weeks of treatment. Improvement may only be apparent in the third and subsequent months of treatment but the end results are spectacular, total remission being achieved in 90% of these selected patients. Long-term benefit can be expected confidently in the majority and it is rare for second courses to be needed.

Rosacea

Rosacea is a disease of unknown aetiology characterized by an eruption of the central areas of the brow, face and chin, and consisting of acneiform papulopustules on a background of erythema and telangiectasiae. It is seen in both sexes in middle and late life and may be complicated by connective tissue and sebaceous hyperplasia of the nose, particularly in elderly men, and by keratoconjunctivitis.

Pathogenesis

Both cutaneous blood vessels and the sebaceous glands seem to be involved but there is no seborrhoea. An abnormal tendency to vasodilatation could explain the observed association with migraine. The response of the papulopustular element to small doses of tetracycline or other antiacne antibiotics suggests that mechanisms similar to those in acne vulgaris may be relevant, a view reinforced by the occasional overlap of acne vulgaris and rosacea in young adults. No pathogenic organism has been demonstrated nor any association with a systemic abnormality, gastrointestinal or otherwise. The histopathology is often granulomatous.

Clinical picture

Rosacea is seen in both sexes. It rarely appears before the fourth decade and the peak of incidence is in the fifth decade. With rare exceptions the disease is strictly confined to the face, particularly the middle longitudinal third, i.e. the central forehead, nose and cheeks and chin. A tendency to flush easily may be an early symptom. Later the affected areas become increasingly red and large telangiectatic venules are seen, especially on the nose and cheeks. Papules of varying sizes or papulopustules develop in some patients. Lymphoedema is a common feature, especially in men, and the turgid red plaques convey a shiny appearance. The disease is well known to the ophthalmologist and ocular symptoms may precede skin problems. Conjunctivitis, keratitis and blepharitis may all be seen. Rhinophyma is an uncommon complication, seen almost exclusively in elderly men in whom sebaceous and connective tissue proliferation occurs in the nose, occasionally producing a grotesque deformity.

Rosacea is a chronic disorder which may persist for years or even decades, although varying in severity. It may be aggravated by bright sunlight.

An iatrogenic variant of the disease has become increasingly common in the last decade due to the use of potent fluorinated corticosteroids in treatment. The picture of a smooth atrophic skin, severe telangiectasia and crops of papulopustules occurring especially when the treatment is temporarily stopped, is characteristic (see also Perioral Dermatitis below).

Differential diagnosis

The comedones and scarring of acne are absent and the age distribution is different. Photosensitive eruptions are seasonal. Contact dermatitis typically affects the eyelids, always spared in rosacea. Rosacea is never atrophic like DLE. Lupus erythematosus is never pustular. Seborrhoeic dermatitis is scaly and affects the brows and scalp margin.

Management

Tetracycline by mouth in very small dosage is the treatment of choice. Almost always 250 mg twice daily promptly suppresses the papulopustular component of the disease but is ineffective in lymphoedematous and rhinophymatous variants. Control can be maintained by 250 mg once daily or even once every second day. The telangiectatic element is less easy to treat but often improves with long-term tetracycline treatment. Rarely, tetracycline fails and one of the other antiacne antibiotics can be substituted. Amoxycillin is also occasionally useful. Isotretinoin is disappointing.

Topical preparations are of limited value. Metronidazole as a 1% gel or 0.5% sulphur in an aqueous cream may sometimes be useful. Potent corticosteroids should never be used. If the patient presents on such steroids they must be withdrawn, tetracycline started orally and the patient warned that the disease will get worse for up to 10 days before improving. Diet,

hormonal therapy and other systemic measures are of no value. Ocular symptoms or signs should never be ignored; appropriate advice should be obtained.

The disease is chronic for decades in some patients but is phasic in others, settling spontaneously. Rhinophyma can be greatly improved by plastic surgery.

Perioral dermatitis

This label has been applied to a clinical picture which has come to prominence in the last 15 years and is thought to be mainly but not entirely iatrogenic.

Clinical picture

The patient is almost always female, in the third, fourth or fifth decade of life, and presents with a striking perioral eruption of small papulopustules. Lesions about the nostrils are common and occasionally around the outer canthi and adjacent cheeks. Often there is erythema, telangiectasia and atrophy of the cheeks, and the history is obtained that a potent corticosteroid has been applied daily for months or even years. Comedones are absent. Such a therapeutic history is almost always obtained, the treatment usually having been started for trivial reasons and continued indefinitely because of the subjective satisfaction obtained. Direct questioning also generally elicits the story that temporary withdrawal of the steroid cream results in rapid 'deterioration' of the skin of the face, leading to prompt restoration of treatment.

Perioral dermatitis has been seen most in countries where drugs are free or subsidized, such as the United Kingdom, where every household in the land has its tube of potent corticosteroid. The disease has become less frequent in the United Kingdom in the 'eighties than in the 'seventies as the hazards of these drugs have gradually impressed prescribing family physicians.

Rarely, the perioral eruption is seen in the absence of such a history and it is a matter of debate whether it then constitutes a localized variant of rosacea.

Management

Treatment is identical to that for steroid-aggravated rosacea. After temporary worsening the prognosis is excellent and the perioral skin usually returns to normal within 3 months. Only a bland local application is needed.

Disorders of the sweat glands

There are two distinct types of sweat gland in man, the eccrine and apocrine glands.

Eccrine sweat glands

These are universal but most profuse in the axillae, palms and soles. The gland secretes a watery sweat containing electrolytes, urea and lactate, which is modified as it passes through the sweat duct to the skin surface. Sweat production is controlled by cholinergic sympathetic fibres of the autonomic nervous system in response to thermal stimuli over most of the body, but also in response to emotional stimuli, on the palms and soles and, to a lesser extent, the axillae, face and brow. Sweating clearly helps thermoregulation, through cooling by evaporation. It also plays a role in maintaining the water content (and therefore the pliability) of the stratum corneum, and the frictional 'grip' of the palms and soles.

Hyperhidrosis

Excessive production of sweat can be localized or diffuse, transient or chronic. Its distribution depends upon the cause. Many systemic disorders may cause hyperhidrosis. These include neurological lesions, particularly in the pontine, medullary and cervical areas; endocrinopathies such as hyperthyroidism; infections causing periodic abnormal temperature variations; and metabolic upsets such as insulin-induced hypoglycaemia or, rarely, phaeochromo-cytoma. Gustatory hyperhidrosis, i.e. sweating on the lips, forehead and nose, may be induced by eating hot spicy foods and is usually physiological; rarely, patho-logical gustatory sweating may be due to disease of the autonomic nervous system or disturbances of the parotid gland.

Notwithstanding this long list of causes, hyper-hidrosis is usually idiopathic. It is most commonly encountered in the second and third decade and in either sex. The hands, especially the palms, and axillae are the commonest sites of troublesome sweating but patients may complain of hyperhidrosis of the feet or face. Anogenital hyperhidrosis seems to be common in middle-aged men whose lives are stressful, for example business executives. There is no doubt that mental or emotional stress evokes sweating of palms, soles and axillae, which can be simply demonstrated. Such stress can also evoke sweating of the forehead, nose, mid-

lines of the chest and the back in some individuals; indeed, generalized sweating may occasionally be pro-voked in this way. However, in many young people minimal physical or mental activity is sufficient to pro-duce palmar or axillary sweating, for example during ordinary social intercourse. In a few unfortunate young people such sweating is almost continuous and may be related to obvious or occult emotional disorders.

Disability is considerable. Axillary sweating rots clothing. The hyperhidrotic foot may be foul-smelling, rots footwear and predisposes to viral warts, tinea and pitted keratolysis. Palmar sweating makes the social grace of shaking hands a torment for many young people. Fortunately, the long-term prognosis for emo-tional or idiopathic hyperhidrosis is good, and the condition usually eventually disappears. Typically, onset is soon after puberty and the condition has cleared by the age of 20–25 years.

Treatment

Management is unsatisfactory. Commercial antiper-spirants containing aluminium salts may be useful in mild cases. Aqueous 4–5% formaldehyde may be useful on the soles, applied as soaks daily for 5–15 minutes. The best treatment for the axillae is 20% aluminium chloride hexahydrate in 70% alcohol, painted on or applied as a roll-on at night and washed off in the morning (Anhydrol forte, Driclor, U.K.). The skin must be dried thoroughly before application, if necessary with a blow-dryer.

Propantheline bromide (Probanthine, U.K.) orally is occasionally useful but usually its anticholinergic action results in side-effects, especially dry mouth, before sweating is suppressed. In a dosage of 15–30 mg it is worth a trial and may act for up to 8 hours.

In severe intractable axillary hyperhidrosis, resistant to medical measures, surgical excision of the sweat gland-bearing skin is effective but leaves a cosmetically unpleasant scar and sometimes some limitation of shoulder movement. It should only rarely be neces-sary. Cervical sympathectomy abolishes palmar sweat-ing but is a major procedure carrying a 4% risk of Horner's syndrome. Endoscopic thoracic sympathec-tomy is safer. Iontophoresis is also effective and can be adapted for axillae, hands and feet, but few physio-therapy departments are suitably equipped. Glyco-pyrronium bromide may be used, but tap water alone is effective, probably by damaging and then blocking the intraepidermal sweat ducts.

Hypohidrosis and anhidrosis

This is reduced or absent sweating even after local pharmacological provocation. It is often unnoticed by the patient but may lead to heat intolerance or itching. Anhidrosis may be congenital, as part of an ectodermal dysplasia associated with absent or sparse hair and eyebrows, and dental abnormalities. Acquired causes include leprosy and diabetes (where there may be autonomic neuropathy), a variety of systemic diseases such as myxoedema, Addison's disease and Sjogren's syndrome, and certain skin diseases, particularly psoriasis and erythroderma. It may be chemically induced, topically by formaldehyde or glutaraldehyde or systemically as in mepacrine-induced lichenoid eruptions.

Bromhidrosis

This is an abnormal or excessive skin odour. Apocrine bromhidrosis is an axillary problem and is due to decomposition of apocrine sweat by surface bacteria; management consists of frequent washing and the local use of antibacterial agents, for example chlorhexidine (Hibitane Cream, U.K.). Eccrine bromhidrosis, induced by the activity of bacteria on sweat-sodden stratum corneum in the feet, can lead to a highly offensive odour. Soap and water are reasonably effective especially in male patients who have previously practised excessive restraint in their use.

Miliaria

Miliaria (prickly heat) is an acute eruption characterized by itching and the development of a papular, vesicular or pustular eruption. It is caused by sweat duct blockage induced by tropical heat and humidity or similar conditions engendered by excessive activity in unsuitable clothing, for example by troops in less extreme climates. Probably overhydration of the stratum corneum is the immediate cause of the sweat duct occlusion.

Treatment includes the encouragement of sweat evaporation by the provision, where possible, of appropriate environmental conditions, such as air-conditioning and loose clothing. Mild topical corticosteroid creams or lotions may relieve itching.

Apocrine Sweat Glands

In the genital and anal regions, the axillae, the nipples and areolae a special variety of sweat gland is found. This is an apocrine type of gland in which the tips of the cells lining the glands disintegrate and mix with the fluid secretion. The apocrine sweat glands are larger than the common, eccrine sweat glands and may open into the hair follicles above the sebaceous glands. Their secretion is odourless until it has been contaminated with bacteria, usually micrococci, when it develops a characteristic smell (varying from race to race) which acquires a sexual significance.

Hidradenitis suppurativa

This is an uncommon chronic inflammation involving the apocrine glands. A genetic factor is sometimes apparent. It may involve one or both axillae or the anogenital region, especially the inguinal creases and adjacent thighs. Papules, nodules, abscesses and cysts form which may lead to sinus formation and later fibrosis and scarring. Pain and tenderness or purulent discharge may be considerable.

The role of secondary bacterial infection is variable, but long-term oral antibiotic therapy is the treatment of first choice. Usually tetracycline, erythromycin or minocycline are tried. At its most severe the disease is disabling and even life-ruining, when extensive surgical extirpation of the whole of the affected apocrine gland-bearing skin is necessary; healing is by secondary intention, i.e. granulation. Radiotherapy may also be effective but is only rarely used, for obvious reasons. Isotretinoin is of little value.

—21—
Disorders of Pigmentation and Pigmented Naevi

Biology of the Melanocyte

The melanocyte is an ectodermal cell whose normal functional position is in the basal layer of the epidermis (Fig. 21.1). It is of neural crest origin and migrates into the epidermis during fetal development. Its functions are to synthesize the pigment melanin and to donate that melanin to surrounding keratinocytes. The maturation of keratinocytes into stratum corneum cells packed with melanin granules confers an ultraviolet light barrier which partly protects the underlying viable epidermis and dermis from the damaging effects of ultraviolet radiation.

Melanin synthesis occurs within a cytoplasmic organelle, the melanosome. Under the influence of tyrosinases, tyrosine is converted to melanin (Fig. 21.2). Fully melanized melanosomes are extruded via the melanocyte's dendritic processes into surrounding keratinocytes by an active interdependent process (Fig. 21.3). The melanin granules concentrate around the nucleus of the recipient cell, possibly thus conferring extra protection on the nuclear DNA. However, in the anuclear corneal cell the granules are uniformly distributed to form an 'ultraviolet screen'.

In different parts of the body melanocytes constitute between 5 and 20% of the basal epidermal cell layer. The races do not differ in total melanocyte populations, only in the rate and quantity of melanin production. The latter is influenced in addition by the effects of ultraviolet light on tyrosinase and by the pituitary lipotrophic hormone (which includes MSH and ACTH). In ordinary sections of skin, basal melanocytes are sometimes recognizable as larger 'clear cells' but special stains are needed to visualize their dendritic nature. Melanin itself appears brown or almost black but may appear blue if deposited in the deeper dermis.

The melanocyte–keratinocyte relationship ('epidermal melanin unit') can be disturbed at various levels (Table 21.1). The important clinical entities characterized by disordered pigmentation are conveniently divided into hypopigmented and hyperpigmented states.

Table 21.1 Disturbances of melanocyte–keratinocyte relationship.

Disturbance	Manifestation
Melanocytes fail to reach epidermis	Blue naevus, moles(?)
Primary melanocyte absence	Piebaldism
Melanocytes present but not functioning	Albinism
Secondary loss of melanocytes	Vitiligo Chemical leucoderma
Shortened melanocyte–keratinocyte contact	Inflammatory dermatoses
Increased melanocyte numbers	Lentigo

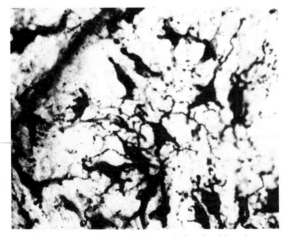

Fig. 21.1 Dopa-positive melanocytes in basal epidermis.

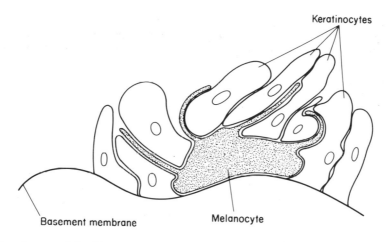

Fig. 21.2 Melanocyte–keratinocyte relationship.

Hypopigmented Disorders

Hypopigmented disorders, are summarized in Table 21.2.

Hypopituitarism

Pale skin is characteristic. There may be loss of axillary and pubic hair and a history of postpartum menstrual failure.

Phenylketonuria

This is an inborn error of phenylalanine metabolism due to deficiency of the enzyme phenylalanine hydroxylase. Tyrosinase is inhibited so the skin is fair and the eyes blue. Mental retardation and eczema occur but can be prevented by a low phenylalanine diet.

Oculocutaneous albinism

This term embraces at least four genetically distinct syndromes, all autosomal and recessive, characterized by hypopigmentation of skin, hair and eyes. Melanocytes are present but function abnormally. In the tyrosinase-positive variant, anagen hair bulbs incubated

Tyrosine ⟶ Dopa ⟶ Dopaquinone

Indole-5,6-quinone ⟵ 5,6-Dihydroxyindole

↓

Melanin

Fig. 21.3 Biosynthesis of melanin.

Table 21.2 Differential diagnosis of hypopigmented lesions.

Generalized hypomelanosis	Phenylketonuria	Babies
	Hypopituitarism	Adults
	Albinism	Nystagmus Pink iris
Patchy hypomelanosis	Vitiligo	
	Achromic naevus	At birth
	Piebaldism	White forelock
	Waardenburg's syndrome	Deafness
	Ash-leaf macules	Babies, 'fits'
	Chemical	Hydroquinone
Patchy hypomelanosis with inflammation	Tinea versicolor	Upper trunk
	Leprosy	Not Europeans
	Pityriasis alba	Itching, flaking(?)
Patchy hypomelanosis with atrophy or induration	Radiodermatitis	
	Morphoea	
	Lichen sclerosus	Vulva(?)
	Burns	

with tyrosine or dopa will darken as melanin is formed. In the tyrosinase-negative type they fail to do so.

The incidence is about 1:20 000. The skin is very fair, the hair white or yellow and the iris pink. In the tyrosinase-positive type, a little pigment may form with increasing age, particularly in negroes who develop striking freckling. The lack of iris pigment leads to photophobia, and habitual squint imparts a characteristic facies. Nystagmus, horizontal or rotatory, is usual and there may be errors of refraction and central scotomata. In the tropics, the depigmentation eventually leads to multiple cutaneous carcinomata due to ultraviolet damage. Prenatal diagnosis is now possible.

Piebaldism

This is an autosomal dominant trait. Patchy areas of completely white skin are present at birth, especially on the forehead and associated with a white forelock. These changes persist throughout life. In the white areas melanocytes are absent. In the hypermelanotic islands which may be seen, melanocytes are present but are abnormal.

Waardenburg's syndrome

Cutaneous changes very similar to those of piebaldism are associated with congenital deafness, abnormalities of hair growth and facial deformities. The condition is rare.

Ash-leaf macules of tuberose sclerosis

Scattered ovoid hypopigmented macules are the first clinical manifestation of this autosomal dominant disease (p. 117). In an infant having 'fits', they point to the diagnosis and are best detected under a Wood's light.

Achromic naevus

Hypopigmented macular naevi are not rare. The lesions are usually on the trunk, unilateral, sometimes dermatomal and occasionally in a bizarre configuration.

Postinflammatory hypopigmentation

Certain inflammatory diseases often lead to loss of pigment, including psoriasis, eczema (see pityriasis alba, p. 111), discoid lupus erythematosus and leprosy. In

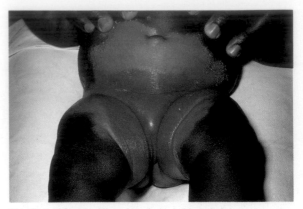

Fig. 21.4 Napkin (diaper) rash in a black baby causing gross hypopigmentation.

tinea versicolor the responsible organism is now known to release a fatty acid which inhibits melanin synthesis. Napkin dermatitis may cause gross temporary hypopigmentation in black babies (Fig. 21.4).

Chemical depigmentation

Hydroquinone, used in photography, by certain chemical workers, and as a skin 'lightening' cream by black women, and tertiary butyl phenols used in disinfectants and glues, may inhibit melanogenesis and even destroy melanocytes causing hypopigmentation, typically of the hands and face.

Vitiligo

Vitiligo is a common (1:200) acquired form of patchy macular loss of pigmentation. The affected areas are sharply defined and there is no inflammation. It may begin in childhood or adult life and tends to last for years. Often the distribution is symmetrical, favoured sites being the eyelids, perioral skin, neck, axillae, hands (especially nail folds), feet and genitalia. Trauma may provoke depigmentation.

In fair Caucasians the disease is apparent only in summer, when the unaffected skin tans or the white areas burn in sunlight. In other white subjects the surrounding normal skin seems to be more pigmented than normal. In brown- or black-skinned subjects the cosmetic impact is dramatic and causes great distress.

Vitiligo varies from the trivial to the near universal. The eyebrow and scalp hair may be depigmented, but sometimes fully pigmented black hairs emerge from vitiliginous skin; the follicular melanocytes seem to be under independent control. In children, halo naevi (p. 183) may be the first manifestation.

Electron microscopy reveals that basal melanocytes disappear. Circumstantial evidence points to an auto-immune cause, particularly clinical associations with thyroiditis, pernicious anaemia and Addison's disease and higher than expected incidences of various organ-specific autoantibodies in the blood. However, a positive family history is not uncommon but the genetics are not understood.

Treatment

Management is unsatisfactory. Prolonged application of a potent corticosteroid cream leads to repigmentation in one-third of patients after many months but may induce skin atrophy according to the site. Photochemotherapy (PUVA) may also be effective in a small proportion but 12 months or more of thrice weekly treatment may be needed and is rarely feasible. Usually cosmetic camouflage is simplest on the face and hands. Protection from sunlight reduces colour contrast between affected and normal skin and is mandatory in tropical climates where the carcinogenic hazard is the same as in albinism. Rarely in near-universal vitiligo it is worthwhile depigmenting small prominent areas of normally pigmented skin, for example on the backs of hands, with 20% hydroquinone ointment (Fig. 21.5).

Hyperpigmented Disorders

There are many well-recognized causes of hypermelanosis other than racial ones. Sun tanning is discussed on p. 124.

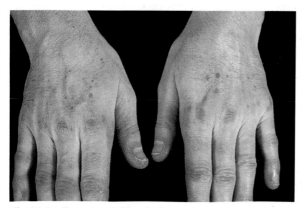

Fig. 21.5 Extensive vitiligo leaving a few disfiguring hyper-pigmented patches.

Postinflammatory pigmentation

Varicella, impetigo, dermatitis, lichen planus and many other diseases may leave hyperpigmentation in their wake, especially in dark-skinned subjects. It is debatable whether or not the curious condition called 'ashy dermatosis' is post-lichenoid.

Hypoadrenalism

Increased ACTH production is probably the cause of the hyperpigmentation of Addison's disease, Cushing's syndrome and after adrenalectomy. In Addison's disease skin subjected to friction, the flexures and palmar creases are particularly affected, as well as the buccal mucosa.

Hyperoestrogenism

In pregnancy the nipples darken and the linea alba becomes a linea nigra. Oestrogen therapy in elderly men for prostatic carcinoma has a similar effect on the nipples.

Chloasma

This is a common symmetrical patterned (Fig. 21.6) form of hyperpigmentation on the face and brow seen in pregnancy and in some women during oral contraception, particularly with the higher oestrogen-containing preparations. It may occur spontaneously in men as well as women, when it is best called melasma. Improvement may only be slow and partial postpartum but sun-screening always helps to lessen the cosmetic impact. In white patients depigmentation with hydroquinone ointment can be attempted; combination of tretinoin, triamcinolone and hydroquinone may also be useful.

Metabolic

Cirrhosis, particularly biliary, malabsorption, haemochromatosis and wasting diseases, for example carcinomatosis, may cause generalized skin darkening. In haemochromatosis the bronzing is due to a combination of iron and melanin. Carotenaemia, sometimes dietary, imparts an orange colour to the skin, especially of the palms and soles. In porphyria cutanea tarda and pellagra, exposed skin darkens.

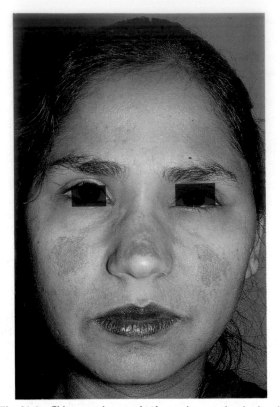

Fig. 21.6   Chloasma; the macular hyperpigmentation is sharply defined but not always so symmetrical.

Chemicals and drugs

Sodium arsenate (Fowler's solution), long abandoned because of its long-term carcinogenicity, caused 'raindrop' pigmentation on the trunk. Silver salts in eye and nose drops led to grey discoloration, especially in exposed areas. Gold pigmentation (chrysiasis) is blue–grey and accentuated on exposed areas.

Other drugs well recognized to discolour the skin (see Chapter 23) include minocycline, amiodarone, clofazimine, chlorpromazine, the antimalarials mepacrine and chloroquine, and busulphan and other cytostatic agents.

Freckles

Freckling appears in childhood on light exposed skin, particularly in fair or red-haired children. It is common in the United Kingdom and in those sunny countries such as Australia and New Zealand with large Celtic populations. The freckles darken in sunlight but do not disappear in winter. Electron micros-

copy shows that although melanocyte numbers are normal, the freckles are due to groups of functionally abnormal cells.

Café au lait macules

Five or more of these sharply defined light-brown macules are pathognomonic of neurofibromatosis, in which axillary freckling is characteristic (p. 116).

Peutz–Jegher syndrome

Multiple guttate melanotic macules of the lips and perioral skin betray intestinal polyposis. This rare disease is an autosomal dominant trait.

Simple lentigo

These melanotic macules are similar to freckles but are less influenced by sun. The basal melanocytes are increased in number.

Actinic (solar) lentigo

These sun-induced lentigines are very common on the exposed parts of elderly Caucasians, especially those more exposed to sunlight.

Pigmented Naevi

A naevus can be defined as a congenitally determined tissue defect. It may be visible at birth or only become apparent later. A 'mole' is a naevus arising from abnormal 'naevocytes' (possibly melanocytes) on the dermal side of the dermoepidermal junction. These are non-functional cells, perhaps related to faulty or arrested migration from the neural crest in embryonic life. The important melanocytic naevi are listed in Table 21.3.

Congenital melanocytic naevus

This lesion is present at or very soon after birth in at least 1% of children and is usually deeply pigmented. Most are small (< 2.0 cm) but occasionally huge areas of skin are involved, as in the 'bear-skin' naevus. Generally macular at first, they may become hyperkeratotic or hairy. Large lesions are not only a major cosmetic problem: lesions over 20 cm in diameter carry a 5–8% hazard of malignant melanoma development before the age of 20 years, and melanoma may even

Table 21.3 Classification of pigmented melanocytic naevi.

Congenital melanocytic naevus—large and small

Acquired melanocytic naevus—moles

Mongolian spot

Acquired blue naevus

Spitz naevus

Halo naevus

develop before 4 years of age. Such naevi should therefore be treated early, and usually serial plastic surgical procedures are necessary. Thorough dermabrasion is an alternative mode of therapy but melanoma has developed in the deeper dermis after superficial dermabrasion.

Small naevi (< 2 cm) can be left alone. The decision to remove or leave intermediate lesions (2–19 cm) must be based on the clinical circumstances; the larger the lesion, the more compelling the need for removal.

Acquired melanocytic naevus

This is the common mole, not present at birth although the naevus cells are doubtless present. It may appear in childhood, adolescence or even early adult life. All humans have moles, rarely less than 20 and occasionally hundreds. Moles initially are very small (2–5 mm), macular and pink-brown. At this stage the naevus cells are congregated near the epidermodermal junction—hence the term 'junctional naevus'. At variable rates moles mature, becoming larger, papular and sometimes protuberant, hyperkeratotic or hairy. These changes reflect increase in the bulk of the naevus as the cell mass expands into the dermis, yet retaining a junctional component—the 'compound naevus'.

Frequently in middle life the junctional component fades away leaving a 'dermal naevus'. Such naevi are common on the face in females, fleshy and lacking pigment—so-called 'cellular naevi'.

These ordinary moles have a fairly regular edge (contour) (although the junctional moles of childhood may have a fuzzy edge) and a regular, smooth profile. Their colour varies from pale brown to almost black but is generally uniform throughout the mole. Some are stippled. They do not bleed unless traumatized and heal quickly if injured. They tend to grow slowly,

although growth may be accelerated in pregnancy and under the influence of oral contraceptives.

The risk of malignant transformation to melanoma is minute, probably less than 1:100 000 for individual moles, but various risk factors are now recognized (see p. 160). The most important is the presence of dysplastic naevi (p. 161).

Ordinary moles should be left alone but may need to be removed for one of the following reasons:
• Constant trauma, for example from shaving or straps
• Cosmesis, especially on the face
• Anxiety (especially fear of malignancy)
• Suspicion of malignant transformation (see p. 162)

In the last case, formal complete excision biopsy is indicated but other moles can be treated satisfactorily by shaving flush with the skin surface followed by light cauterization.

Mongolian spot

A grey–blue extensive macular discoloration of the skin in the lumbosacral area, present at birth, is extremely frequent in East Asians (mongoloids) and rather less so in black Africans (congoids). It is rare in caucasoids. It tends to disappear spontaneously and is due to sheets of deep, mid-dermal melanocytes.

Acquired blue naevus

This is an uncommon, usually solitary, symptomless blue papule seen in adults usually on the extremities or head. Lesions are rarely bigger than 7–8 mm and are smooth and regular. Collections of pigment-producing melanocytes are seen deep in the mid-dermis. Blue naevi are harmless. They should not be confused with benign glomangioma which is vascular, tender or painful.

Spitz naevus

This is a very uncommon solitary nodule seen in children (juvenile melanoma) and young people on the face or elsewhere. The nodules may reach 1 cm in diameter and are smooth, domed and reddish-brown in colour, with a 'vascular' appearance. They are benign but have a characteristic histology. If left alone they resolve slowly.

Halo naevus

This is an uncommon disorder of children sometimes

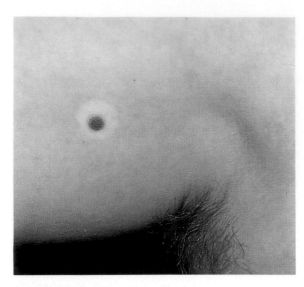

Fig. 21.7 Halo naevus.

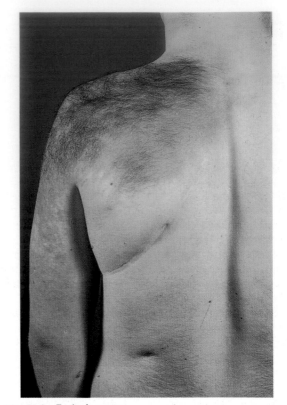

Fig. 21.8 Becker's naevus.

called Sutton's naevus or leucoderma centrifugum acquisitum (Fig. 21.7). A 'halo' of depigmentation appears around one or more small acquired moles, usually on the trunk. If the lesion is observed the central mole is seen to change colour slowly and disappear after many months, following which repigmentation may occur. If the lesion is excised early a lymphocytic infiltrate is seen around the mole, implying an immune reaction to it, a notion supported by the finding of circulating antimelanocytic antibodies similar to those described in malignant melanoma. Nevertheless, halo naevi are entirely benign and should be left alone. However, a proportion of patients later develop vitiligo.

Pigmented hairy epidermal naevus

This is a common acquired lesion also known as Becker's naevus, usually developing in males in the second or third decade. An irregular macular area of hyperpigmentation develops usually around one shoulder (Fig. 21.8) and the adjacent areas. Later, coarse terminal hair growth is superimposed and the epidermis may become slightly thickened. Basal melanocytes are not increased and 'naevus' cells are absent from the dermis.

The condition persists, but there is no tendency to malignant change.

Diseases of the Scalp, Hair and Nails

Hair Follicle Biology

Hair is epithelial in origin. In the embryo, downgrowths of epidermal cells into the dermis and subcutis canalize to form the hair follicle. Outer and inner root sheaths enclose the hair shaft (Fig. 22.1). At the base of the follicle is an expanded hair bulb enclosing a dermal papilla which is vascularized and innervated. Mitotic activity in the hair bulb results in the growth of the hair shaft.

Hair follicles are found all over the body except on the palmar and plantar skin, the glans penis and vulval introitus. By the sixth month in utero the foetus is coated in soft *lanugo* hair which is shed before birth except on the scalp, eyebrows and eyelashes. The infant then grows soft, downy, short non-medullated *vellus* hair but the scalp, lashes and brows evolve into longer medullated *terminal* hairs.

Profuse terminal hair growth occurs after puberty in the pubis and axillae of both sexes and on the legs, face and chest of males over the following decade. Many females also develop terminal hair on the legs and, to a

lesser extent, the arms. Terminal hair is very straight in mongoloids, straight or wavy in caucasoids and curled in congoids. The shaft, consisting of packed keratinized cells, has an outermost *cuticle* covering a *cortex* and an inner *medulla* (absent in *lanugo* and *vellus* hair) (Fig. 22.1).

The external root sheath cells contain glycogen; the inner root sheath and hair bulb contain melanocytes. The arrector pili muscles pass from the superficial dermis downwards into the outer root sheath: slow contraction erects the hair follicle, leading to 'goose pimples'.

Endocrine influence on hair follicles

Scalp, eyebrow and eyelash hair follicles are independent of androgens. The axillary and lower pubic triangle follicles are testosterone-dependent, whereas the upper pubic triangle and rest of the body follicles are dihydrotestosterone-dependent. Dihydrotestosterone can convert vellus to terminal hairs.

However, genetic factors operating on a prolonged time-scale modify follicular response to androgens so that male hairiness evolves over a decade or more, and a marked increase in hairiness of nostrils and ears only appears in men in later life. Conversely, male balding also evolves over several decades.

The hair follicle cycle

Unlike epidermal or nail growth, hair follicle activity and hair growth are cyclic throughout the animal kingdom. Each follicle undergoes alternating phases of growth (*anagen*) and rest (*telogen*) (Fig. 22.2). The length to which hair can grow is determined by the daily rate of growth (usually about 0.45 mm per day on the scalp) and the length of the anagen phase. The latter may be 3–5 years (occasionally up to 8 years; Fig. 22.3) on the scalp, but only 2–4 months on the eyebrows. The resting (*telogen*) phase tends to be much more constant, at about 3 months. Each follicle has a constitutional 'time clock' controlling the cycle. When

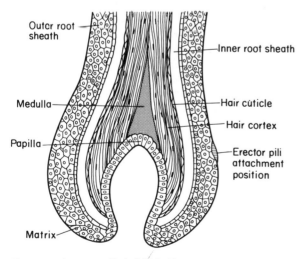

Fig. 22.1 Anatomy of hair follicle (deep part).

Outer root sheath

Inner root sheath

Medulla

Hair cuticle

Hair cortex

Papilla

Erector pili attachment position

Matrix

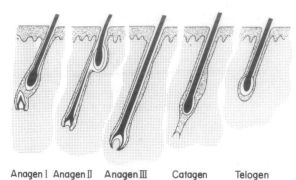

Anagen I Anagen II Anagen III Catagen Telogen

Fig. 22.2 The hair follicle cycle.

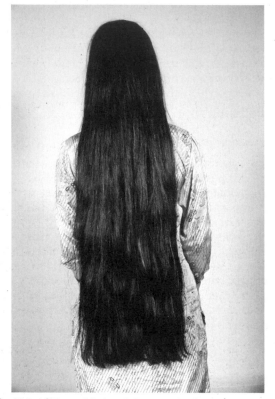

Fig. 22.3 Chinese girl whose hair grew to her knees (anagen phase of about 8 years).

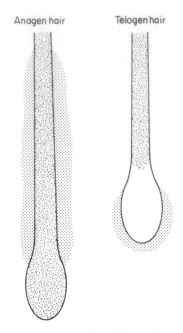

Fig. 22.4 Anagen and telogen hairs. The 'club' of the telogen hair is not pigmented.

the clock switches *anagen* off, a short involutional phase, *catagen*, follows in which mitosis in the hair bulb ceases and its matrix is enveloped by a shortening outer root sheath so that the resulting telogen hair is 'clubbed' at its base. When anagen starts again a new matrix is formed and with its underlying papilla descends to its anagen level. The new anagen hair soon pushes out the old telogen hair and the follicle has gone full circle (Fig. 22.2).

Loss of dislodged telogen hair is thus normal. Such club hairs are easily recognized on the pillow or hairbrush, as the club is depigmented as well as expanded (Fig. 22.4). In contrast, an anagen hair, obtained by traction, is fully melanized. In the human scalp, containing perhaps 100 000 follicles, 5–10% are in telogen at any time, i.e. 5–10 000. Since their individual 'time clocks' are randomized and telogen lasts approximately 3 months, say 100 days, the number of telogen hairs pushed out each day is 50–100. In contrast, certain animals have synchronized follicles resulting in periodic 'moults'.

Alopecia

Alopecia means hair loss. It may be patchy or diffuse, partial or complete, transient or prolonged or even permanent. There are two fundamentally different forms.

Cicatricial (scarring) alopecia

Inflammatory disease of the skin destroys hair follicles in its wake. The resulting alopecia is irreversible and the affected skin is shiny, atrophic and devoid of

Table 22.1 Causes of cicatricial alopecia.

Uncommon	Chemical or thermal burns
	X-irradiation
	Trigeminal zoster (first division)
	Discoid lupus erythematosus
	Kerion (see tinea capitis, p. 64)
	Favus (p. 65) in Asia
Rare	Lupus vulgaris
	Lichen planus
	Tertiary syphilis (gumma)
	Chronic staphylococcal folliculitis
	Idiopathic

Table 22.2 Classification of non-scarring alopecia.

Diffuse	Localized
Common baldness	Alopecia areata
Androgenic alopecia in women	Tinea capitis
Telogen alopecia	Traumatic alopecia
Anagen alopecia	Secondary syphilis
Metabolic alopecia	
Drug-induced	

follicular orifices. The important causes are listed in Table 22.1.

Non-cicatricial (non-scarring) alopecia

Here the follicle itself is disordered as a primary event, not secondary to surrounding skin disease. There are many recognizable causes of non-scarring alopecia but in general the skin looks and feels normal and the alopecia is reversible. It is convenient to divide non-scarring alopecia into diffuse and localized patterns, the important causes of which are listed in Table 22.2.

The Cicatricial Alopecias

Burns. Chemical or thermal burns may destroy hair follicles. Low doses of X-ray may cause only a temporary epilation (previously utilized in treatment of tinea capitis) but heavy dosage may induce a scarring radiodermatitis.

Zoster. When a severe zoster affects the whole dermatome of the first division of the trigeminal nerve, healing may leave a unilateral frontal scarring alopecia in its wake.

Discoid lupus erythematosus. In the United Kingdom this is probably the commonest cause. Slowly spreading areas of erythema and alopecia gradually give way to paler scar tissue. Any part of the scalp may be affected but the frontal areas and crown are most at risk (Fig. 22.5).

Kerion. An intensely inflammatory tinea capitis of animal origin may heal with scarring.

Favus. This is cicatricial tinea capitis due to *Trichophyton* schoenleinii (see p. 65).

Lupus vulgaris. A century ago cutaneous tuberculosis was a common cause. Now it is very rare in Europe but is still seen in the Third World.

Lichen planus. Lichen planus is rare on the scalp but can rapidly devastate the head when it does occur, causing irretrievable follicular loss in a few weeks. If diagnosed early, prompt oral prednisolone (30–40 mg daily) may save the hair. Lichenoid gold eruptions are particularly liable to affect the scalp.

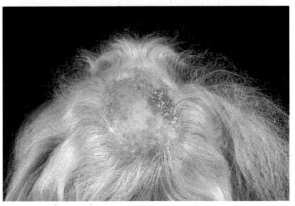

Fig. 22.5 Cicatricial alopecia due to discoid lupus erythematosus.

Syphilis. Gummatous scarring of scalp is now rare in Europe.

Chronic staphylococcal folliculitis. In preantibiotic days, a slowly destructive coccal folliculitis was not uncommon, especially in the debilitated. Today it is rare in Europe and can be arrested promptly by oral antistaphyloccal antibiotics.

Idiopathic. Cicatricial alopecia, developing without obvious cause, is known as pseudo-pelade. Shiny white atrophic areas (Fig. 22.6) appear very slowly, often leaving islands of sparse terminal hairs.

Diagnosis

Wood's light examination should always be undertaken. Usually a biopsy for histopathology and sometimes microbial culture is necessary.

Treatment

Apart from the use of oral antimalarials and potent

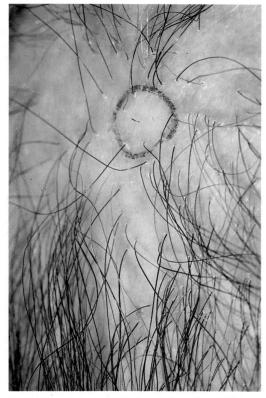

Fig. 22.6   Idiopathic cicatricial alopecia (pseudo-pelade).

topical corticosteroids for discoid lupus erythematosus, prednisolone for active lichen planus, prompt oral griseofulvin for tinea and early acyclovir for zoster, little can be done.

Diffuse Non-Scarring Alopecia

Common baldness

Male balding (male-pattern alopecia) is determined genetically but requires adequate androgen levels and the march of time for its expression. Its earliest manifestation is the altering of the straight anterior hairline of childhood by temporal recession, followed slowly by thinning on the crown and eventually the whole frontal scalp and crown. It may never occur or it may be complete by 20 years of age, with all gradations of speed and extent in between these extremes.

Other primates exhibit balding and it was the classical studies of Montagna in the stump-tailed macaque monkey which demonstrated the progressive transformation of *terminal* back to *vellus* follicles, with gradual shortening of the anagen phase and follicular and hair shaft involution. Balding is universal but is more prevalent and severe in caucasoids than in black people.

The precise genetics are not yet understood but the role of androgens is clear. Prepubertal castrates do not go bald but may do so later if given testosterone injections. Plasma testosterone levels are normal in bald men. Possibly, relative lack of androgens explains the absence of balding in premenopausal females but some elderly women do slowly go bald, half a century later than their menfolk.

Treatment

Most men require none. There is new evidence that topical application of a 2% minoxidil lotion (Regaine, U.K.) can slow the progression of balding and can induce the growth of terminal hairs in some men, but the effect lasts only so long as treatment is continued. The cost of years of therapy is great and long-term safety is not established. Punch hair grafting in skilled hands is a rational, safe and effective permanent treatment but the technical difficulties in obtaining cosmetically good results may be formidable and the cost is very high. Nevertheless, it is the treatment of choice for those men professionally exposed to the scrutiny of the camera lens. Radical flap transposure of hair-bearing skin from the side of the head across the frontal region is also feasible but is a painful major procedure. Topical antiandrogens are of no value.

Androgenic alopecia in women

Some premenopausal women, probably genetically predisposed and perhaps with marginally raised blood or tissue androgen levels, exhibit a somewhat different pattern of diffuse thinning over the frontovertical region, usually with preservation of the anterior hairline. Involuted vellus follicles are interspersed amongst reasonably preserved terminal ones, a pattern sometimes preserved for many years. However, very high androgen levels, for example from an androgen-secreting ovarian tumour, will induce recession at the temples and baldness of the crown as in male-pattern loss. Androgenic alopecia may be accompanied by hirsutism and acne in young women.

A similar pattern of diffuse alopecia in premenopausal women may be 'idiopathic', in the complete absence of any evidence of androgenism.

Treatment

Endocrine investigation may be needed. Oral administration of the antiandrogen, cyproterone acetate, combined with ethinyloestradiol is of established value but side-effects may be troublesome. In severe cases a wig may be necessary. The value of topical minoxidil is not established as yet. Spironolactone, 100–200 mg daily, may be worth trying.

Telogen alopecia

Certain stresses on the follicle can prematurely terminate anagen without inflicting further disturbance on the hair cycle. The result is a diffuse shedding (effluvium) about 3 months later when temporarily synchronized follicles resume the growth phase and push out telogen hairs, the severity being precisely proportional to the number of affected follicles. The disease is quite common.

Childbirth (postpartum alopecia), severe acute infections (e.g. pneumonia), withdrawal of oral contraception, 'crash' dieting and severe emotional stress may all be responsible. However, the 3 months' interval means that patients rarely recognize cause and effect. Diagnosis depends upon establishing that the effluvium is entirely of telogen hairs and obtaining the appropriate history. The prognosis is for complete recovery.

Anagen alopecia

The anagen follicle is vulnerable to antimitotic agents which damage the hair shaft, which breaks easily. Cyclophosphamide and other cytostatic agents are well known to cause hair loss. Hypervitaminosis A and synthetic retinoid treatment modify hair growth and may cause loss.

Metabolic alopecia

Severe iron deficiency at any age can cause diffuse hair loss (Fig. 22.7), as may hypothyroidism, hypopituitarism and hypoadrenalism. Malnutrition reduces hair growth, as may malabsorption.

Drug-induced alopecia

Apart from anagen alopecia, heparin, heparinoids, the coumarins, dextran sulphate and antithyroid drugs may cause alopecia by inducing premature telogen.

Localized Non-Scarring Alopecias

Alopecia areata

This is an extremely common condition characterized by complete hair loss from patches of the scalp. It has a rapid onset but a strong tendency to spontaneous reversal.

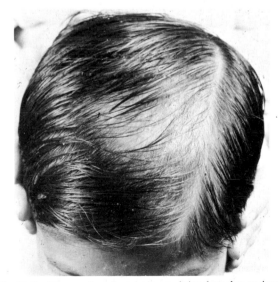

Fig. 22.7 Non-scarring alopecia in an Asian boy due to iron-deficient diet.

The condition is of unknown aetiology but there appears to be an ill-defined genetic factor. There is a clinical association with vitiligo, and organ-specific autoantibodies may be found. A lymphocytic infiltrate is present around the hair follicle, suggesting that alopecia areata itself is due to autoimmune mechanisms. Some atopic subjects develop alopecia areata and in such cases the prognosis for regrowth is poor. There is an increased incidence in Down's syndrome.

The disease may first appear at any age but usually does so in the second or third decades, affecting both sexes equally. Sharply defined bald patches of any size develop rapidly. Usually there are no local symptoms but itching and slight tenderness may be elicited. The disease is rarely total on the scalp or universal, affecting every hair follicle on the body including eyebrows and eyelashes.

On examination the affected skin looks normal. Sometimes dystrophic 'exclamation-mark' hairs are seen, especially at the margins of lesion. These are very short hairs tapering and becoming depigmented as the scalp is approached. Plucking reveals such hairs to be in the telogen phase. Pitting of the fingernails may also be seen. Histologically some dystrophic anagen follicles can be found. The transition from telogen to anagen appears to be terminated prematurely, leading to hasty return to telogen so that the cycle is truncated.

In the localized forms of the disease the prognosis is generally for complete recovery to occur after many weeks or even months. When the hair does regrow it is usually depigmented at first but later hair growth is completely normal. The prognosis is poor when alopecia areata is extensive around the ears and posterior scalp (opheasic pattern). It is also poor when total or universal alopecia develops in early life. Nevertheless, potential follicular function is retained even after decades of inactivity, as can be demonstrated by local steroid injection.

Treatment

Local steroid therapy, given by needle injection or 'spray gun', is the most effective form of treatment but its results are only temporary and it is only appropriate or possible in localized disease. The deliberate induction of allergic contact dermatitis on the affected scalp using dinitrochlorbenzene or squaric acid dibutyl ester has been advocated, as has induction of a primary irritant dermatitis using dithranol (anthralin)-containing creams but these manoeuvres are rarely rewarding. PUVA therapy may be rarely effective. High dose oral prednisolone is effective but side-effects are inevitable if treatment is continued and the hair falls out if it is stopped. Its use should be firmly resisted.

Tinea capitis

The various patterns are described in Chapter 9. *Microsporum* and most *Trichophyton* infections are non-scarring.

Traumatic alopecia

Babies often have occipital alopecia caused by rubbing the head on the pillow. Older children frequently develop a 'nervous' habit of twiddling and pulling a lock of hair until a bald patch is induced. Psychotic adults rarely rub or pull out large masses of hair—and may even swallow it. Marginal traction alopecia is common in black women who straighten the hair and pull it into a bun (Fig. 22.8). Hot comb usage to straighten or wave hair may damage and break hair shafts.

Syphilis

Patchy 'moth-eaten' alopecia without scarring can occur in secondary syphilis.

Diseases of the Scalp Skin

Pityriasis capitis (dandruff)

A fine flaking exfoliation from the scalp is common in young adults and is best regarded as a minor form of

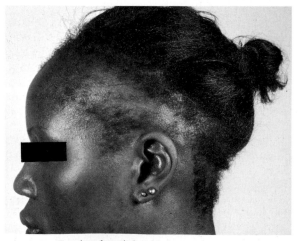

Fig. 22.8   Traction alopecia in a black woman who pulled her hair into a 'bun' after straightening it.

seborrhoeic dermatitis. Pityrosporum yeasts are probably causative. Shampoos containing selenium sulphide or zinc pyrithione reduce the yeast population to good effect.

Psoriasis and seborrhoeic dermatitis

These are discussed in Chapter 12 and 11, respectively.

Pityriasis amiantacea

This is an uncommon but singular disease of children's scalps in which adherent scale forms a cuff around the hair. Hair loss may follow or be caused by treatment. It is usually reversible. It may be a manifestation of eczema or psoriasis. Salicylic acid 4% in emulsifying ointment and frequent shampooing and combing will remove most adherent scale but topical steroids may be needed in addition for the underlying inflammation. The condition eventually clears completely.

Acne keloid

Acne keloid is discussed in Chapter 20.

Seborrhoeic folliculitis

This uncommon chronic acneiform folliculitis of the scalp may be provoked by pityrosporum yeasts and may respond to topical imidazole lotions or creams.

Acne varioliformis

This uncommon but characteristic picture is invariably seen in young or middle-aged women under emotional stress. Follicular itching leads to excoriation and sometimes secondary infection. Varioliform hypopigmented scars may be evident at the anterior hairline and are invariably profuse on the upper back, shoulders and V of neck. Treatment is ineffectual.

Hirsutism and Hypertrichosis

Women with beards have fascinated artists since ancient times. *Hirsutism* is male hair pattern in the female and is androgen-induced. In contrast, *hypertrichosis* is the growth of hair abnormal and excessive for the site and age in either sex.

Hirsutism

Causes

Adrenal disease. In congenital adrenal-genital syndrome there is an enzymatic block limiting the synthesis of cortisol. This results in increased secretion of pituitary ACTH, in turn resulting in overproduction of androgenic steroids and consequent pseudo-hermaphroditism in the female child. In adult life adrenal tumours or Cushing's syndrome may cause hirsutism together with other symptoms and signs of virilization.

Ovarian disease. The polycystic ovary syndrome (Stein–Leventhal) is common and presents as secondary amenorrhoea, obesity, acne or infertility as well as hirsutism. The abnormal ovaries can usually be visualized by ultrasound but laparoscopy is occasionally needed. The ratio of LH to FSH is raised and blood androstenedione, dehydroepiandrosterone sulphate, testosterone and oestrone are all raised. Androgen-secreting malignant ovarian tumours occur but are rare.

Drug-induced. Prolonged corticosteroid therapy, androgens and attenuated androgens and progestogens may cause hirsutism, as may phenytoins.

Idiopathic. This is much the commonest type of hirsutism. Often it has an ethnic basis and is particularly seen in Mediterranean, West Asian and Indian women. It begins in adolescence and tends to worsen steadily with age. Terminal hair on the chin and upper lip is least acceptable but excessive body hair may also cause distress depending on the cultural influences at play and the woman's psychological make-up. It is a cause of great distress in many affected women in Western cultures (probably at least 3% of caucasian females have terminal hairs on the upper lip and 6% on the chin) and a lucrative source of income for the practitioners of bleaching, waxing and electrolysis.

The degree of hirsutism correlates poorly with blood androgen levels although, statistically, testosterone and androstenedione are significantly elevated in hirsute women. Increased activity of the enzyme $5\text{-}\alpha$-reductase in the skin around affected hair follicles may explain the poor correlation. This enzyme converts testosterone to the more potent androgen dihydrotestosterone. Conversely, low activities of this enzyme may explain absence of hirsutism in some women with late-onset adrenal hyperplasia who have a very high serum testosterone level.

Diagnosis and investigation of hirsutism

If other symptoms or signs of androgen excess are absent and menstruation is normal, investigation is not worthwhile. If they are present, appropriate referral is essential.

Management of idiopathic hirsutism

Attention to the psyche is crucial; boosting the feelings of femininity and playing down perceptions or fears of masculinization are invaluable. Simple bleaching using hydrogen peroxide or use of depilatory cream may be adequate in mild cases, although the latter may be irritant. Waxing or shaving are best for the legs but will need to be repeated regularly. Skilled electrolysis is the best approach to long-lasting treatment of the face. Combined oral treatment with cyproterone acetate (an antiandrogen) and ethinyl oestradiol is slow, disappointing and not without side-effects.

Hypertrichosis

Anorexia nervosa in adult women and severe malnutrition in children of either sex cause hypertrichosis if prolonged. Porphyria cutanea tarda typically causes increased bushiness of the eyebrows in men and facial hair growth in women. Conversely, it may also cause cicatricial alopecia. There are rare congenital causes and 'hypertrichosis lanuginosa' is a rare cutaneous marker of malignancy (p. 37).

A number of drugs may be responsible, particularly diazoxide, minoxidil, cyclosporin, hydantoins and penicillamine.

Localized hypertrichosis is seen in hairy pigmented naevi, prolonged localized inflammatory disease and after prolonged use of potent topical steroids. A lumbosacral tuft of hair (faun tail) suggests underlying spina bifida.

Diseases of the Nails

The anatomy of nail and related structures

The nail (Fig. 22.9) is a plate of tough, dense, hard keratin, produced by mitotic division and differentiation in a specialized zone of epidermis, the *matrix*. The distal part of the matrix is visible as the *lunula*. The root of the nail is covered by the proximal nail fold which becomes the lateral nail folds on each side of the nail plate. The edge of the posterior nail fold is the thin *eponychium* (*cuticle*) which partly covers the lunula.

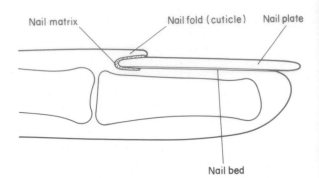

Fig. 22.9   The anatomy of the nail and related tissues in vertical section.

The nail plate lies on the *nail bed* which is very vascular. Distally the nail bed becomes the *hyponychium*, the thickened epidermis under the free end of the nail plate. Cell division and keratinization in the matrix produce the nail plate which moves forward, taking with it keratinized cells of the nail bed to which it is firmly bound.

Fingernail grows at 0.1–0.15 mm per day; toenail growth is much slower. In psoriasis and in onycholysis fingernail growth is speeded up; digital ischaemia slows nail growth and an acute toxic illness may almost halt growth temporarily. In the latter situation the temporary defects are seen later as Beau's lines as the nail grows out.

Nail disease may affect the nail fold, the underlying nail matrix itself, the more distal nail plate or the nail bed (Table 22.3). The common and important less common abnormalities are described below.

Diseases of the Nail Fold

Acute paronychia

This is an acute coccal infection with pus formation, usually originating at the junction of the posterior and lateral folds. Incision and drainage are indicated and sometimes erythromycin or flucloxacillin orally.

Table 22.3   Components of the nail to be considered separately in nail disease.

The nail fold
The nail matrix
The nail plate
The nail bed

Chronic paronychia

This is a very common condition usually seen in women. Excessive maceration is the usual cause due to constant immersion of the hands in water in young mothers, housewives, kitchen and canteen workers and barmaids. Male bakers, chefs and barmen are equally at risk.

The cuticle which is normally sealed to the nail plate becomes detached, allowing access to the space under the posterior nail fold of food, dirt, soap powders, etc, and micro-organisms, especially *Candida albicans*. Less commonly, circulatory disease which devitalizes the nail fold may have the same effect, for example in Raynaud's phenomenon and systemic sclerosis.

The result is inflammation of the posterior and posterolateral nail folds which are swollen, red and tender ('bolstering'). The cuticle retracts and may disappear and the subcuticular gap is apparent and may discharge a small amount of cheesy material. Secondary involvement of the matrix results in an abnormal ridged nail and *Candida* species may invade the nail plate.

Treatment is not easy. Avoiding wet work and wearing rubber or plastic gloves when possible are essential. Simple antiseptic and anti-*Candida* applications such as clotrimazole lotion or cream (Canesten, U.K.) or amphotericin B lotion (Fungilin, U.K.) may be useful. Gentian violet or brilliant green 1% in spirit are also valuable but messy and staining. Resort to cauterization of the subcuticular space by inserting a fine cottonwool wick soaked in pure phenol for one minute is valuable in resistant cases. Oral griseofulvin is valueless and antibiotics are contraindicated.

Miscellaneous

'Palisading' of dilated nail fold capillaries is seen in the fingers in dermatomyositis and lupus erythematosus. Small (2–3 mm) infarcts at the posterior or lateral folds are seen in the vasculitis of rheumatoid disease and in polyarteritis nodosa.

Diseases of the Nail Plate

Discoloration

White nails (leuconychia). White nails are seen in portal cirrhosis and other systemic disorders. Small white spots are idiopathic and unrelated to any nutritional deficiencies.

Blue–black nails. These are almost always due to trauma and subungual bleeding. The haematoma can be observed to grow out. Blue–black or dark-brown pigmentation is rarely a sign of malignant melanoma of the nail bed. Here the pigment does not separate from the matrix and may invade the nail fold. Rarely pigmentation is absent in subungual melanoma which may present as ulceration, nail distortion or paronychia. The diagnosis may be missed for months or longer and not be established until full longitudinal biopsy (p. 163) has been carried out.

Longitudinal coloured bands. These are common in coloured races but, if acquired in a Caucasian over 35 years, melanoma should be suspected.

Greenish discoloration. Greenish discoloration with onycholysis is often due to *Pseudomonas aeruginosa* infection of the subungual space.

Splinter haemorrhages. These are often due to trauma but may be an important sign in infective endocarditis.

Yellow nails. Yellow nails with irregular colour change are seen in psoriasis and onychomycosis (tinea unguium). In the rare *yellow nail syndrome* all the nails are thickened, curved, yellow and slow-growing. There is an underlying defect of lymphatic drainage and lung disease may be associated.

Coloured half-moons. The lunula may be red in heart failure and brown in chronic renal failure.

Koilonychia

Thinning and concavity, producing a spoon-shaped nail, are seen in iron-deficiency anaemia but also occur in lichen planus and are rarely congenital.

Clubbing

Clubbing consists of increased curvature of the nails in both directions with loss of the angle between the posterior nail fold and nail plate. Eventually the whole end of the finger enlarges. Additional periostitis of distal bones is seen in *hypertrophic pulmonary osteoarthropathy*. The important causes of clubbing are bronchial carcinoma, chronic pulmonary infection, cyanotic congenital heart disease and infective endocarditis, but it may also be seen in thyroid acropachy, biliary cirrhosis and colitis.

Onycholysis

This is separation of the nail plate from the nail bed distally. The resulting subungual space cannot be kept dry and contamination with various micro-organisms is common, often producing green or black discoloration. It is common in psoriasis but is often idiopathic in adult women, involving one or more finger nails and often being intermittent for many years. Photo-onycholysis may be due to drugs. Demethylchlortetracycline is the best known cause but other tetracyclines may be implicated if the dose is high enough and solar exposure is intense. Usually the thumb nail is spared because it is less exposed. The onset may be very painful. The anti-inflammatory analgesic benoxaprofen (now withdrawn) often caused photo-onycholysis.

Pitting

Pin-head saucer-shaped depressions in the nail plate are seen in psoriasis and, less commonly, in eczema and alopecia areata.

Ridging

Horizontal ridges and grooves extending to part or all of the middle of the nail are common in psoriasis. Trauma to the matrix from a nervous tic is a common cause of partial ridging. Rarely an idiopathic symmetrical median dystrophy of the thumb nail produces a herring-bone pattern of ridging.

Subungual hyperkeratosis

Thickening of the nail due to accretion of hyperkeratotic material from the nail bed is common in the toes. Psoriasis and tinea are common causes but trauma and ischaemia may be important. *Onychogryphosis* is a dramatic extreme form where the nail thickens and curves like a ram's horn.

Congenital Nail Dystrophies

Nail-patella syndrome

This syndrome is inherited as a Mendelian dominant trait. The nails are absent or rudimentary. Not all digits are necessarily involved but thumb changes are always found. The patellae are absent or rudimentary and tend to sublux. Other defects may occur.

Pachyonychia congenita

In this autosomal dominant disorder the nails are thickened and discoloured from birth. Later there may be palmo-plantar keratoderma, sometimes associated with hyperhidrosis. In one variant, potentially malignant mucosal dysplasia may supervene.

Dystrophic epidermolysis bullosa

Nail dystrophy is characteristic of this inherited disease in which the skin blisters readily in response to trauma (p. 120).

Dyskeratosis congenita

Finger and toe nails are grossly abnormal in this very rare sex-linked recessive disorder in which mucosal dysplasia and pancytopenia also occur.

Miscellaneous Related Disorders

Mucous (synovial) cysts

These 3–7-mm grey–white semitranslucent fluctuant papules occur on the dorsum of a finger over the terminal interphalangeal joint. Their proximity to the matrix may result in a central depressed longitudinal groove in the nail; a clear gel is obtained if the cyst is opened. Whether they arise in synovial folds or are the result of mucinous degeneration within the dermis remains controversial. Injecting a very small amount of triamcinolone into the cyst is often curative.

Ingrowing toenails

Trauma is fundamental: firstly, unsuitable shoes lead to deformities of the feet; secondly, incorrect cutting of the nails leaves sharp spicules of nail which damage the lateral nail fold. Sometimes congenital malalignment of the nails is the cause. Usually the hallux nail is involved, less often the nail of the second toe. Initial inflammation and infection of the lateral nail fold are aggravated if hyperhidrosis is present, especially if occlusive footwear is used. Swelling of the nail fold intensifies the ingrowing and granulation tissue may form in the lateral fold. Discomfort may be severe.

Treatment has several strands. Occlusive, tight shoes should be avoided. The nail should be cut at 90° to its long axis. In mild cases antibiotic ointment or powder may suffice. Potassium permanganate soaks are valuable in more severe cases and a coarse of oral antibiotic may be needed. Resistant granulation tissue can be cauterized with a silver nitrate stick. Spicules of nail should be removed.

Occasionally surgery is needed, usually curettage of granulation tissue and partial or total removal of the nail plate. Once cured, foot hygiene and care must be meticulous.

Subungual exostosis

This benign proliferation of bone dorsally from the distal phalanx presents as a characteristic small hard swelling of the hyponychium with slight hyperkeratosis overlying it. The free end of the nail may be pushed upwards. Verruca plantaris is often misdiagnosed. A lateral radiograph confirms the diagnosis, and excision of the exostosis is curative (see Figs 7.9 and 7.10).

—23

Adverse Reactions to Drugs

Adverse reactions may be due to systemic or topical drug therapy or indeed unwitting exposure to chemicals in foods, drinks, etc. The sheer diversity of drugs available ensures that drug reactions are extremely common. It has been estimated that one-quarter of all symptoms in industrialized societies are now drug-induced.

The undesirable and unwanted effects of drugs are of various types (Table 23.1).

Overdosage

This may be absolute (as in attempted suicide) or relative. Thus, one-quarter of the normal dose of methotrexate may cause grave marrow depression if renal function is grossly impaired.

Intolerance

Here the characteristic effects are produced by an abnormally low dose. Some subjects, for instance, are abnormally sensitive to sleeping tablets and need a half or quarter of the usual dose to achieve the desired effect.

Idiosyncrasy

This implies an uncharacteristic effect. A good example is the haemolytic anaemia induced by sylphonamides in subjects who are genetically deficient in the enzyme, glucose-6-phosphate dehydrogenase.

Side-effects

These are simply unwanted pharmacological reactions

Table 23.1 Undesirable effects of drugs.

Overdosage	Facultative effects
Intolerance	Teratogenicity
Idiosyncrasy	Hypersensitivity reactions
Side-effects	

which can become useful if the purpose of the drug is different. Thus, the sedative side-effect of certain antihistamines may be of value in the restless child with atopic dermatitis.

Facultative effects

Such effects depend upon the alteration of a biological balance. Candidosis, induced by wide-spectrum antibiotics, is the best known example.

Teratogenicity

The thalidomide disaster alerted the whole world to this potential danger 25 years ago. The new retinoids are teratogenic, as are most of the antimitotic drugs.

Hypersensitivity reactions

Any of the four types of allergic hypersensitivity may be involved.

History

Laboratory aids are almost valueless in the diagnosis of drug eruptions. Analysis of the history and the findings on examination are all-important. All drugs taken in the 3 weeks prior to an acute eruption must be listed and the date of onset of therapy noted. The patient may have to be asked about medication several times to 'jog' the memory. Drugs taken routinely for months or years may be forgotten. It is useful to make specific enquiry about various classes of drugs, for example hypnotics, laxatives, antibiotics, analgesics, etc. Asking the patient (or relative) to bring up the contents of bathroom cupboards, bedside tables, etc, is invaluable. Most revealing is a domiciliary consultation, when a veritable pharmacy is often found. Over-the-counter drugs may be important and not only prescribed medicines should be considered. In the United Kingdom, *Martindale's Extrapharmacopoeia* has an invaluable alphabetical listing of over-the-counter medications and their ingredients.

Drugs introduced 7–14 days before the onset of rash

are most suspect and must be arranged in rank order of suspicion on the basis of their known predilection to cause eruptions. Thus some commonly prescribed drugs virtually never cause rashes: these include digoxin, diazepam, salbutamol, frusemide and paracetamol. Ideally, drugs under suspicion should be withdrawn but this must depend partly on therapeutic imperatives and whether chemically unrelated alternatives are available.

Patterns of Reaction

Drug reactions can mimic most diseases of the skin. The commonest offending drugs are listed in Table 23.2.

Urticaria

Several mechanisms are involved in the production of urticaria. Morphine, codeine, aspirin and atropine act directly as histamine liberators from the mast cells in the dermis. Aspirin or penicillin may also cause allergic urticaria either by a Type I IgE-mediated reaction or a Type III IgG complement-fixing reaction. Rarely, more severe and complex serum sickness and anaphylactic reactions are seen. Other drugs causing urticaria are serum, toxoids, pollen vaccines, meprobamate and imipramine.

Table 23.2 Drugs commonly causing adverse reactions.

Ampicillin
Aspirin
Beta-blockers
Gold
Hydantoins
Lithium
Non-steroidal anti-inflammatory drugs
para-Aminosalicylic acid
Penicillin
Penicillamine
Sulphonamides (including co-trimoxazole)
Sulphonylureas
Tetracyclines

Purpura

This may be due to either drug-induced thrombocytopenia, for example by quinine, or to a capillaritis as a result of stimulation of antibody to a drug–capillary endothelial cell complex, as seen with the sedatives carbromal and meprobamate. It may follow a Type III-induced vasculitis, for example from sulphonamides.

Lupus erythematosus-like syndrome

This syndrome differs from systemic lupus erythematosus in that renal disease does not occur and rashes are less common. Causative drugs include hydralazine, isoniazid, penicillamine and procainamide.

Photosensitivity

Drug reactions may be phototoxic or photoallergic. A phototoxic non-immune reaction occurs when photoactive drugs are present in the skin in adequate concentration and are then exposed to sufficient light of appropriate activating wavelength.

Potentially phototoxic drugs include tetracyclines, sulphonamides, naproxen, nalidixic acid, psoralens and griseofulvin. In the very high dosages used in renal failure, frusemide is phototoxic. Some phototoxic drugs may induce blistering, scarring reactions, mimicking porphyria cutanea tarda.

In contrast, the photoallergic response depends upon an immune reaction. The mechanism probably involves the alteration of the drug by light, and the attachment of the new compound to a protein, which then acts as an antigen. Chlorpromazine, sulphanilamide and promethazine may all cause photoallergic reactions. Amiodarone causes photosensitivity frequently followed by characteristic pigmentation.

Fixed eruptions

This is a rare but remarkable reaction in which each exposure to the offending drug produces areas of inflammation and even blistering whose borders are sharply defined, fixed, constant and exactly reproducible. The hands, forearms, penis and mouth are the usual sites. Tetracyclines, barbiturates, sulphonamides, phenazone, salicylates, dapsone, phenolphthalein (in laxatives), oxyphenbutazone and chlordiazepoxide are the commonest causes. The mechanisms involved are not understood.

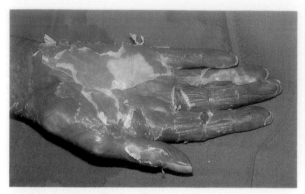

Fig. 23.1   Scarlatiniform peeling.

Exanthematic eruptions

This is the commonest drug reaction. It may be erythematous and macular (scarlatiniform) or maculopapular (morbilliform), and is symmetrical. Associated fever is common. Peeling may follow (Fig. 23.1). The underlying mechanism is usually allergic. Ampicillin is the commonest cause of a morbilliform reaction today but sulphonamides, barbiturates, phenylbutazone, *para*-aminosalicylic acid and many others may be responsible. Atropine and meprobamate characteristically can cause scarlatiniform exanthemata. Cotrimoxazole may induce a rubella-like (rubelliform) erythema.

Eczematous eruptions

These may be caused by sulphonamides, sulphonylureas, phenylbutazone, methyldopa and gold. Sometimes the primary sensitization is topical, i.e. contact dermatitis can be provoked by systemic administration of a drug, previously used topically. Examples of drugs used both topically and systemically include antibiotics, for example tetracyclines, fusidic acid, gentamicin; other antiseptics, such as iodoquinolines; and local anaesthetics of the procaine series, for example benzocaine and amethocaine. Ethylenediamine, contained in certain creams (e.g. Tri-Adcortyl, U.K.), is a contact sensitizer and is used parenterally in aminophylline (see Chapter 11; Table 11.9).

Exfoliative dermatitis

This variant of dermatitis is one of the most dangerous drug-induced reactions and may prove fatal. Causative drugs include gold, phenylbutazone, indomethacin, allopurinol, hydantoins, sulphonylureas, *para*-aminosalicylic acid and captopril.

Pigmentation

Heavy metals such as gold and silver may form pigmented deposits in skin. Certain antimalarials, such as chloroquine and mepacrine, chlorpromazine and hydantoins may cause hypermelanosis, as may oral contraceptives (facial chloasma). Fixed eruptions may show pigmented relics between exacerbations. Inorganic arsenic causes 'rain-drop' pigmentation of the trunk. Recently amiodarone, used in cardiac dysrhythmias, has been recognized as a cause of blue–grey pigmentation in exposed areas, especially the face. Rarely, minocycline causes similar pigmentation.

Acneiform eruptions

Corticotrophin, corticosteroids, androgens in females, isoniazid, lithium salts, bromides and iodides may induce rashes resembling acne vulgaris.

Bullous eruptions

There are several types of bullous eruptions. The sparse large bullae seen on pressure areas after barbiturate overdosage are distinctive and are not due to immunological mechanisms. Fixed eruptions may be bullous if very intense. Sulphonamides, halides and barbiturates may induce allergic bullous reactions. Phototoxic bullae can be caused by nalidixic acid and high dose frusemide. A pemphigus-like reaction can be caused by penicillamine, captopril and rifampicin, and a porphyria-like reaction by tetracyclines, naproxen and pyridoxine.

Lichenoid eruptions

Drug rashes mimicking lichen planus are well recognized. The mucosae and skin may both be involved. The causes include mepacrine, chloroquine, quinine, quinidine, thiazides, chlorpropamide, gold and various beta-blockers.

Psoriasiform eruptions

Methyldopa, beta-blockers, gold and phenylbutazone may induce rashes with some features suggestive of psoriasis. Lithium salts and the antimalarials, mepacrine and chloroquine, may aggravate pre-existing psoriasis.

Erythema multiforme

This hypersensitivity reaction can be caused by barbiturates, salicylates, sulphonamides (particularly the long-acting ones), penicillin, hydantoins and sulphonylureas.

Toxic epidermal necrolysis

This particularly dangerous reaction can occur in adults or children and is usually due to a sulphonamide, hydantoin, penicillin or non-steroidal anti-inflammatory drug. Diffuse erythema of dramatic onset is followed by skin tenderness and blistering due to epidermal necrosis. The mucosae are almost always involved. Intensive care is required, particularly intravenous fluid and electrolyte replacement, intranasal feeding and protein replacement, and prompt antibiotics for infection. Low dose heparin should be given to prevent thrombosis. Mouth and eye toilet may be required hourly. Even so, synechiae formation and keratoconjunctivitis sicca are liable to develop. The mortality is at least 25%, even with skilled care.

Drug-induced alopecia

Cytotoxic drugs, particularly cyclophosphamide and synthetic retinoids, interfere with the growth or anagen phase of the hair follicle cycle. Heparin, coumarins, dextran sulphate and possibly oral contraceptive withdrawal can induce a premature resting, or telogen, phase which leads to loss of hair 3 months later when growth recommences. Antithyroid drugs may have a similar action.

Nail dystrophy

Photo-onycholysis may be one manifestation of tetracycline phototoxicity. Benoxaprofen, now withdrawn, frequently caused onycholysis.

Vasculitis

Blood vessel involvement is probably due to drug-induced immune complex deposition in the small vessels. The skin and kidneys are most likely to be affected. Purpuric and necrotic papules, ulceration, etc, may be seen. Sulphonamides, thiouracils, guanethidine, diuretics and phenytoin have been implicated.

Erythema nodosum

This is a type of vasculitis with a characteristic pattern (see p. 132). Sulphonamides, including salazopyrin, and oral contraceptives may induce this reaction.

Diagnosis and Management

In general, discontinuation of the offending drug will lead to clearance of the rash in 1–3 weeks. Exceptions are penicillin urticaria, which may take months to disappear, and exfoliative dermatitis of any cause. Where several suspect drugs have been withdrawn simultaneously, readministration may be the only way of making certain of the diagnosis. This procedure is safe with fixed, lichenoid, photosensitive or acneiform eruptions but may be dangerous or even fatal with urticaria, erythema multiforme, toxic epidermal necrolysis or exfoliative dermatitis. Patch testing is rarely of value and intradermal testing is likely to give false negative results since the offending drug is rarely a complete antigen. Patch and intradermal testing may also be dangerous, causing anaphylactic shock, for example tests with penicillin and streptomycin. There is no reliable in vitro test although eosinophilia, basophilopenia or low serum complement point towards a drug reaction. Skin biopsy is rarely helpful.

Systemic reactions to topical applications

Many substances applied to the surface of damaged or intact skin may be absorbed and may produce systemic effects which are unwanted or dangerous. The quantity absorbed in relation to body weight is greatest in infancy. Potentially dangerous therapeutic substances include boric acid, cantharidin, hexachlorophane (which is neurotoxic), lead and mercury. Neomycin, absorbed from ulcerated areas, has caused severe ototoxicity and deafness. Oestrogenic hormones may feminize male infants accidentally exposed. Other potentially dangerous substances include phenol, podophyllin (used to treat genital warts) and salicylates.

Tropical Diseases Imported into Temperate Countries

Since earliest times people have moved about the world but slowly and usually locally. The advent of mass air travel, its relative cheapness, the growth of tourism and business travel have led to huge and rapid movements so that the tropics are only hours away from Europe.

In addition, the legacy of empire has left the United Kingdom, France, Portugal and Holland with substantial numbers of immigrants from Asia, Africa, Central and South America. The search for work has brought Turks, Moroccans and others to Germany and other northern European countries. All these factors have led to an increasing incidence of several diseases hitherto regarded as tropical or subtropical in temperate countries.

Leprosy

Leprosy (Hansen's disease) is a chronic disease caused by *Mycobacterium leprae*. Although it eventually may involve many systems, the peripheral nervous system and then skin are affected very early. The disease is no longer endemic in northern Europe but is found in Portugal, southern Italy and Greece as well as throughout the tropics and subtropics. The clinicopathological manifestations are determined by the immunological response to invasion by *M. leprae*.

Tuberculoid leprosy

If immunity is high, bacilli in nerves are phagocytosed by cells which become fixed epithelioid cells, later aggregating into giant cells. This process is initially in peripheral nerves but bacilli may reach the dermis, leading to cutaneous granulomata.

Lepromatous leprosy

If immunity is low, bacilli disseminate throughout the body in wandering macrophages (lepra cells).

Borderline leprosy

Here immunity is intermediate, as are the pathological changes.

Indeterminate leprosy

This is the earliest stage of the disease lasting months or years, giving way to one of the other patterns as the immune status is determined.

Skin lesions in leprosy

In tuberculoid leprosy, lesions are few or even solitary. Typically a raised erythematous plaque with a well-defined edge may have a flattened hypopigmented central area. The surface is dry and hairless, and sensory impairment can be demonstrated. Less often, macular hypopigmented lesions occur. Thickened nerves may be palpable in the area or elsewhere.

In lepromatous leprosy early skin lesions are less likely to be noticed by the patient who may have nasal stuffiness and discharge. The skin shows varying combinations of macules, plaques, papules and later nodules. The lesions are less inflammatory, not well defined and sensory impairment is difficult to demonstrate. The nasal mucosa is red, eroded and bleeds easily. If untreated, gross cutaneous changes with skin thickening, loss of outer eyebrows ('madarosis') and dryness occur.

Borderline lesions are intermediate between these two extremes. Indeterminate lesions are only macular.

Diagnosis

Skin smears or nasal scrapes establish the diagnosis in lepromatous leprosy. Skin or nerve biopsy is necessary in tuberculoid patterns. Occasionally the histamine and lepromin tests may be useful.

Treatment

This can only be summarized. Antileprosy drugs are now never used alone. The latest recommended regime for multibacillary (lepromatous or borderline lepromatous) leprosy consists of rifampicin 600 mg once monthly taken under supervision, together with dapsone 100 mg daily, and clofazimine 300 mg monthly (supervised) and 50 mg daily. Treatment is given for at least 2 years and until smears are negative.

Paucibacillary (tuberculoid and borderline tuberculoid) disease is treated with rifampicin 600 mg once monthly (supervised) and dapsone 100 mg daily for 6 months.

Reactional states in leprosy

These occur either due to rapid increase or lessening of cell-mediated immunity (Type I), or due to immune complex formation (Type II). The latter occurs only in lepromatous leprosy and is called *erythema nodosum leprosum*.

In Type I reactions skin lesions rapidly become more inflamed and nerve swelling and pain develop, sometimes with nerve abscess formation. In Type II reactions multiple widespread erythematous nodules and plaques develop associated with fever and malaise. Oral prednisolone may be needed to control reaction.

Leishmaniasis

This disease is due to a protozoon transmitted by the bite of sand flies (*Phlebotomus*).

Cutaneous leishmaniasis

This disease (oriental sore) is due to *Leishmania tropica*. It is endemic in the dry deserts around the shores of the Mediterranean and Western Asia, where infection is common in childhood leading to subsequent immunity. It is occasionally seen in northern Europeans after Mediterranean holidays.

The incubation period is 1–12 months and the lesion is usually on the face (Fig. 24.1). An enlarging nodule may or may not ulcerate and heals spontaneously after a year or more. Uncommonly, a chronic form develops closely resembling lupus vulgaris.

Diagnosis depends on microscopy of scrapings and biopsy for histopathology and culture. Sodium stibogluconate (pentavalent antimony) (Pentostam, U.K.) is the treatment of choice, given intralesionally. Pento-

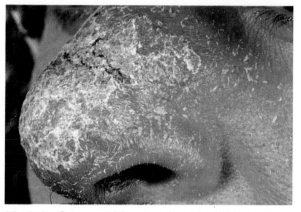

Fig. 24.1 Cutaneous leishmaniasis due to *L.tropica* in an Arab.

stam 100 mg/ml can be diluted 1:3 with 1% lignocaine. Usually, 2–4 ml of diluted solution is needed to infiltrate the whole lesion. Pentostam may also be given intramuscularly, 600 mg daily for 10 days for an adult.

American leishmaniasis

This disease affects the skin and upper respiratory tract and is due to *L. braziliensis*. It is endemic in the tropics of Central and South America, particularly in the rainy season and in forest workers or soldiers campaigning in jungle areas. Unlike *L. tropica*, primary infection does not induce permanent immunity, hence the later mucosal spread, sometimes years after the initial 'sore'. Antimony, amphotericin B and metronidazole have all been used in treatment.

Visceral leishmaniasis

This disease (kala-azar) is due to *L. donovani*. Dermal involvement is particularly seen in the Indian form of the disease, with spreading nodules appearing years after first infection. Differential diagnosis is from leprosy.

Larva Migrans

This condition is no longer rare now that hundreds of thousands of Europeans holiday on tropical beaches. It is due to filaria-like hookworm larva emerging from eggs deposited in the sand in the faeces of infested dogs and cats.

The larva usually penetrates the skin of the foot.

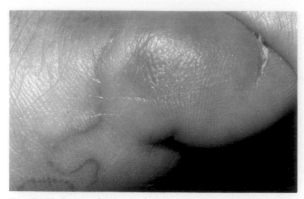

Fig. 24.2 Larva migrans.

Uncommonly, the disease occurs elsewhere, for example on the trunk. Within a day or two the site itches. Migration in the skin begins within a few days to produce distinct raised red erratic tortuous tracks which are easily visible (Fig. 24.2). Itching may be intense. The larva cannot complete its life-cycle in man and dies in a few weeks, producing spontaneous cure.

Oral albendazole 400 mg twice daily for 3 days is effective and well tolerated. Thiabendazole (5%) in dimethyl sulphoxide applied topically has been used. Oral thiabendazole is effective but too toxic for routine use.

Deep mycoses

The important systemic mycoses are described in Chapter 9.

Onchocerciasis

This is a filarial disease caused by *Onchocerca volvulus*. It is extremely common in tropical Africa and America. The adult worm is 2–7 cm long. Microfilariae are transmitted by the bite of gnats.

Worms and microfilariae are found in granulomatous dermal nodules. Microfilariae are more widespread in the dermis and may invade the eye, leading to blindness.

Clinical features

Pruritus and excoriated erythema are the first features. The dermatitis is chronic, lichenified and papular and in Africans is most marked on the flanks and thighs. Hyperpigmentation and eventually skin atrophy ensue.

The nodules are painless, non-itching and usually occur in the pelvic area in Africans. The risk of eventual blindness is high.

Diagnosis

Scabies must be excluded. Skin snips should be immersed in normal saline and examined microscopically. Nodules can be excised for histology. Eosinophilia is usual. Intradermal tests and filarial complement fixation tests are occasionally useful.

Treatment

Diethylcarbamazine citrate (Banocide, U.K.) is given orally in increasing doses over 3 or 4 weeks. Several courses may be needed. Great care is required to avoid a Jarisch–Herxheimer type of reaction if the eyes are involved. Suramin, given intravenously, kills adult worms but it very nephrotoxic.

Psychogenic Disorders

The concept of psychosomatic disease is well established. It can apply to many organs and is widely believed to be particularly important in skin disease. The solid evidence that this is so appears less convincing and the mechanisms, other than autonomic ones, are not understood. However, on the basis of such obvious phenomena as flushing induced by embarrassment, or pallor due to fear or anger, the ability of emotions to influence the skin is accepted, particularly by the lay mind. The following discussion is confined to those few clinical situations where a psychic disorder unequivocally underlies cutaneous symptoms or signs.

Psychogenic pruritus

Itching, localized or generalized, may be entirely psychogenic in origin. The diagnosis must be based on exclusion of organic disease and the presence of positive factors pointing to anxiety, depression or psychosis. Physical signs may be entirely absent or there may be frictional erythema, scratch marks or skin thickening. One variety of pruritis induces pinching or localized rubbing of the skin to produce hyperkeratotic nodules (nodular prurigo).

The scalp is a common site and there may be associated symptoms, such as vertical headache or 'feelings of pressure', on the top of the head. Pruritus due to depression may occasionally be associated with tingling or discomfort of the tongue, mouth or lips. Typically, the symptoms are said to be constant and unremitting. Characteristically, depression is attributed by the patient to the pruritus, whereas the opposite is the case.

Delusions of parasitism

Psychotic subjects with various forms of schizophrenia and paranoia may have unshakeable delusions that insects are crawling in or under the skin. Such patients complain of itching and may produce tiny fragments of dirt, hair or stratum corneum as evidence of such infestation. This is a rare condition and has to be distinguished from the more common symptom, formication, where the patient has a sensation 'as though insects are crawling in the skin' but is prepared to accept after examination that this is not so. Members of the household and even neighbours may be drawn into the delusions. Expert psychiatric help is needed; pimozide orally may be of value.

Acne excorieé

It is not uncommon for adolescent girls or young women with or without acne vulgaris to have an irresistible desire to pick at and excoriate 'spots' on the face. The resultant lesions are characteristic artefactual erosions which may leave scarring. There seems to be a strong correlation between the presence of this condition and obvious emotional disturbance. Control of the acne may help the situation but treatment can be very difficult and psychiatric help may be needed.

Cholinergic urticaria

This is a common pattern of urticaria characterized by the development of numerous pin-head weals surrounded by large erythematous flares and precipitated by heat, exercise and particularly emotional stress. It is relatively unresponsive to antihistamines but eventually undergoes spontaneous remission (see p. 139).

Dermatitis artefacta

This is a self-inflicted skin lesion whose morphology is variable. The application of heat, for example from a cigarette-end, may induce burns. Chemical application can induce areas of erythema, erosion and crusting which may heal leaving scarring. Gouging of the skin is less common but results in ulceration, occasionally gross. Intermittent application of a tourniquet to a finger or limb may induce chronic oedema.

The lesions, usually multiple, occur on parts of the body which are easily reached by the patient's own hands. The face (Fig. 25.1), neck, arms and breasts in women are the commonest sites. Discomfort is minimal and, characteristically, the lesions do not

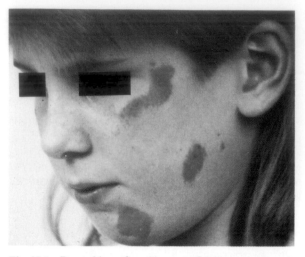

Fig. 25.1 Dermatitis artefacta; bizarre artificial lesions on face of a young girl.

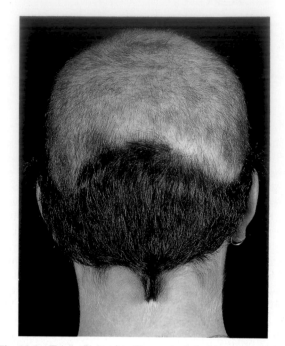

Fig. 25.2 Trichotillomania. Traumatic hair loss in a young woman.

induce the obvious alarm and anxiety in the patient which such florid pathology would generate in those of healthy mind. Confrontation with the diagnosis invariably produces a blank denial, in which close relatives may share.

The disease is most commonly seen in young girls or women whose subconscious aim may be to manipulate a mother, boyfriend or even employer. Some such young women are emotionally immature; others are hysterical and 'angry' and the symptom is attention-seeking. Many seem to have dominating mothers. In adults of either sex the subconscious aim may be to deceive for gain, for example legal compensation after a minor accident at work or in a motor car, or to avoid work or, in a tramp, to obtain admission to hospital. A few are frankly psychotic.

The diagnosis is usually obvious because of the bizarre, artefactual nature of the lesions but finding the precise mechanism may be difficult. Psychiatric help is needed but often resented, so that cooperation is poor.

Hair pulling and rubbing

The habit of twisting a lock of hair and so producing a patch of alopecia is common in nervous children (trichotillomania). Recovery is usually spontaneous. Perpetual rubbing of the hair, resulting in uniformly short fractured hairs, is a symptom of a more deep-seated psychiatric disorder (see also p. 190) (Fig. 25.2).

Hyperhidrosis

There is no doubt that excessive sweating of any part of the body can be psychogenic in origin (see Chapter 20).

— Appendix I

Sport and the Skin

The worldwide rising popularity of sport impinges on the dermatologist as well as the orthopaedic surgeon. Below are briefly mentioned the main cutaneous hazards.

Sunburn. (see p. 123).

Insect bites. Papular urticaria is common.

Cholinergic urticaria and pruritus. Itching and wealing are commonly precipitated by exercise (p. 139).

Phytophotodermatitis. Contact with meadow weeds by joggers on very sunny days (p. 125).

Black heel. Traumatic purpura of the heel can simulate melanoma.

Tennis toe. Traumatic subungual haemorrhage in a big toe.

Jogger's nipple. Soreness of the nipple can occur in both sexes due to friction on a tracksuit during exercise.

Perniosis. Chilblains are common in winter, for example on the upper outer thighs of plump girls who ride horses (p. 131).

Tinea. Fungal infections of the feet and groin are very common in young male sportsmen, acquired in changing rooms and showers.

Scrum-pox. This is coccal impetigo spread by the proximity of the rugby football scrum.

Herpes gladiatorum. Wrestlers slavering over each other may transmit *Herpes simplex* virus.

Verruca plantaris. Plantar warts are common in adults and children who use public swimming baths, changing rooms, etc (p. 45).

Miliaria. Intense exercise in tropical heat and inappropriate clothing can lead to sweat duct occlusion and the intensely pruritic papular or vesicular rash of miliaria.

Swimming-pool granuloma. A solitary cutaneous nodule or ulcer due to an atypical mycobacterium, caused by an abrasion sustained in a swimming pool (p. 57).

Swimmer's ear. Otitis externa due to constant wetting.

Molluscum contagiosum. Commonly acquired from swimming pools or changing rooms.

— Appendix II

Drug Interactions Important to the Dermatologist

Drug	Potentiators	Inhibitors	Drug	Potentiators	Inhibitors
Methotrexate	Aspirin Naproxen Frusemide		Digoxin	Thiazide diuretics Quinidine Verapamil	
Cylosporin A	Erythromycin	Phenytoin	Beta-blockers	Cimetidine	
Zidovudine	Paracetamol		Theophyllines	Erythromycin Cimetidine	
Azathioprine	Allopurinol		Phenytoin	Isoniazid Cimetidine Sulphonamides	Carbamazepine
Oral contraceptives		Rifampicin Anticonvulsants			
Warfarin	Cimetidine Aspirin Sulphonamides	Phenytoin Rifampicin			

— Appendix III

A Formulary of Useful Topical Preparations

Antiseptics well tolerated by normal or inflamed skin

1:8000 potassium permanganate (aqueous solution)
(Permitabs, U.K.-one tablet dissolved in 3 litres of water provides a 1:7500 solution)

10% povidone iodine (aqueous solution) (Betadine Antiseptic solution, U.K.)

1% chlorhexidine cream (Hibitane Cream, U.K.)

0.65% aluminium acetate (aqueous solution)

Anti-bacterial creams and ointments

Neomycin and bacitracin cream (Cicatrin Cream, U.K.)

Neomycin and gramicidin ointment (Graneodin Ointment, U.K.)

Framycetin and gramicidin cream (Soframycin Cream, U.K.)

Polymyxin B and bacitracin ointment (Polyfax Ointment, U.K.)

Silver sulphadiazine cream (Flamazine Cream, U.K.)

Chlortetracycline 3% cream (Aureomycin Cream, U.K.)

Fusidic acid 2% (Fucidin Cream, ointment and gel, U.K.)

Mupirocin 2% ointment (Bactroban ointment, U.K.)

Desloughing and antiseptic agents for ulceration

1.5% stabilized hydrogen peroxide cream (Hioxyl, U.K.)

0.9% cadexomer iodine (Iodosorb, U.K.)

0.5% brilliant green and 0.5% lactic acid (aqueous) (Variclene, U.K.)

Note: Preparations containing neomycin or framycetin should never be applied to ulcerated lesions.

Compound preparations containing hydrocortisone

Hydrocortisone 1% with urea 10% for dry dermatitis (Alphaderm Cream, U.K.; Calmurid HC Cream, U.K.)

Hydrocortisone 1% with crotamiton 10% (Eurax HC Cream, U.K.)

Hydrocortisone 1% with an imidazole 1% (Canesten HC Cream, U.K.; Daktacort Cream, U.K.; Econacort Cream, U.K.)

Hydrocortisone 1% with oxytetracycline 3% (Terra-Cortril Ointment, U.K.; Terra-Cortril Nystatin Cream, U.K.) (Stains clothing yellow)

Hydrocortisone 1% with clioquinol 3% (Vioform — HC ointment and cream, U.K.) (Stains clothing yellow)

Topical corticosteroid preparations (see Table 4.1, p.28)

Potency I   0.05% clobetasol propionate (Dermovate ointment, cream and scalp lotion, U.K.)
0.1% halcinonide (Halciderm Cream, U.K.)

Potency II   0.1% hydrocortisone butyrate (Locoid ointment, cream, fatty cream and scalp lotion, U.K.)
0.025% beclomethasone dipropionate (Propaderm ointment and cream, U.K.)
0.1% betamethasone valerate (Betnovate ointment, cream and scalp lotion, U.K.)
0.05% betamethasone dipropionate (Diprosone ointment cream and scalp lotion, U.K.)
0.025% fluocinolone acetonide (Synalar ointment, cream and scalp gel, U.K.)
0.1% triamcinolone acetonide (Adcortyl ointment and cream, U.K.)
0.05% fluocinonide (Metosyn ointment and scalp lotion, U.K.)

Potency III   0.025% betamethasone valerate (Betnovate RD ointment and cream, U.K.)
0.05% clobetasone butyrate (Eumovate ointment and cream, U.K.)
0.00625% fluocinolone acetonide (Synalar 1 in 4 Dilution, U.K.)
0.1% fluocortolone hexanoate (Ultradil Plain ointment and cream, U.K.)
0.0125% flurandrenolone (Haelan ointment and cream, U.K.)

Potency IV   Hydrocortisone 1% (Efcortelan, U.K.; Hydrocotisyl, U.K.: creams and ointments)
Hydrocortisone 0.1% (Dioderm cream, U.K.)

Corticosteroid — anti-microbial preparations

(See also 'Compound preparations containing hydrocortisone')

0.1% hydrocortisone butyrate with 3% chlorquinaldol (Locoid C ointment and cream, U.K.) (Stains clothing)

0.025% beclomethasone diproprionate with 3% chlortetracycline HCl (Propaderm-A ointment, U.K.) (Stains clothing)

0.1% betamethasone valerate with 3% clioquinol (Betnovate-C ointment and cream, U.K.) (Stains clothing)

0.1% betamethasone valerate with fusidic acid 2% (Fucibet cream, U.K.)

0.05% clobetasone butyrate with 3% oxytetracycline and nystatin (Trimovate ointment and cream, U.K.) (Stains clothing)

0.025% fluocinolone acetonide with clioquinol 3% (Synalar C ointment and cream, U.K.) (Stains clothing)

0.0125% flurandrenolone with 3% clioquinol (Haelan-C ointment and cream) (Stains clothing)

0.1% triamcinolone acetonide with 0.025% gramicidin and 0.25% neomycin (Adcortyl with Graneodin ointment)

0.1% triamcinolone acetonide with 0.025% gramicidin, 0.25% neomycin and nystatin (Tri-Adcortyl ointment, U.K.) (The cream preparation contains ethylenediamine (see Table 11.9) and should be avoided.)

Note: Preparations containing neomycin should never be used on eczematized skin for more than five days.

Preparations for psoriasis

Tar preparations

5% coal tar with allantoin (Alphosyl, U.K., cream and lotion)

10% coal tar solution (Carbo-Dome Cream)

6% coal tar with 0.4% lecithin (Psoriderm Cream, U.K.)

5% coal tar extract with 0.5% hydrocortisone (Tarcortin Cream, U.K.)

Bath additives

Polytar Emollient

Psoriderm Bath Emulsion

Dithranol (Anthralin) preparations

Dithranol 0.01% to 1.0% in Lassar's paste (see p. 25) — only suitable for in-patient or day care centre use.

Dithranol 0.1%–2.0% in soft-yellow paraffin (mineral oil). (Suitable for 10–30 minute applications daily (short-contact treatment)).

Dithranol 0.1%–2.0% in a cream (Dithrocream range, U.K.)

Preparations for acne vulgaris

2.5% benzoyl peroxide cream (Acetoxyl 2.5 gel, U.K.)

5.0% benzoyl peroxide cream or lotion gel (Acetoxyl 5 gel, U.K.; Benzoyl 5 cream and lotion, U.K.; Benzagel 5 U.K.; Panoxyl 5 gel, U.K.)

10.0% benzoyl peroxide cream or lotion gel (Benoxyl 10 lotion, U.K.; Benoxyl 10 with sulphur, U.K.; Benzagel 10, U.K.; Panoxyl 10 gel, U.K.)

5% and 10% benzoyl peroxide with potassium hydroxyquinoline sulphate 0.5% cream and lotio-gel (Quinoderm, U.K.)

0.05% tretinoin as cream (Retin A Cream, U.K.)

0.025% tretinoin as gel or lotion (Retin A gel and lotion, U.K.)

Tretinoin preparations are irritant and should be used sparingly and for very short periods of 1-2 hours daily initially.

Preparations for viral warts

Salicylic acid, lactic acid and copper sulphate gel (Cuplex gel, U.K.)

Salicylic acid and lactic acid in flexible collodion (Salactol, U.K.; Duofilm, U.K.)

50% salicylic acid in paraffin (Verrugon, U.K.)

1.5% formaldehyde in a gel (Veracur, U.K.)

10% glutaraldehyde solution (Glutarol, U.K.)

0.5% podophyllotoxin solution (Warticon solution, U.K.) — used for penile warts

Shampoos for scalp psoriasis and seborrhoeic dermatitis

4% povidone-iodine (Betadine shampoo Solution, U.K.)

0.5% benzalkonium chloride (Capitol Shampoo, U.K.)

10% cetrimide (Ceanel concentrate Shampoo, U.K.)

17.5% cetrimide (Cetavlon PC shampoo, U.K.)

Various tar-containing shampoos (Gelcotar, U.K.; Genisol, U.K.; Ionil T, U.K.; Polytar, U.K.; T-Gel, U.K.)

2.5% selenium sulphide (Lenium Cream shampoo; Selsun, U.K.)

Anti-viral preparations

5% acyclovir cream (Zovirax, U.K.)

40% idoxuridine in dimethylsulphoxide (Iduridin 40%, U.K.)

Anti-fungal Preparations

For candidosis only

3% amphotericin cream, ointment, lozenges, pessaries (Fungilin, U.K.)

Nystatin 100,000 μ/g (Nystan cream, pessaries, U.K.)

For candidosis and tinea infections

Whitfield's ointment: benzoic acid 6% salicylic acid 3% in emulsifying ointment (use at half-strength if groin is to be treated)

1% clotrimazole cream, solution and powder (Canesten, U.K.)

1% econazole cream, lotion and powder (Ecostatin; Pevaryl, U.K.)

2% ketoconazole cream (Nizoral, U.K.)

2% miconazole nitrate cream, powder (Daktarin, U.K.)

Parasiticidal preparations for scabies

1% lindane cream (Lorexane, U.K.)

1% lindane lotion (Quellada, U.K.)

25% benzyl benzoate emulsion (Ascabiol, U.K.) (Never use for more than two days)

10% crotamiton cream and lotion (Eurax, U.K.)

25% monosulfiram in alcohol (Tetmosol, U.K.) (To be diluted before use)

Parasiticidal preparations for pediculosis

0.5% malathion aqueous (Derbac — M, U.K.)

0.5% malathion alcoholic (Prioderm; Suleo — M, U.K.)

0.5% carbaryl alcoholic (Carylderm lotion, U.K.)

0.5% carbaryl aqueous (Clinicide lotion, U.K.)

Index

Page references in *italics* indicate figures, whereas those in bold face refer to tables.

Abscess
  definition, 16
  "Pautrier", 169
  perianal, 32
Acantholysis, 153
Acanthosis, 36, 83, 99, 160
Acanthosis nigricans, 36
Achromic naevus, 180
Acne conglobata, 172
Acne excorieé, 203
Acne fulminans, 172
  treatment, 174
Acne keloid, 149
Acne varioliformis, 191
Acne vulgaris, 171
  acneiform eruptions, 172–173
    chlorinated hydrocarbons, 173
    corticosteroids, 172
    drug-induced, 198
    in infants, 173
    isoniazid, 172
    oil, 173
    treatment, 173–174
    topical therapy, 173, 209
Acral lentiginous malignant melanoma,
    162
Acral psoriasis, 100
Acrodermatitis chronica atrophicans, 56
Acrodermatitis enteropathica of
    Danbolt, 32, 97, 109
Acropustulosis of infancy, 109
Acrosclerosis, *see* Sclerosis, systemic
Actinic dermatitis, chronic, 128
Actinic lentigo, 124
Actinic prurigo, 128
Actinomyces infections, 71–72
Actinomycosis, 70–71
Acyclovir, use, 22, 39, 91
  herpes simplex, 43
  herpes zoster, 42
Addison's disease, 30, 181
Adenoma sebaceum, 117
Adrenal disease
  hirsutism cause, 191
Adrenal-genital syndrome, congenital
  hirsutism cause, 191
Adrenaline, use, in angioedema, 140
Ageing
  and sunlight exposure, 124
AIDS, 50–51
AIDS-related complex, 50–51
Allergic contact dermatitis
  causes

cosmetics, 86–87
  medicaments, 87
  metals, 85
  organic dyes, 86
  plants, 86
  plastics, 86
  resins, 86
  rubber, 86
  clinical features, 85
  cross-sensitization, 88
  diagnosis, 87–88
    patch testing, 87–88
  irritant differential diagnosis, 84
  management, 88
  pathogenesis, 84–85
Allergic hypersensitivity, *see*
  Hypersensitivity
Alopecia
  definition, 16
  forms, 186–187, *see also* Cicatricial
    alopecia; Non-cicatricial
    alopecia
Alopecia areata, 189–190
  "exclamation-mark" hairs, 190
Aluminium acetate solution, 25
Amiodarone
  pigmentation effects, 198
Amniocentesis, 116
  detectable diseases by, 116
Amphotericin B, use, 22, 70
Anagen alopecia, 186, 189
Analgesics, use, 22
Anchoring fibrils
  collagen type, 6
Anderson-Fabry disease, 121
Androgens
  alopecia in women, 189
  influence on hair follicles, 185
Angioedema, 138, 140
  hereditary, 140
Angiokeratoma corporis diffusum
  (Anderson-Fabry disease), 121
Angiomatosis, eruptive disseminated,
    113
Angiosarcoma, 168
Angular stomatitis, 69
Anhidrosis, 177
Ankylosing spondylitis
  HLA antigens and, 116
Anogenital area
  differential diagnosis of lesions, 16
  lichen sclerosus et atrophicus, 147
Anthrax, 55–56

Antibiotics
  systemic use, 22
  topical preparations, 207
Antifungal agents
  systemic use, 22
  topical use, 27–28, 210
Antihistamines, use, 22, 26, 139–140
Anti-infective chemotherapeutic agents,
    22
Antipruritic drugs, use, 22
Antiseptics, 26, 207
Anti-viral topical preparations, 210
Apocrine sweat glands, 1, 2, 177
  hidradenitis suppurativa, 177
Aquagenic urticaria, 139
Arachidonic acid pathways
  in psoriasis, 98
  inflammation mediators generation, 10
ARC (AIDS-related complex), 50
Arsenic, inorganic
  carcinomas and, 38, 158
  keratosis, 165
  "rain drop" pigmentation cause, 198
Arterial disease
  large vessel, 133, 134–135
    management, 136
    see also under individual names
  small vessel, 133, *see also under*
    individual names
Arterial emboli, 135
Arthus reactions, 8
"Ashy dermatosis", 181
Aspirin
  drug interactions and, 206
  urticaria cause, 139
Asteatotic dermatitis, 96
Astemizole, 22
Atherosclerosis
  large-vessels of leg, 135
Atopic dermatitis, 89–92
    complications
      coccal infections, 91
      contact dermatitis, 91
      eczema herpeticum, 91
      viral warts and mollusca, 91
    management, 91–92
"Atrophie blanche", 136
Atrophy
  definition, 15
  occurrence in neonates, 144
Autoimmune diseases
  collagen-vascular
    dermatomyositis, 147–149

lupus erythrematosus, 141, *see also
    under individual names*
scleroderma, 144, *see also under
    individual names*
lymphoma aetiological factor, 168
Autosomal inheritance
    explanation of term, 115
Axillae
    differential diagnosis of lesions, **16**
    digitate warts, 45
    erythrasma eruptions, 55
    freckling, 116
    molluscum contagiosum, 44
    pemphigus vegetans eruptions, 154
    sweating, 176
Azathioprine
    drug interactions, 206
    use, 148, 154

B-cells
    immune response role, 8
        activation, 8–9
        interleukin-induced proliferation, 7
        recognition, 8
    lymphoma, 38, 170
Babies, skin of
    disorders, 109
    post-term, 109
    pre-term, 109
Bacille Calmette-Guerin infections
    (BCG), 57
Bacillus anthracis infection, 55–56
Bacitracin, use, 26
Bacterial diseases
    actinomyces infections, 71–72
    bacillus infections, 55–56
    borrelia infections, 56
    chlamydia infections, 62
    congenital, 113
    corynebacterial infections, 55
        granuloma inguinale, 61–62
    erysipelothrix infections, 55
    haemophilus infections, 62
    micrococcal infections, 55
    mycobacterial infections, 58
        acute tuberculous ulceration, 57
        diagnosis, 57
        lupus vulgaris, 56
        mycobacterium marinum, 57–58
        scrofuloderma, 57
        treatment, 57
        tuberculides, 57
        tuberculosis of skin, 56
        warty tuberculosis, 57
    non-venereal treponemal, 61
    sexually transmitted
        gonorrhoea, 58
        syphilis, 58–61
    staphylococcal infections, 52
        boils and carbuncles, 53
        ecthyma, 53
        folliculitis, 53
        impetigo, 52–53

"scalded skin" syndrome, 53
streptococcal infections
    cellulitis, 54
    erysipelas, 53–54
    infected fissures, 55
Bactroban, use, 26
Balanitis xerotica obliterans, 147
Balanoposthitis, 69
Baldness, common, 188
    in females, 188
Basal cell carcinoma, 158–159
    microscopic preparation (cytology), 19
Basal cell layer, 2
    cytolysis, 120
    degeneration, 142
Basal cell naevus syndrome, 159
Basal cell papilloma, 157
Basement membrane, 4
    antigens, 4
    collagen type, **6**
Basidiobolus meristosporus infection, 73
Bazin's disease, 57, 133
Beard, ringworm of, 67–68
Becker's naevus, 184
Bed bug bites, 80–81
Bee stings, 140
Benign mucous membrane pemphigold,
    155
Benoxaprofen, reactions to, 125
Benzyl benzoate, use, 77
Benzyl penicillin G, use, 22
Berlocque dermatitis, 125
Bilateral acoustic central
    neurofibromatosis, 117
Biliary cirrhosis, 30
Black heal, 205
Blackheads
    definition, 15
    occurrence
        acne vulgaris, 171, 172
        DLE, 141
Blastomyces dermatitidis infection, 74
Blastomycosis, 74
Bleomycin, side-effects, 147
Blistering
    anatomy, 151
        levels of cleavage, 151
    common conditions, 151, *see also under
        individual names*
    pathogenesis, 151
    uncommon diseases, 152, *see also
        under individual names*
Blood vessels of skin, 6
    drug-induced vasculitis, 199
    extremities, 6
    monoclonal antibodies in
        immunoperoxidase studies, **21**
Bloom's syndrome, 120
Blue rubber bleb naevus syndrome, 113
Boils, 53
    management, 53
    occurrence, 29
Bombesin, 5
Bone cysts, occurrence, 30

Borrelia bergdorferi infection, 56
Bournville's disease, *see* Tuberose
    sclerosis
Bowenoid papulosis, 47
Bowen's disease, 165
    penis, 166
    treatment, 165
Breasts, lesions of
    ductal carcinoma, 36
    jogger's nipple, 205
    morphoea lesions, 144
    Paget's disease, 166
Bromhidrosis
    apocrine, 177
    eccrine, 177
Bromides, side-effects, 172
Bronchial carcinoma, 37
Buccal mucosa
    hyperpigmentation, 30
    Kaposi's sarcoma eruptions, 51
    "Koplik's spots", 39
    lichen planus eruptions, 107
    "mucous patches", 59
    varicella lesions, 39
Buerger's disease, 136
Bullae
    definition, 15
    see also Blistering
Bullous dermatitis, childhood benign
    chronic, 156
Bullous ichthyosiform erythroderma,
    119
Burkitt's lymphoma, 170
Burns
    blistering cause, 152
    cicatricial alopecia cause, 187
Burow's solution, 25, 26
Burrows, definition, 16
Buttocks
    dermatitis herpetiformis rash, 156
    eruptive xanthomata, 31
    type II herpes simplex eruptions, 43
    warty nodules, 72

Calamine, use, 24, 25, 39
Callus, definition, 16, 46
Campbell de Morgan spot (cherry
    angioma), 167
Candida albicans infections, 69
    and granuloma gluteale infantum, 109
    clinical patterns, 69
        angular stomatitis and cheilitis, 69
        balanoposthitis, 69
        chronic paronychia, 69
        intertrigo, 69
        onychia, 70
        thrush, 69
        vulvovaginitis, 69
    clinical situations involvement, 69
    differential diagnosis, 70
    microscopic preparation, *19*
    treatment, 70

Candidosis, *see Candida albicans*
  infections
Capillaritis, 131
Carbuncles, 53
Carcinoid syndrome, 32
Carotenaemia, 181
Cat-Scratch Disease, 51
Caterpillar rash, 81
Cavernous haemangioma, 112
CD1 antigen
  Langerhans' cell expression, 5
CD4 antigen
  immune response role, 9
  Langerhans' cell expression, 5
CD8 antigen
  immune response role, 9
Cellular naevus, 183
Cellulitis, 54
Chancroid, 62
Cheilitis, 69
Cherry angioma (Campbell de Morgan
      spot), 167
Chicken-pox, *see* Varicella
Chilbain lupus, 144
Chilbains, 131–132
Chlamydia infections,
  and Reiter's disease, 106
Chloasma, 181
Chloracne, 173
Chloramphenicol, side-effects, 87
Chlortetracycline, use, 26
Cholinergic urticaria, 139, 203
Chromate
  allergic contact dermatitis cause, 85
Chromoblastomycosis, 72
Chromasomes
  explanation of term, 115
Chrysiasis, 182
Cicatricial alopecia, 186–187
  burns, 187
  chronic staphylococcal folliculitis, 188
  DLE, 187
  favus, 65, 187
  idiopathic, 188
  kerion, 187
  lichen planus, 187
  lupus vulgaris, 187
  syphilis, 188
  zoster, 187
Cicatrix, *see* Scars
Cimex lenticularis bites, 80–81
Cladosporum infection, 72
Clear cell acanthoma, 158
Clofazimine, use, 22
Clotrimazole, use, 28
Clubbing, 30, 193
Cobalt
  allergic contact dermatitis cause, 85
Coccidioides immitis infection, 74
Coccidioidomycosis, 74
Codeine, side-effects, 139
Collagen
  disorders, 149–150
    autoimmune, 141–149

helical structure, 6, 141
  human skin types, 6
  synthesis, 6
Collagenase, 6
"Collodion baby", 119
Comedones, *see* Blackheads
Common warts
  clinical picture, 45
  treatment, 47
Complement, 10
  activation pathways, 10
Compound naevus, 183
Condylomata acuminata, *see* Genital
      warts
Condylomata lata, 59
C1 inhibitor deficiency, 140
Congenital aplasia cutis, 113
Connective tissue disorders
  cutis laxa, 118
  Ehlers-Danlos syndrome, 118
  pseudo-xanthoma elasticum, 118
Contact urticaria, 139
Corns, explanation of term, 46
Corticosteroids
  side-effects
    acneiform eruptions, 172
    iatrogenic rosacea, 175
    perioral dermatitis, 175
    striae, 150
    widespread topical exposure, 27
  systemic use, 23
    disadvantages, 23
    dosage, 23
    patient supervision, 23
    withdrawal and post-drug period,
      23
  topical use, 27
    dilution, 27
    disadvantages, 27
    local side-effects, 27
    potency classification, 27
    preparations containing, 208
    use, 88, 91, 105, 142, 181
Corticotrophin, 23
Corynebacterial infections
  C. minutissimum, 55
  granuloma inguinale, 61–62
Cosmetics, allergic contact dermatitis
      cause, 86–87
Co-trimoxazole, use, 22
"Crabs", 78
Creams, 24
Crohn's disease, 32
Crosti's indolent lymphoma, 170
Crotamiton, use, 77
CRST syndrome, *see* Sclerosis, systemic
Crusts, 39, 41, 76
  definition, 15
  removal, 24
Cullen's sign, 33
Cushingoid features, 27
Cushing's syndrome, 30
Cutaneous nerves, 7
  monoclonal antibodies in

immunoperoxidase studies, **21**
Cuticle, 192
  detachment, 193
Cutis laxa, 118
Cutis marmorata, 109
Cyanosis, 109, 135, *see also* Livedo
      reticularis
Cysts
  acne, 172
    treatment, 174
  definition, 16
  epidermal
    epidermoid, 158
    milia, 158
    pilar, 158
  "millet seed", 109
  mucous, 194
  of bone cysts, 30
  subcutaneous epidermoid, 37
  translucent, white, 159
Cytokines, 7, 9

Dactylitis, 34
Dandruff, 190–191
Dapsone
  side-effects, 156
  use, 22
Darier's disease, 121
Deep vein thrombosis
  and leg venous disease, 136
Degos' acanthoma (clear cell
      acanthoma), 157
7-Dehydrocholesterol metabolism, 4
Depigmentation
  chemical, 180
  hydroquinone-induced, 28
  in pityriasis versicolor, 71
  streaky in incontinentia pigmenti, 120
Depression
  as pruritis cause, 203
Dermal naevus, 183
Dermatitis, 82
  basal clinical features, 82–83
  childhood, 110, *see also under*
        individual names
  clinical classification, 83
    miscellaneous, 97
    see also under individual names
  in leg venous disease, 136
    treatment, 137
  pathology, 83
Dermatitis artefacta, 203–204
Dermatitis herpetiformis, 32, 156
  variants
    childhood benign chronic bullous
          dermatitis, 156
    linear IgA disease, 156
Dermatofibroma, 166
Dermatoliposclerosis, 136
Dermatomyositis, 37, 147–149
Dermatopathic lymphadenitis, 97
Dermatophyte fungus, microscopic
      preparation, *19*

Dermis
  "accessory cells", 8
  atrophy, 15
  benign tumours
    fibroblast derivation, 166
    lymphatic tissue derivation, 167
    vascular tissue derivation, 166–167
  blisters, **152**
  cell populations
    fibroblasts, 7
    lymphocytes, 7
    macrophages (monocytes), 7
    mast cells, 7
  elastic tissue loss, 118
  function, 6
  granulomatous infiltration, 35
  lymphocyte and histiocyte infiltration, 142
  malignant tumours
    angiosarcoma, 168
    Kaposi's sarcoma, 167–168
    lymphangiosarcoma, 168
    secondary deposits, 167
  psoriatic changes, 99
  structure, 5–6
    cutaneous nerves, 7
    epidermodermal junction, 4
    lymphatics, 7
Dermographism, 138
  "white", 89
"Desert ear", 93
Detergents, 25
Diabetes mellitus
  arterial disease, 29
  candidosis, 29
  granuloma annulare, 30
  necrobiosis lipoidica, 29–30
  neuropathy, 29
  staphyloderma, 29
  xanthomata, 29
Diagnosis
  examination, 12–16
  linear differential, 18
  patient history, 11–12
  regional differential, 16–18
    axillae, 17
    face, 18
    feet, 16
    glans penis, 17–18
    groin, 17
    hands, 16–17
    nails, 18
    scalp, 18
  see also Investigative techniques
Diaper dermatitis, 110
Diet
  manipulation for dermatitis, 92
Digitate warts
  clinical picture, 45
  treatment, 47
Dinitrochlorbenzene
  allergic contact dermatitis cause, 85
Discoid dermatitis, 96–97
Discoid lupus erythrematosus, chronic,

see DLE
Discoid psoriasis, clinical picture, 99
Dithranol
  use in psoriasis, 104–105
Diuretic therapy
  asteatotic dermatitis development, 96
DLE, 141–142
  cicatricial alopecia, 187
DNA probes, use, 21
Down's syndrome, 113
Drugs
  commonest reactive drugs, **197**
  diagnosis, 199
    systematic reactions to topical therapy, 199
  history of medication, 196–197
    onset of rash, 196–197
  interactions, 206
  patterns of reaction
    acneiform eruptions, 198
    allergic contact dermatitis, 87
    alopecia, 189, 199
    bullous eruptions, 152, 198
    eczematous eruptions, 198
    erythema multiforme, 199
    erythema nodosum, 199
    exanthematic eruptions, 198
    exfoliative dermatitis, 198
    fixed eruptions, 197
    hirsutism, 191
    hyperpigmentation, 182
    lichenoid eruptions, 198
    lupus erythematosus-like syndrome, 142, 197
    nail dystrophy, 199
    photosensitivity, 197
    pigmentation, 198
    psoriasiform eruptions, 198
    purpura, 197
    scleroderma, 147
    sedation, 22
    toxic epidermal necrolysis, 199
    urticaria, 139, 197
    vasculitis, 199
  unwanted effects, 196
    facultative effects, 196
    hypersensitivity reactions, 196
    idiosyncrasy, 196
    intolerance, 196
    overdosage, 196
    side-effects, 196
    teratogenicity, 23, 196
    timing of onset, 11–12
Dupuytren's contracture, occurrence, 30
Dusting powders, 25
Dyskeratosis congenita, 194
Dysplastic naevus syndrome, 161–162
Dystrophic epidermolysis bullosa, 121

Ears
  blue-red coloration, 34
  red-brown eruptions, 33
Eccrine sweat glands, 1, 2, 176

disorders
  anhidrosis, 177
  bromhidrosis, 177
  hyperhidrosis, 176, 204
  hypohidrosis, 177
  miliaria, 177, 205
Ecthyma, 53
Ectodermal dysplasias, 121
  Darier's disease, 121
  hypohidrotic, 121
  keratoderma of palms or soles, 121–122
  Kyrle-Flegel disease, 121
Eczema, see Dermatitis
Eczema cracquelé, 96
Eczema herpeticum, 39, 43
  atopic dermatitis complication, 90–91
  treatment, 91
Eczematoid dermatitis, infective, 97
Ehlers-Danlos syndrome, 118
Elastin, 6
Electrical resistance of skin, 1
Electron microscopy, use, 21
Elephantiasis neuromatosa, 117
Emotional stress
  urticaria cause, 139
Endothelium
  collagen type, 6
Eosinophilic fasciitis, 147
Epidermis
  atrophy, 15, 145, 147
  barrier function, 4
  basal layer degeneration, 142
  benign tumours
    basal cell papilloma, 157
    clear cell acanthoma, 157
    cysts, 158
    squamous papilloma, 157
  blisters, **152**
  cell populations, 2
  cornification disorder, 118–119
  hyperpigmentation, 36
  IgG staining, 153
  intermediate tumours, 164
    actinic keratosis, 164
    arsenical keratosis, 165
    Bowen's disease, 165
    erythroplasia of Queyrat, 166
    hydrocarbon keratosis, 165
    keratoacanthoma, 166
    leukoplakia, 165
    Paget's disease of breast, 166
    thermal keratosis, 165
    x-irradiation keratosis, 164–165
  malignant tumours, 158
    basal cell carcinoma, 158–159
    basal cell naevus syndrome, 159
    melanoma, 160–164
    squamous cell carcinoma, 159–160
  oedema and vesicle formation, 83
  psoriatic, 98–99
  shedding in "scalded skin" syndrome, 53
  structure, 2

basal layer, 2
  epidermodermal junction, 4
  granular layer, 3
  horny layer, 3–4
  Langerhans' cells, 4–5
  melanocytes, 2, 5
  Merkel cells, 5
  prickle cell layer, 3
  sunlight-induced hyperplasia, 124
  thickening, 36, 83, 99, 160
  vitamin D3 metabolism, 4
Epidermodermal junction, 4
  basement membrane antigens, 4
  blisters, **152**
  C3 and IgG bands, 142, 155
  granular IgA deposition, 156
  loss, 160
  "saw-toothed", 108
  structure, 4
Epidermodysplasia verruciformis, 46
Epidermoid cysts, 158
Epidermolysis bullosa, **120**
  dominant dystrophic, 121
  junctional, 120–121
  recessive dystrophic, 121
  simplex, 120
Epidermolytic hyperkeratosis, 119
Epidermophyton infections, **63**, 66
Epilepsy, occurrence, 117
Epiloia, *see* Tuberose sclerosis
Epstein-Barr virus, 168
Erosions, definition, 15
Eruptive xanthomata, 31, 32
Erysipelas, 53–54
Erysipeloid, 55
Erysipelothrix insidiosa infection, 55
Erythema, 130
  definition, 14
  dermatitis in infancy, 110
  palms, 29, 30
  UVB cause, 123
Erythema ab igne, 131
Erythema chronicum migrans, 56
Erythema gyratum repens, 36–37
Erythema induratum, 57, 133
Erythema infectiosum, 49–50
Erythema multiforme, 132–133
  after herpes simplex attack, 43
  drug-induced, 199
  symmetry, 13
Erythema nodosum, 33, 132
  drug-induced, 199
Erythema nodosum leprosum, 201
Erythrasma, 55
Erythroderma, 37, 38, 97
  with Sezary cells, 169, 170
Erythromycin, use, 22
Erythroplasia of Queyrat, 166
Ethambutol, use, 22
Etretinate, use, 23, 106
Eumelanin, 124
Euproctis chrysorrhoea
  caterpillar rash, 81
Eusol, toxicity, 26

Exanthema
  drug-induced, 198
    morbilliform, 198
    scarlatiniform, 198
  of hand, foot and mouth disease, 48
  of pityriasis rosea, 49
Exanthema subitum, 50
"Exclamation-mark" hairs, 190
Excoriations
  definition, 15
  in dermatitis, 82
Exfoliation, definition, 15
Exfoliative dermatitis
  drug-induced, 198
  generalized, *see* Erythroderma
Exudation
  common causes, 11
  in dermatitis, 82
Eyebrows, loss, 30
Eyelids
  digitate warts, 45
  puffy red upper outer, 147
  "salmon patch", 111
  waxy, translucent eruptions, 35
Eyes
  herpes simplex infection, 43
  xanthelasma palpebrarum, 31

Face
  allergic dermatitis eruptions, 85
  atopic dermatitis eruptions, 89
  basal cell carcinoma, 158
  Bloom's syndrome lesions, 120
  blue-red coloration, 34
  "butterfly eruption", 143
  congenital syphilitic rash, 61
  cutaneous leishmaniasis eruptions, 201
  dermatitis herpetiformis rash, 156
  differential diagnosis of lesions, 17, 18
  DLE lesions, 141
  "en coup de sabre", 144
  eruptive xanthomata, 31
  erysipelas lesions, 54
  flat, plane warts, 47
  flat-topped yellowish papules, 45
  flushing, 32
  hyperpigmentation, 30
  Kaposi's sarcoma eruptions, 50, 51
  lentigo maligna pigmentation, 161
  lupus vulgaris lesions, 56
  milia papules, 158
  pemphigus erythematosus eruptions,
    154
  pemphigus vulgaris eruptions, 153
  red-brown eruptions, 33
  reddish-yellow papules, 37
  ringworm of glabrous skin, 68
  rosacea eruptions, 174
  roundness, 30
  "salmon patch", 111
  seborrhoeic dermatitis lesions, 92–93
  "slapped cheek" appearance, 49–50
  squamous cell carcinoma, 159

telangiectasiae, 145
Facultative effects of drugs
  explanation of term, 196
Fat necrosis, subcutaneous, 109
Fatty acids deficiency, essential
  stratum corneum function
    impairment, 4
Faun tail, 192
Favus, 65, 187
Feet
  atopic dermatitis eruptions, 90
  blisters, 151–152
  congenital syphilitic rash, 61
  cutaneous sporting hazards, 205
  dermatitic lesions, 82
  differential diagnosis of lesions, 16
    ulceration in elderly, 29
  Kaposi's sarcoma eruptions, 167
  keratolysis plantare, 55
  maduramycosis, 73
  ringworm, *see* Tinea pedis
  secondary syphilis rash, 59
  warty nodules, 72
  see also Plantar dermatitis; Plantar
    warts
Fetoscopy, 116
Fibroblasts, 7
  origin, 7
Fibrocytes, 7
Fifth disease, 49–50
Filaggrin, 3
Filiform warts, 45, 47
Fingers
  chilblains, 131
  dilated capillaries, 143
  irritant contact dermatitis, 84
  orf lesions, 49
  psoriatic arthritis, 103
  scaly dermatitis of backs, 32
  see also Dactylitis
Fish tank granuloma, 58
Fissures, definition, 15
Flea bites, 80–81
  treatment, 81
Flexural psoriasis, clinical picture, 100
5-Fluorouracil, use, 164
Flurandrenolone, 25
Flushing, 32, 130, 174
  definition, 14
  generalized in rubella, 40
Focal dermal hypoplasia, 114, 120
Fogo selvagem, 154
Folliculitis, 51, 53
  definition, 16
Food
  urticaria cause, 139
    oral test dosing, 139
Food additives
  urticaria cause, 139
Formaldehyde solution, use, 48, 176
Fowler's solution
  hyperpigmentation cause, 182
Framycetin, use, 26
Freckles, 182

Friction blisters, 151–152
FTA-ABS test, 61
Functions of skin, 1
  as barrier, 1
  electrical conductivity restriction, 1
  frictional resistance, 1
  immune system role, 1
  nervous systems roles, 1
  protection, 1
    mechanical injury, 1
    micro-organisms, 1
  thermoregulation, 1
  vitamin D formation, 1
  see also Nails; Hair
Furuncles, definition, 16
Fusidic acid
  systemic use, 22, 26
  topical use, 26

Gangrene
  definition, 16
  zoster, 41
Gardner's syndrome, 37
Gastrointestinal tract
  carcinoma, 36
  secondary dermatoses, 32–33
Gels, 24
Genes, 115
Genetic counselling, use, 116
Genetic diseases
  characteristics of inheritance, 115–116
  HLA antigens, 116
  prenatal diagnosis, 116
    amniocentesis, 116
    fetal skin biopsy, 116
  see also under individual names
Geniculate zoster, 41
Genital warts
  clinical picture, 45–48
Genodermatoses
  involving vascular tissue
    Anderson-Fabry disease, 121
    Osler's disease, 121
  with photosensitivity, 120
    Bloom's syndrome, 120
    congenital poikiloderma, 120
    xeroderma pigmentosum, 120
Genotype
  explanation of term, 115
Gentamicin
  systemic use, 26
  topical use, 26
Gentian violet lotion, use, 27
German measles, see Rubella
Gianotti Crosti syndrome, 50
Gingivostomatitis, primary herpetic, 42
Glabrous skin
  location, 1
  ringworm, 65–66
    facial, 68
Glans penis
  differential diagnosis of lesions, 17–18
    lichen sclerosus et atrophicus, 147

primary syphilis, 58
  type II herpes simplex infection, 43
Glomangioma, 167
Glomus bodies, 6
Glucagonoma, 37
Glucagonoma syndrome, 33
Goltz's syndrome, 114, 120
Gonococcal septicaemia, 58
Gonorrhoea, 58
Gorlin's syndrome, 159
Gramicidin, use, 26
Granular cell layer, 3
  absence, 118–119
Granuloma annulare, 34
  in diabetes mellitus, 30
Granuloma gluteale infantum, 109
Granuloma inguinale, 61–62
Granuloma telangiectaticum, 166–167
Grey Turner's sign, 33
Griseofulvin, 28
  use, 22, 65
Gummata
  cutaneous, 60
  mucosal, 60
Guttate psoriasis, clinical picture, 99

Haem biosynthesis, disorders, see
    Porphyrias
Haemangioma simplex, 167
Haemochromatosis, 33, 181
Haemophilus ducreyi infection, 62
Haemorrhage, cutaneous, 33, 35
Haemorrhagic sarcoma, idiopathic, see
    Kaposi's sarcoma
Haemorrhagic telangiectasia, hereditary
    (Osler's disease), 121
Hair
  absence, 32
  daily growth rate, 185
  development of fine, lanugo, 37
  fine, discoloured, 32
  functions, 1
    see also Cicatricial alopecia; Non-
      cicatricial alopecia
  premature greying, 51
  pulling and rubbing, 204
  shaft monitering, 21
  see also Hair follicles
"Hair brushing", technique, 20
Hair follicles, 185
  cycle, 185–186
    anagen, 185, 186
    catagen, 186
    telogen, 185–186
  dermatophyte penetration and growth,
    63–64
  endocrine influence, 185
  keratoacanthoma, 166
  nervous system, 7
Halo naevus, 183–184
Hand, foot and mouth disease, 48
Hands
  common warts, 45

dermatitic lesions, 82, 94–95
  allergic contact, 85
  differential diagnosis, 95
  irritant contact, 84
  pompholyx, 94–95
  scaly dermatitis of backs, 32
  treatment, 95–96
dermatomyositis rash on backs, 147
differential diagnosis of lesions, 16–17
  orf lesions, 49
  plane warts, 45
  ringworm, 68
  scabetic lesions, 76
  streptococcal infection of fissures, 55
Hansen's disease, see Leprosy
Hartnup disease, 127
HDLs, 31
  increased, 32
  levels in hyperlipidaemia types, 31
Hemidesmosome attachment plaques, 4
Henoch-Schoenlein syndrome, 133
Hepatitis B, 30, 50
"Herald patch", 48–49
Herpes gestationis, 155–156
Herpes gladiatorum, 205
Herpes simplex, 42–43
  aggravation by sunlight, 128
  eczema herpeticum, 43
Herpes Zoster, 40–42
Herpetic whitlow, 42–43
Heterozygous
  explanation of term, 115
Hidradenitis suppurativa, 177
"Hirsuties papillaris penis", 18
Hirsutism, 191–192
  suprarenal disease, 30
Histamine release
  and urticaria, 138
Histiocytoma, 166
Histiocytosis X, 114
Histocompatibility (HLA) antigens, 116
HIV disease, see Human
    immunodeficiency virus disease
HLA antigens, 116
  B8 antigen, 116, 156
  B27 antigen, 106, 116
  DR3 antigen, 155
  DR4 antigen, 155
Homozygous
  explanation of term, 115
Horn, definition, 16
Horny layer, see Stratum corneum
Human immunodeficiency virus disease,
    50
  classification of HIV infection, 50
  HIV-related syndromes, 50, 50–51
    AIDS, 50
    ARC, 50
    Kaposi's sarcoma, 50–51, 167–168
    oral candidosis, 51
    other mucocutaneous
      manifestations, 51
    PGL, 51
Human papilloma viruses (HPV)

clinical association of subtypes, 44
Hutchinson's summer prurigo, 128
Hydrocarbons
    acne from chlorinated, 173
    keratosis, 165
Hydrocortisone
    topical preparations containing, 207
Hydroquinone
    chemical depigmentation by, 180
    topical use, 28
Hydroxychloroquine
    side-effects, 142
    use, 35, 143
Hydroxyurea
    use in psoriasis, 105–106
Hypercholesterolaemia, familial, 31–32
Hyperhidrosis, 176
    gustatory, 176
    psychogenic, 204
Hyperkeratosis, 142
Hyperlipidaemia, 30
    classification, 30
    genetic, 31–32
Hyperoestrogenism, hyperpigmentation
        of, 181
Hyperparathyroidism, 30
Hyperpigmentation, causes of, 181–182
    acanthosis nigricans, 36
    Addison's disease, 30, 181
    lichen planus, 108
    neurodermatitis, 96
Hypersensitivity
    drug-induced, 196
    immunological, 8–10
    see also Allergic contact dermatitis
Hypertrichosis, 191, 192
Hypertrichosis lanuginosa, acquired, 37
Hypertriglyceridaemia, familial, cause,
        32
Hypoadrenalism, hyperpigmentation of,
        181
Hypohidrosis, 177
Hypohidrotic ectodermal dysplasia, 121
Hypoparathyroidism
    onychia in, 70
Hypoparathyroidism, idiopathic
        childhood, 30
Hypopigmentation, 179
Hypopituitarism
    hypopigmentation in, 179
Hypothyroidism,
    asteatotic dermatitis development, 96

Ichthyoses, 118
    acquired in malignant lymphoma, 37
    classification, 118, see also under
        individual names
    management, 119
Ichthyosis vulgaris, 118–119
"Id" reaction, 67
Idiosyncrasy, drug
    explanation of term, 196
Idoxuridine in dimethyl sulphoxide,

(Iduridin) use, 41–42
IgE
    high serum levels, 89
    infant seborrhoeic dermatitis levels,
        110
    receptors, 7
Immunofluorescence techniques, use, 20
Immunological hypersensitivity, 8
    classification, 8
    drug-induced, 196
    inflammation, 9
        mediators, 9–10
    see also Allergic contact dermititis
Immunoperoxidase studies, 20
    principal monoclonal antibodies, 20
Immunosuppression
    UVB radiation, 124
Impetigo, 52
    neonatorum, 109
    secondary, 79
    treatment, 52–53
Incontinentia pigmenti, 119
Indeterminate leprosy, 200
Infantile acne, 173
Infarcts, definition, 16
Ingrowing toenails, 194–195
Inoculation primary herpes, 42
Insect bites, 81
    bed bugs, 80–81
    caterpillar rash, 81
    fleas, 79–80
        treatment, 80
γ-Interferon, 9
    immune response role, 9
Interleukins, 7, 10
Interstitial tissue
    collagen type, 6
Intertrigo, 67, 69
    neonatal, 109
    seborrhoeic, 93
Intolerance, drug
    explanation of term, 196
Intradermal testing, use, 199
Intraepidermal carcinoma, see Bowen's
        disease
Investigative techniques
    cytology, 20
    DNA probes, 21
    electron microscopy, 21
    "hair brush", 20
    hair shaft microscopy, 21
    stratum corneum scrapings, 19
    surgical biopsy, 20
    swabbing, 19
    Wood's light examination, 20
Involucrin, 3
Iodides
    acneiform eruptions cause, 172
Iodoquinolines, use, 26
Irritant contact dermatitis, 83–84
Isomorphic (Köbner) phenomenon, 18,
        107
Isoniazid
    acneiform eruptions cause, 172

use, 22
Isotretinoin, use, 22
Itching
    causes, 11, 29
        actinic prurigo, 128
        bed bug bites, 80
        chronic actinic dermatitis, 128
        dermatitis herpetiformis, 156
        in pregnancy, 29
        larva migrans, 202
        lichen planus, 107
        main systemic diseases, 11
        malignant lymphoma, 37
        miliaria, 177
        neurodermatitis, 96
        pityriasis rosea, 49
        scabies, 75–76
        sunburn, 123
        T-cell lymphoma, 169
    classification of complaints, 11

Jaundice, 30
Jogger's nipple, 205
Junctional epidermolysis bullosa, 120–
        121
Junctional naevus, 183

Kala-azar, 201
Kaposi's sarcoma, 50–51, 167–168
Kasabach-Merritt syndrome, 112
Kawasaki disease, 114
Keloid, 149
Keratinocytes, 2
    acantholytic cells, 153
    as light barrier, 123
    melanocytes relationship, 178
    separation, 83
    steroid sulphatase deficiency, 119
    structure of epidermis, 2–4
    vitamin D3 receptors on, 4
Keratins of epidermal cells, 2–4
Keratoacanthoma, 166
Keratoderma
    blennorrhagicum, 106
    palms and soles, 122
Keratohyalin, 3
Keratolysis plantare, 55
Keratosis
    actinic, 164
    arsenical, 165
    follicularis, 121
    hydrocarbon, 165
    thermal, 165
    x-irradiation, 164–165
Kerion, 64–65, 187
Ketoconazole, use, 22
Klippel-Trenaunay-Weber syndrome,
        112
Köbner (isomorphic) phenomenon, 18,
        107
Koilonychia, 193
"Koplik's spots", 39

Kwashiorkor, 32
Kyrle-Flegel disease, 121

Lamellar granules, function, 3
Lamellar ichthyosis, 119
Lamina densa, 4
   antigens, 5
   collagen type, 6
Lamina lucida, 4
   antigens, 5
   C3 localization, 155
   separation, 120–121
Langerhans' cells, 2
   characteristics, 5
   functions, 5, 8
   histiocytosis, 114
   monoclonal antibodies for
         immunoperoxidase studies, 21
   origin, 5
   structure, 4–5
      surface antigens, 5
      surface receptors, 5
   UVB radiation effect, 124
Larva migrans, 201–202
LDLs, 31–32
   receptor gene abnormalities, 31–32
Legs
   asteatotic dermatitis lesions, 96
   chilbains, 131–132
   chromoblastomycotic nodules, 72
   clear cell acanthoma, 157
   erysipelas lesions, 54
   erythema ab igne, 131
   erythema nodosum lesions, 132
   golden-brown colour, 131
   Kaposi's sarcoma eruptions, 167
   Kyrle-Flegel disease eruptions, 121
   leucocytoclastic vaculitis lesions, 133
   lichen planus eruptions, 107
   ringworm of calves, 68
   SLE lesions, 143
   superficial thrombophlebitis, 37
   ulceration causes, 135
   venous disease, 136–138
Leishmaniasis, 201
Lentigo
   actinic, 182
   maligna, 160–161
      melanoma, 162
   simple, 182
Leprosy, 200
   clinicopathological manifestations
      borderline, 200
      indeterminate, 200
      lepromatous, 200
      tuberculoid, 200
   reactional states
      type I, 201
      type II, 201
   treatment, 201
Leucocytoclastic vasculitis, 133–134
Leucoderma centrifugum acquisitum
      (Halo naevus), 183–184

Leuconychia, 30, 193
Leukaemia
   aetiological factors, 168
   skin lesions in, 170
Leukoplakia, 165
   differential diagnosis, 60, 165
   "hairy", 51
Leukotrienes
   B4 excess, 98
   generation, 10
Lichen planus, 107–108
   cicatricial alopecia, 107, 187
   glans penis, 17
clinical variants, 107–108
   Köbner phenomenon, 107
Lichen sclerosus et atrophicus, 147
Lichen scrofulosorum, 57
Lichenification
   definition, 15
   in dermatitis, 82, 84, 89, 94
Lichenoid eruptions, drug-induced, 198
Lick dermatitis, 114
Lignocaine, 26
Linaments, 24
Lindane, use, 76
Linear IgA disease, 156
Lipid metabolism, 31
Lips
   lichen planus eruptions, 107
   pigmentation, 37
   squamous cell carcinoma, 159, 160
   type I herpes simplex infection, 43
Livedo reticularis, 131, 134
Liver disease, 30
Local anaesthetics, 26
   side-effects, 87
Lotions, 24
Lunula, 192
   coloration and systemic diseases, 192
Lupus erythematosus, 128, 141, 144
   lupus erythematosus-like syndrome
      drug-induced, 197
   neonatal, 144
   subacute cutaneous, 144
   see also DLE; SLE
Lupus erythematosus profundus, 144
Lupus pernio, 34
Lupus vulgaris, 56, 187
Lutzner cells, 169
Lyme disease, 56
Lymphadenopathy, persistent
      generalized (PGL), 50
Lymphangioma, diffuse, 167
Lymphangioma circumscriptum, 167
Lymphangiosarcoma, 168
Lymphatic dysplasias, congenital, 97
Lymphatics of skin, 7
Lymphogranuloma venereum, 62
Lymphoid cells
   monoclonal antibodies for
         immunoperoxidase studies, 21
Lymphoma, 168–170
   B-cell, 170
   Burkitts, 170

Crosti's indolent, 170
cutaneous T-cell, 168–170
lymphomatoid papulosis, 170
malignant
   acquired icthyosis, 37
   arsenic-induced changes, 38
   erythroderma, 38
   itching, 37
   pigmentation, 37
   poikiloderma atrophicans vasculare,
      37–38
Pagetoid, 170
Sezary syndrome, 170
Lymphomatoid papulosis, 170

Macrophages
   monoclonal antibodies for
         immunoperoxidase studies, 21
Macules
   "ash leaf patches", 117
   blue-black, 30
   brown, blue-grey, 119
   cafe au lait, 116, 182
   definition, 14
   fawn, scaling, 70–71
   "herald patch", 48–49
   large, pigmented on babies, 113
   multiple, small, erythematous, 154
   pale-pink, discrete, 59
   pin-head, erythematous, 40
   plane xanthomata, 31
   transient, 33
Madura foot, 73
Maduramycosis, 73
   treatment, 73
Madurella infections, 73
Malassezia furfur infection, 70–71
Malathion, use, 77, 79
Male-pattern alopecia, 188–189
Malignant diseases
   cutaneous manifestations, 36–38
   see also under individual conditions
Marginal traction alopecia, 190
Mast cells, 7
   naevus, 113
Mastocytosis
   adult-onset, 113
   in babies, 113
Measles, 39–40
MED (Minimal erythema dose), 123
Meissner's corpuscles, 7
Melanin, 2, 123
   coloration, 178
   function, 1
   synthesis, 124, 178
Melanocyte naevus
   acquired, 183
   congenital, 182–183
Melanocytes, 2, 5
   anatomy, 178
   damage, 124
   hydroquinone effect, 28
   keratinocyte relationship, 178

monoclonal antibodies for
   immunoperoxidase studies, **21**
tumour, *see* Melanoma, malignant
Melanoma, juvenile, 183
Melanoma, malignant, 160–163
  acral lentiginous, 162
  diagnostic procedures, 163
  differential diagnosis, 163
  lentigo maligna, 162
  nodular, 162
  pathology, 163
    Breslow thickness, 163
    Clarke's levels, 163
  prognosis, 163
    clinical staging, 163
    relation to Breslow thickness, 163
  risk factors, 160–162
  subungual, 163
  superficial spreading, 162
  treatment, 163–164
Melasma, 181
Membrane-coating granules, function, 3
Mental handicaps, syndromes with
  congenital infections, 113
  Down's syndrome, 113
  phenylketonuria, 113
Mepacrine, side-effects, 142
Mepyramine maleate, use, 22
Merkel cells
  function, **2**, 5
  structure, 5
Metabolic alopecia, 189
Metabolic diseases
  hyperpigmentation cause, 181
  light-aggravated
    erythropoietic protoporphyria, 126
    Hartnup disease, 127
    pellagra, 127
    porphyria cutanea tarda, 126–127
    porphyrias, 126
    variegate porphyria, 127
Metals
  allergic contact dermatitis cause, 85
Metencephalin, 5
Methotrexate
  drug interactions, 206
  side-effects, 105
  use, 35, 105
Methyl dopa, side-effects, 97
Miconazole, use, 28
Micrococcus sedentarius infection, 55
Microsporum infections
  M. audouini, **63**, 64
  M. canis, **63**, 64
Milia, 109, 158
Miliaria, 177, 205
  neonatorum, 109
  treatment, 177
Minimal erythema dose, 123
Minoxidil lotion, use, 188
Mole, common, 183
  clinical patterns, 183
Moles
  definition, 182

in pregnancy, 29
see also Mole, common
Molluscum contagiosum, 43–44
  atopic dermatitis complication, 91
  treatment, 44
Molluscum fibrosum, 116–117
Molluscum sebaceum, 166
Mongolian spot, 183
Moniliasis, *see Candida albicans*
  infections
Monoclonal antibody investigative
  studies, 20
Monomorphic eruption
  explanation of term, 13
Monosulfiram, use, 77
Morbilli, *see* Measles
Morgan-Dennie folds, 90
Morphoea, 144–145
Mouth
  cheilitis and angular stomatitis, 69
  pemphigus vulgaris blisters, 153
Mucocutaneous diseases, **12**
Mucocutaneous lymph node syndrome,
  114
Mupirocin, use, 26
Mutations
  explanation of term, 115
Mycobacterial diseases
  acute tuberculous ulceration, 57
  atypical, 58
    BCG infections, 57
    M. marinum, 57–58
    M. ulcerans, 58
  diagnosis, 57
  lupus vulgaris, 56
  scrofuloderma, 57
  treatment, 57
  tuberculides, 57
  tuberculosis of the skin, 56
  warty tuberculosis, 57
Mycobacterium leprae infection, *see*
  Leprosy
Mycobacterium marinum infection, 57–58
Mycobacterium ulcerans infection, 58
Mycoses
  classification, 63
  see also under individual names
Mycosis fungoides, *see* T-cell
  lymphoma, cutaneous
Mycostatin, use, 22
Myxoedema, 30
  pretibial, 30

Naevi
  definition, 182
  hypopigmented
    achromic, 180
  pigmented, 182
    acquired blue, 183
    atypical, 161–162
    classification, **183**, *see also under*
      individual names
  vascular in childhood, 111–113

Naevus flammeus, 111–112
Naevus simplex, 111
Nail-patella syndrome, 194
Nails, 30
  anatomy, 192
    cuticle, 192
    daily growth rate, 192
    lunula, 192
    matrix, 192
  "beaking", 145
  differential diagnosis of lesions, **17**, 18
    lichen planus, 107–108
  diseases of fold, 193
    acute paronychia, 192
    chronic paronychia, 193
    palisading, 193
    periungual fibromata, 117
  diseases of plate
    blue-black coloration, 193
    clubbing, 193
    coloured half-moons, 193
    greenish coloration, 193
    koilonychia, 193
    longitudinal coloured bands, 193
    onycholysis, 125, 194, 199
    pitting, 194
    ridging, 107–108, 194
    splinter haemorrhages, 193
    subungual hyperkeratosis, 194
    white coloration, 30, 193
    yellow coloration, 193
  dystrophy, 34
    Darier's disease, 121
    drug-induced, 199
  functions, 1
  fungal infections, 68–69
  genetic dystrophies
    dyskeratosis congenita, 194
    dystrophic epidermolysis bullosa,
      194
    nail-patella syndrome, 194
    pachyonychia congenita, 194
  miscellaneous disorders
    ingrowing toenails, 194–195
    melanoma, 163
    mucous cysts, 194
    subungual exostosis, 47, 195
  psoriasis lesions
    growth rate, 98
    matrix, 102
    nail bed, 102
Napkin dermatitis, 110
  treatment, 110
Napkin psoriasis, clinical picture, 99
Necrobiosis lipoidica, occurrence, 29–30
Necrolytic migratory erythema, 37
Neisseria gonorrhoeae infection, 58
Neomycin, 138
  side-effects, 87
  use, 26
Neonatal disorders, 109
Neonatal intertrigo, 109
Neurodermatitis, 96
  differential diagnosis, 96

disseminated, *see* Atopic dermatitis
  management, 96
Neurofibromatosis
  bilateral acoustic central, 117
  Von Recklinghausen's peripheral,
    116–117
Neuropathy, occurrence, 29
Nickel
  allergic contact dermatitis cause, 85
Nicotinic acid deficiency, 127
Nikolsky's sign, 153
Nocardia infections, 73
Nodular prurigo, 96
Nodular vasculitis, 134
Nodules
  definition, 14
  diffuse, blue-red, 132
  domed, firm, 166
  of actinomycosis, 71, 72
  of chromoblastomycosis, 72
  of Kaposi's sarcoma, 50–51
  of sporotrichosis, 72
  Lisch, 117
  painless, non-itching, 202
  painless, red-brown, 56
  red, red-blue, 35
  red-brown, 30, 33, 183
  reddish-yellow, 37
  small, hard, 73, 158
  squamous cell carcinoma onset, 160
  see also Molluscum fibrosum; Tendon
    xanthomata; Xanthelasma
    palpebrarum
Non-bullous ichthyosiform
    erythroderma, 119
Non-cicatricial alopecia
  causes of diffuse, **187**
    anagen alopecia, 189
    common baldness, 188–189
    drug-induced alopecia, 189, 199
    female androgenic alopecia, 189
    HIV disease, 51
    metabolic alopecia, 189
    telogen alopecia, 189
    thyroid disease, 30
  causes of localized, **187**
    alopecia areata, 189–190
    secondary syphilis, 190
    tinea capitis, 190
    traumatic alopecia, 190
  definition, 187
Non-scarring alopecia, *see* Non-
    cicatricial alopecia
Norwegian scabies, 76
Nummular dermatitis, 96–97
Nutritional dermatoses, 32
Nystatin, use, 70

Oculocutaneous albinism, 179–180
Odland bodies, function, 3
Oil acne, 173
Ointments, 25
Onchocerca volvulus infestation, 202

Onchocerciasis, 202
Onychia, 70
Onychogryphosis, 194
Onycholysis, 125, 194
  drug-induced, 199
Onychomycosis, 68
  treatment, 69
Ophthalamic zoster, 41
Oral mucosa
  corrugations, 33
  multiple punctate telangiectases, 121
Oral warts, 47
Orf, 49
Organic dyes
  allergic contact dermatitis cause, 86
Oriental sore, 201
Osler's disease, 121
Otitis externa, chronic, 93
Ovarian disease
  hirsutism cause, 191
Overdosage, drug, 196

Pachyonychia, congenita, 194
Pacinian corpuscles, 7
Pagetoid lymphoma, 170
Paget's disease of breast, 166
  extramammary, 166
"Palisading", 147, 193
Palmer erythema, occurrence, 29, 30
Palpation
  importance in diagnosis, 13
    peripheral arterial pulses, 13
    regional lymph glands, 13
Pancreatic carcinoma
  cutaneous manifestations
    necrolytic migratory erythema, 37
    thrombophlebitis migrans, 37
Pancreatic disease
  secondary dermatoses, 33
Panniculitis, 33
Papillary dermis, 7
  collagen type, 6
Papillomata
  definition, 16
  in yaws, 61
  multiple warty, 36
Papular acrodermatitis of childhood, 50
Papular urticaria, 139
Papules
  blue, 183
  clustering in herpes Zoster, 41
  conical, orange-yellow, 100
  "coral bead", 37
  definition, 14
  erythematous itching, 128
  flat-topped, blue-red, 107
  flat-topped, yellowish, 45
  friable, easily bleeding, 167
  glistening white, 158
  hyperkeratotic plugs, 121
  linear urticated, 80
  of dermatitis, 82
  of Gianotti Crosti syndrome, 50

red, 35, 49
red, vascular, 167
red-brown, 33
reddish-yellow, 37
satellite pigmented, 163
smooth, yellow or red-brown, 114
solitary, blue-red, 167
strawberry naevus, 112
translucent, 44
warty, 119
waxy, translucent, 35
yellow, 31
yellow-brown, 121, 166
Papulonecrotic tuberculide, 57
Parakeratosis, 83, 99
Paraphenylenediamine
  allergic contact dermatitis cause, 86
Parasitic infections, 75
  urticaria cause, 139
  see also under individual names
Parasitism, delusions of, 203
Parathyroid disease, 30
Parathyroidectomy, 30
Paronychia
  acute, 192
  chronic, 193
Pastes, 25
Patch testing, 87–88
  standard contact allergens, **88**
  use, 199
Pediculosis, 77
  capitis, 78–79
  corporis, 77–78
  parasiticidal topical preparations for,
    210
  pubis, 78
Pediculus humanus infestation, 77–79
Pellagra, 127
Pemphigoid, 154–155
  variants
    benign mucous membrane
      pemphigoid, 155
    herpes (pemphigoid) gestationis,
      155–156
Pemphigus erythematosus, 154
Pemphigus foliaceus, 154
  Brazilian, 154
Pemphigus neonatorum, 109
Pemphigus vegetans, 154
Pemphigus vulgaris, 152–153
  diagnosis, *21*, 153
  prognosis, 153
  treatment, 153–154
Penicillins
  side-effects, 87
  systemic use, 22, 25
Penis
  chancroid ulcers, 62
  primary syphilis site, 58
  shaft
    genital warts clinical picture, 45
    lichen planus eruptions, 107
    scabetic lesions, 76
    type II herpes simplex infection, 43

see also Glans penis
Peri-anal area
  abscesses, 32
  ulcers, *15*
  warts, 45–46
Peri-oral area
  dermatitis, 175
    lick dermatitis, 114
    type I herpes simplex infection, 43
Peripheral pulses, absence, 135
Perniosis, *see* Chilbains
Peutz-Jegher syndrome, 37, 182
PGL, 51
Phaeomelanin, 124
Phenotype
  explanation of term, 115
Phenoxymethyl penicillin, use, 22
Phenylalanine metabolism, defective, *see*
        Phenylketonuria
Phenylketonuria, 97, 179
Phialophora infection, 72
Philadelphia chromosome, 168
Photoallergy
  dermatitis, 125
  drugs, **125**
Photochemotherapy, see PUVA
Photodermatoses, 124–125
  idiopathic
    actinic prurigo, 128
    chronic actinic dermatitis, 128
    facial, *14*
    polymorphic light eruption, 128
    solar urticaria, 128
  photoallergy, 125
  photosensitization, 125
  phototoxicity, 125
  phytophotodermatitis, 125
Photosensitivity
  dermatitis, 125
  drug-induced, 125, 197
    Berlocque dermatitis, 125
    phytophotodermatitis, 125
  genodermatoses with, 120
Phototoxicity
  dermatitis, 125
  drugs, **125**
Phycomycosis, subcutaneous, 73
Piebaldism, 180
Pigmentation
  of back in pediculosis, 78
  "bronze", 33
  delayed, 124
  drug-induced, 198
  increased in pregnancy, 29
  in malignant lymphoma, 37
  patchy, 37
  see also Jaundice
Pigmented hairy epidermal naevus, 184
Pilar cysts, 158
Pinta, 61
"Pitch wart", 165
Pitted keratolysis, 55
Pitting of nails, 194
Pityriasis alba, 111

Pityriasis amiantacea, 191
Pityriasis capitis, 190–191
Pityriasis rosea, 48–49
Pityriasis rubra pilaris, 97
Pityriasis versicolor, 70–71
  treatment, 71
Pityrosporum ovale, 92
Plane warts, clinical picture, 45
Plane xanthomata, 31
Plantar dermatosis, juvenile, 111
Plantar warts
  clinical picture, 45
  treatment, 48
Plants, effects of
  allergic contact dermatitis, 86
  photodermatoses, 125
Plaques
  annular-patterned, 107
  definition, 14
  eczema-like, 165
  erythematous, scaly, 141
  horse-shoe shape, 169
  hyperkeratotic mosaic-like, 45
  multiple, blue-red, 167
  orange-yellow velvety, 114
  psoriasis-like, 165
  raised, ovoid, 96
  raised, erythematous, 200
  red-brown, 30, 33
  red, scarred, 159
  salmon-red, 99
  "shagreen patch", 117
  thickish, whitish-grey, 165
  waxy, translucent, 35
  see also Plane xanthomata;
        Xanthelasma palpebrarum
Plasma cell balanitis of Zoon, 18
Plastics
  allergic contact dermatitis cause, 86
Pleomorphic eruption
  explanation of term, 13
Plexiform neuroma, 117
Podophyllin, use, 47
Poikiloderma, congenital, 120
Poikiloderma atrophicans vasculare
  in malignant lymphoma, 37–38
Poison ivy
  allergic contact dermatitis cause, 86
Polyarteritis, chronic cutaneous, 134
Polyarteritis nodosa, 134
Polycystic ovary syndrome
  hirsutism cause, 191
Polymixin, use, 26
Polymorphic light eruption, 128
Polymyositis, 148
Pompholyx, 94–95
Porphyrias, 126
  erythropoietic protoporphyria, 126
  porphyria cutanea tarda, 126–127
  variegate, 127
"Port wine stain", 111–112
Portal cirrhosis, 30
Postinflammatory pigmentation
  hyperpigmentation of, 181

hypopigmentation, 180
Postpartum alopecia, 189
Potassium permanganate, use, 26, 27–
    28, 88
Povidone iodine, use, 26
PPD (Paraphenylenediamine), 86
Prednisolone
  dosage, 23
  use, 32, 88, 95, 133, 143, 148
    herpes zoster, 42
    lichen planus, 108
    pemphigus vulgaris, 153–154
    sarcoidosis, 35
Pregnancy, 29
  alopecia, 29
  chloasma in, 181
  examinations in, 116
  gonococcal septicaemia risk, 58
  herpes gestationis and, 155–156
  hyperpigmentation of, 181
  incidence of warts, 47
  increasing pigmentation, 29
  parvovirus B19 infection, 49–50
  rashes, 29
  spider naevi incidence, 130
Pressure, effects of
  urticaria, 138
    treatment, 139
Prickle cell layer, 3
Prickly heat, 177, 205
Primula obconica
  allergic contact dermatitis cause, 86
Procollagen, formation, 6
Promethazine hydrochloride, use, 22
Propantheline bromide, use, 176
Protein energy malnutrition, 32
Protoporphyrin IX, accumulation, 126
Pruritis, *see* Itching
Pruritis, psychogenic, 203
  depression as cause, 203
  physical signs, 203
Pruritis ani, 93–94
  occurrence, 100
Pruritis vulvae, 94
Pseudo-pelade, 188
Pseudo-xanthoma elasticum, 118
Pseudoacanthosis nigricans, 36
Pseudomonas infection
  nail plate discoloration, 193
Psoralens
  photosensitive reactions, 125
Psoriasiform eruptions, drug-induced,
    198
Psoriasis, 98
  aetiology, 29, 98
    aggravation by sunlight, 128
    distribution, *13*
    glans penis, *17*
  arthritis, 103
  clinical picture, 99–100
  complications, 102
    erythrodermic psoriasis, 102
    generalized pustular, 102
  HLA antigens and, 116

localized patterns, 100
management, 104
metabolic complications
  erythrodermic psoriasis, 102–103
of nails, 102
pathogenesis and pathology, 98–99
provocative factors, 98, 128
systemic treatment, 105
  etretinate, 106
  hydroxyurea, 106
  methotrexate, 105
  miscellaneous, 106
  PUVA, 106
topical therapy, 104
  bath additives, 209
  corticosteroids, 105
  dithranol, 104–105, 209
  tar, 104, 208–209
Psoriatic arthritis, 103
Psychogenic disorders, 203
  acne excorieé, 203
  cholinergic urticaria, 203
  delusions of parasitism, 203
  dermatitis artefacta, 203–204
  hair pulling and rubbing, 204
  hyperhidrosis, 204
  psychogenic pruritis, 203
Pthirus pubis infestation, 78
Punctate purpura, definition, 14
Purpura, 130–131
  definition, 14
  drug-induced, 197
  occurrence, 32, 78
Pustular psoriasis, clinical picture, 100,
  102
Pustules
  causes in infancy, 109
  definition, 15
  whorled-patterning, 119
PUVA, use, 181
  hazards of long-term, 106
  psoriasis, 106
  T-cell lymphoma, 170
Pyoderma gangrenosum, 32
Pyogenic granuloma, 166–167

Race
  and hirsutism, 191
Radioallergoabsorbent testing, 89
RAST testing, 89
Raynaud's phenomenon, 131
Refsum's syndrome, 119
Reiter's disease, 106–107
  HLA antigens and, 116
Resins
  allergic contact dermatitis cause, 86
Reticular dermis
  collagen type, **6**
Reticulohistiocytosis, multicentric, 37
Retinoids, 22–23
Rhagades, 61
Rheumatic fever, 149
Rheumatoid arthritis, *14*, 134, 149

Ridging of nails, 194
Rifampicin, use, 22
Ringworm, *see* Tinea
Rosacea, 174–175
  aggravation by sunlight, 128
Roseola infantum, 50
Rothmund-Thomson syndrome, 120
Rowell's syndrome, 144
Rubber
  allergic contact dermatitis cause, 86
Rubella, 40
Rupioid psoriasis, clinical picture, 100

Salicylic acid, 25
"Salmon patch", 111
Saquet-Hoyer canal, 6
Sarcoidosis, 33
Sarcoptes scabiei hominis, 75
Scabies, 75–77
  parasiticidal topical preparations, 210
"Scalded skin" syndrome, 53
Scale
  "carpet-tack", 141
  definition, 15
  ichthyoses, 119
  psoriatic, 99
  removal, 24
Scarring alopecia, *see* Cicatricial alopecia
Scars
  blue, spongy, 118
  definition, 15
  depigmented in pinta, 61
  DLE, 141
  in sarcoidosis, 34
  porphyria cutanea tarda, 127
  varioliform, 39
Scleredema of Buschke, 147
Scleroderma, 144
  drug-induced, 147
  eosinophilic fasciitis, 147
  lichen sclerosus et atrophicus, 147
  mixed connective tissue disease, 147
  occupational, 146–147
  see also Morphoea; Sclerosis, systemic
Sclerosis, systemic, 145–146
Scrofuloderma, 57
Scrum-pox, 205
Scurvy, 32
Sebaceous cysts, 158
Sebaceous naevus, 114
Seborrhoea
  and acne vulagaris, 171
Seborrhoeic dermatitis, 92–93
  chronic otitis externa, 93
  of infancy, 110
  pruritis ani, 93–94
  pruritis vulvae, 94
  topical shampoos, 209–210
Seborrhoeic folliculitis, 191
Seborrhoeic intertrigo, 93
Seborrhoeic keratoses, 157
Seborrhoeic warts, 157
Sebum constituents, 171

Sedatives, 22
Senear-Usher syndrome, 154
Senile purpura, definition, 14
Senile warts, 157
Sex-linked characteristics
  explanation of term, 115
Sexually transmitted bacterial diseases,
  see Gonorrhoea; Syphilis
Sezary cells, 170
Sezary syndrome, 170
Shampoos, 25
Shingles, *see* Herpes Zoster
Side-effects, drug
  explanation of term, 196
  see also Drugs
Silver salts, side-effects, 182
Sixth disease, 50
Sjögren's syndrome, 149
"Slapped cheek", 49–50
SLE, 142–144
Small vessel disease
  diabetic dermopathy cause, 29
Smoking
  and Buerger's disease, 136
Sneddon's syndrome, 134
Soaps, 25
Sodium hypochlorite solution, toxicity,
  26
Solar elastosis, 150
Solar lentigo, 124
S100 antibodies,
  immunoperoxidase studies use, **21**
Sphingolipid metabolism, disorder, 121
Spider naevi, 14, 29, 30, 130
Spitz naevus, 183
Splinter haemorrhages, 193
Spongiosis, 83
Sporotrichosis, 72–73
Sporotrichum schenckii infection, 72
Sport
  main cutaneous hazards, 205
Squamous cell carcinoma, 159–160, 164,
  165
  chronic lupus scarring supervention,
    56
Squamous papilloma, 157
Staphylococcal infections
  atopic dermatitis complication, 90
  boils, 53
  carbuncles, 53
  ecthyma, 53
  folliculitis, 53, 188
  impetigo, 52–53
  infective eczematoid dermatitis, 97
  psoriasis complication, 102
  "scalded skin" syndrome, 53
  see also Staphylococcus aureus
Staphylococcus aureus, 52
  infections
    antibiotic treatment, 22
    ecythemas, *53*
    impetigo, 52–53
Staphyloderma, 29
Steatorrhoea, 97

Stein-Leventhal syndrome, 191
Steroid-induced purpura, definition, 14
Steroid sulphatase deficiency, 119
Stewart-Treves syndrome, 168
Still's disease, 149
Stratum corneum
  functions
    barrier, 4
    mechanical injury protection, 1
  hydration, 24
  investigatory scrapings, 19
  M. furfur mycelial attack, 70
  psoriatic appearance, 98
  structure, 3–4
    intercellular material, 3–4
  water content variations, 4
Strawberry naevus, 112
Streptococcal infections
  atopic dermatitis complication, 90
  cellulitis, 54
  erysipelas, 53–54
  erythema multiforme cause, 133
  infected fissures, 55
  see also Streptococcus pyogenes
    infections
Streptococcus pyogenes infections
  erysipelas, 53–54
  impetigo, 52
  of fissures, 55
Streptomycin, side-effects, 87
Striae, 149–150
  Wickham's, 107
Structure of skin, 1
  regional variations, 1–2
  surface dryness role, 1
  see also Dermis; Epidermis
Sturge-Weber syndrome, 112
Subungual exostosis, 46–47, 195
Subungual hyperkeratosis, 194
Subungual melanoma, 163
Sulphapyridine, side-effects, 156
Sulphonamides
  drug interactions and, 206
  side-effects, 87, 125
  use, 26
Sulphur, use, 77
Sun filters, 128
Sun protection factors, 128–129
  UVA, 129
  UVB, 128–129
Sunburn, 123–124
  prevention, 123–124
Sunlight
  biological effects on skin, 123–124
  cutaneous barrier, 123
  diseases aggravated by, 128
  external protection, 128, 129
  malignant melanoma risk factor, 162
  photobiology, 123
    solar spectrum, **123**
  photodermatoses, 124–125
Sunscreens, 25, 128
Suprarenal disease, 30
  Addison's disease, 30

Cushing's syndrome, 30
Sutton's naevus, 183–184
Swabbing technique, 19
Sweat glands, *see* Apocrine sweat glands;
    Eccrine sweat glands
"Swimming pool ear", 93
Swimming pool granuloma, 58
Sycosis barbae, 53
Syphilis, 58–61
  biological false-positive tests, 61
  cicatricial alopecia cause, 188
  congenital, 60–61
  cutaneous gumma, 60
  endemic, 61
  late, 60
  latent, 59
  mucosal gumma, 60
  primary, 58–59
  secondary, 59
    non-cicatricial alopecia cause, 190
  serological tests, 61
    FTA-ABS test, 61
    TPHA test, 61
    TPI test, 61
    VRDL test, 61
  treatment, 61
Systemic amyloidosis, 35
Systemic diseases
  cutaneous manifestations, 29–35
Systemic lupus erythematosus, *see* SLE
Systemic therapy
  analgesia, 22
  anti-infective chemotherapeutic
      agents, 22
  antibiotics, 22
    Staphylococcus aureus infection, 22
    streptococcal infections, 22
  antifungal agents, 22
  antipruritic drugs, 22
  corticosteroids, 23
  retinoids, 22–23

T-cell lymphoma, cutaneous, 168–170
T-cells
  immune response role, 8, 9
    helper cells, 8
  interleukins origins, 7
  see also T-cell lymphoma, cutaneous
Tar
  hydrocarbon keratosis development,
      165
  use in psoriasis, 104, 208–209
Telangiectasia, 37, 120, 130
  definition, 14
  multiple punctate, 121
Telogen alopecia, 186, 189
Temperature-related vascular
      abnormalities
  cold
    chilbains, 131–132
    livedo reticularis, 131
    Raynaud's phenomenon, 131
    urticaria, 138, 139

heat
  erythema ab igne, 131
  urticaria, 139
Temporal arteritis, 134
Tendon xanthomata, 31, 32
Tennis toe, 205
Teratogenic drugs, 196
Terfenadine, 22
Tetracosactrin zinc, 23
Tetracyclines, use
  acne vulgaris, 173–174
  rosacea, 175
  photosensitive reactions, 125
Thermal keratosis, 165
Thermoregulation
  eccrine sweat glands role, 176
Thrombophlebitis migrans, 33, 37
Thrush, 69
Thyroid disease, 30
  gross myxoedema, 30
Thyrotoxicosis, 30
Tinea
  and sport, 205
  barbae, 67–68
  capitis, 64–65
    favus, 65
    microsporum infections, 64
    trichophyton infections, 64–65
  corporis, 65
  cruris, 66
  facei, 68
  follicular of calves, 68
  hair penetration and growth, 63–64
    ectothrix infection, 64
    endothrix infection, 64
  incognito, 66–67
  main pathogenic species, 63
  manuum, 68
  pedis, 67
  unguium, 68–69
  versicolor, 70–71
Tioconazole, use, 28
Titanium dioxide, 25
Toes
  chilbains, 131
  ingrowing nails, 194
  juvenile plantar dermatosis, 111
  psoriatic arthritis, 103
Tonofibrils of epidermal cells, 2–3
Topical therapy
  aims, 24
  antibacterial creams and ointments,
      207
  antibiotics, 25–26
  anti-fungal preparations, 27–28, 210
  antiseptics, 207
  anti-viral preparations, 210
  corticosteroids, 27, 208
  for pediculosis, 210
  for scabies, 210
  for ulceration, 207
  hydrocortisone-containing, 207
  hydroquinone, 28
  psoriasis preparations, 208–209

shampoos, 209–210
systemic reactions, 199
vehicles, 24–25
   allergic dermatitis side-effect, 87
viral warts preparations, 209
Toxic epidermal necrolysis, 199
Toxic erythema of newborn, 109
TPHA test, 61
TPI test, 61
Trauma, effects of
  alopecia, 190
  urticaria, 138
Treatment, *see* Systemic therapy;
     Topical therapy
Treponemal diseases
  non-venereal
    endemic syphilis, 61
    pinta, 61
    yaws, 61
  venereal, *see* Syphilis
Trichilemmal cysts, 158
Trichophyton infections
  T. interdigitale, **63**, 67, 68
  T. mentagrophytes, **63**, 64, 66, 67, 68
  T. rubrum, **63**, 66, 67, 68
  T. schoenleinii, **63**, 65
  T. soudanense, **63**
  T. tonsurans, **63**
  T. verrucosum, **63**, 64, 67
  T. violaceum, **63**, 64
Trichotillomania, 204
Trisomy 21, 113
Tropocollagen, 6
Tryptophan metabolism, abnormal, 127
Tuberculides, 57
  Bazin's disease, 57
  erythema nodosum, 57
  lichen scrofulosorum, 57
  papulonecrotic tuberculide, 57
Tuberculoid leprosy, 200
Tuberculosis of skin, 56
Tuberculosis verrucosa cutis, 57
Tuberose sclerosis, 117–118
Tuberose xanthomata, 31, 32
"Tulip fingers", 86
Tumours of skin
  benign dermal, 166–167
  benign epidermal, 157–158
  carcinogens, 157
    sunlight, 124
  intermediate epidermal, 164–166
  leukaemia, 168–170
  lymphomas, 168–170
  malignant dermal, 167–168
  malignant epidermal, 158–164
Tzanck test, 20, 153

Ulcerative colitis, 33
Ulcers
  blue-red edged, shallow, 57
  causes of leg, **135**
  crateriform, 158
  definition, 15

of chancroid, 62
of diabetes mellitus, 29
of ecythema, 53
oral mucosa, 33
"punched-out", 60
topical preparations for, 207
venous, 136–137
  treatment, 137–138
Ultrasound imaging, 116
Ultraviolet light
  chemical filters, 129
  collagen degradation, 6
  dermatitis association, 97
  skin protective role, 1
  sunscreens, 25
  vitamin D3 skin metabolism, 4
  xeroderma pigmentosum hazard, 120
  see also PUVA
Uroporphyrinogen III, accumulation,
  126–127
Urticaria, 138–139
  drug-induced, 197
  solar, 128
  occurrence, 30
  treatment, 139–140
Urticaria pigmentosa, 113
UVA, 123
  protection factor assessment, 129
  see also PUVA
UVB, 123
  abnormal responses to, 128
  intermittent therapy for lymphoma,
    170
  protection factor assessment, 128–129
  psoriasis therapy, 104, 105
  sunburn cause, 123
  vitamin D metabolism, 123
UVC, 123

"Vagabond's itch", 78
Vaginal warts, 46–47
Vancomycin, use, 22
Varicella, 39
Varicose veins, 136
Vascular disorders
  angioedema, 138, 140
  erythema induratum, 57, 133
  erythema multiforme, 43, 132–133,
    199
  erythema nodosum, 33, 132, 199
  erythemas and other small vessels,
    130–131
  large-vessel arterial disease, 134–136
  leg venous disease, 136–138
  small-vessel arterial disease, 133–134
  temperature-related, 131–132
  urticaria, 138–140
Vascular naevi, childhood, 111
  blue rubber bleb naevus syndrome,
    113
  cavernous haemangioma, 112
  eruptive disseminated angiomatosis,
    113

Kasabach-Merritt syndrome, 112
Klippel-Trenaunay-Weber syndrome,
    112
naevus flammeus, 111–112
naevus simplex, 111
strawberry naevus, 112
Sturge-Weber syndrome, 112
Venereal warts, 45–48
Venous dermatitis, 94
"Venous stars", 130
Verruca digitata, 45, 47
Verruca filiformis, 45, 47
Verruca plana, 45
Verruca plantaris, 45, 48, 205
Verruca vulgaris, *see* Common warts
Vesicles
  definition, 14
  "frogspawn-like", 167
  of dermatitis, 82, 83
  of hand dermatitis, 94–95
  of herpes simplex, 43
  of impetigo, 52
VIN (Vulval intraepithelial neoplasia),
  165
Vinyl chloride
  scleroderma cause, 146–147
Viral infections
  lymphoma aetiological factor, 168
  urticaria cause, 139
  see also under individual diseases
Viral warts
  atopic dermatitis complication, 91
  topical preparations for, 209
Vitamin C
  collagen formation role, 6
  deficiency, 32
Vitamin D3
  formation in skin, 4, 123
  functions, 4
Vitiligo, 180–181
  treatment, 181
VLDLs, 31
  increased, 32, **32**
  levels in hyperlipidaemia types, **31**
Von Recklinghausen's peripheral
    neurofibromatosis, 116–117
  cutaneous neurofibromata, 116–117
  Lisch nodules, 117
VRDL test, 61
Vulva
  chancroid ulcers, 62
  primary syphilis site, 58
  VIN, 165
  vulvovaginitis, 69
    primary herpetic, 42
  warts, 46
Vulval intraepithelial neoplasia, 165

Waardenburg's syndrome, 180
Warts, 44
  clinical picture
    common, 45
    digitate, 45

genital, 45–47
plane, 45
plantar, 45
differential diagnosis, 47
epidermodysplasia verruciformis, 47
HPV types, 44
immunology, 44–45
treatment, 47–48
Warty tuberculosis, 57
Wasp stings, 140
Water
urticaria cause, 139
regional variation of loss, 2
Wegener's granulomatosis, 134
"Wens" (Pilar cysts), 158

Wheals
definition, 14
see also Urticaria
"White dermographism", 89
Whiteheads
in acne vulgaris, 171, 172
Wickham's striae, 107
Wiskott-Aldrich syndrome, 97
Wood's light examination, 20
Woringer-Kolopp disease, 170

X-linked ichthyosis, 119
X-rays
cicatricial alopecia cause, 187

Xanthelasma palpebrarum, 31, 32
Xanthogranuloma, juvenile, 114
Xanthomata, 29, 30–31
Xeroderma pigmentosum, 120

Yaws, 61
Yellow nail syndrome, 193

Zinc malabsorption, 32, 109
Zoster
cicatricial alopecia cause, 187
herpes, see Herpes zoster